Editors

ASIF M. ILYAS
SHITAL N. PARIKH
SAQIB REHMAN
GILES R. SCUDERI
FELASFA M. WODAJO

ORTHOPEDIC CLINICS OF NORTH AMERICA

www.orthopedic.theclinics.com

July 2014 • Volume 45 • Number 3

ELSEVIER

1600 John F. Kennedy Boulevard • Suite 1800 • Philadelphia, Pennsylvania, 19103-2899.

http://www.orthopedic.theclinics.com

ORTHOPEDIC CLINICS OF NORTH AMERICA Volume 45, Number 3
July 2014 ISSN 0030-5898, ISBN-13: 978-0-323-31167-0

Editor: Jennifer Flynn-Briggs
Developmental Editor: Stephanie Carter

Orthopedic Clinics of North America (ISSN 0030-5898) is published quarterly by Elsevier Inc., 360 Park Avenue South, New York, NY 10010-1710. Months of issue are January, April, July, and October. Business and Editorial Offices: 1600 John F. Kennedy Blvd., Suite 1800, Philadelphia, PA 19103-2899. Customer Service Office: 3251 Riverport Lane, Maryland Heights, MO 63043. Periodicals postage paid at New York, NY and additional mailing offices. Subscription prices are $310.00 per year for (US individuals), $596.00 per year for (US institutions), $365.00 per year (Canadian individuals), $727.00 per year (Canadian institutions), $450.00 per year (international individuals), $727.00 per year (international institutions), $150.00 per year (US students), $220.00 per year (Canadian and international students). Foreign air speed delivery is included in all *Clinics* subscription prices. All prices are subject to change without notice. **POSTMASTER:** Send change of address to *Orthopedic Clinics of North America*, **Elsevier Health Sciences Division, Subscription Customer Service, 3251 Riverport Lane, Maryland Heights, MO 63043. Customer Service (orders, claims, online, change of address): Elsevier Health Sciences Division, Subscription Customer Service, 3251 Riverport Lane, Maryland Heights, MO 63043. Tel: 1-800-654-2452 (U.S. and Canada); 314-447-8871 (outside U.S. and Canada). Fax: 314-447-8029. E-mail: journalscustomerservice-usa@elsevier.com (for print support); journalsonlinesupport-usa@elsevier.com (for online support).**

Reprints. For copies of 100 or more, of articles in this publication, please contact the Commercial Reprints Department, Elsevier Inc., 360 Park Avenue South, New York, NY 10010-1710. Tel.: 212-633-3874; Fax: 212-633-3820; E-mail: reprints@elsevier.com.

Orthopedic Clinics of North America is covered in *MEDLINE/PubMed* (*Index Medicus*), *Cinahl, Excerpta Medica,* and *Cumulative Index to Nursing and Allied Health Literature.*

PROGRAM OBJECTIVE

Orthopedic Clinics of North America offers clinical review articles on the most cutting-edge technologies and techniques in the field, including adult reconstruction, the upper extremity, pediatrics, trauma, oncology, and sports medicine.

TARGET AUDIENCE

Practicing orthopedic surgeons, orthopedic residents, and other healthcare professionals who specialize in orthopedic technologies and techniques for adult reconstruction, the upper extremity, pediatrics, trauma, oncology, and sports medicine.

LEARNING OBJECTIVES

Upon completion of this activity, participants will be able to:

1. Review five polyostotic conditions that general orthopaedic surgeons should recognize.
2. Discuss orthopedic conditions in the upper extremities including the shoulder and elbow.
3. Recognize techniques for the surgical treatment of distal tibia fractures.

ACCREDITATION

The Elsevier Office of Continuing Medical Education (EOCME) is accredited by the Accreditation Council for Continuing Medical Education (ACCME) to provide continuing medical education for physicians.

The EOCME designates this enduring material for a maximum of 15 *AMA PRA Category 1 Credit*(s)™. Physicians should claim only the credit commensurate with the extent of their participation in the activity.

All other health care professionals requesting continuing education credit for this enduring material will be issued a certificate of participation.

DISCLOSURE OF CONFLICTS OF INTEREST

The EOCME assesses conflict of interest with its instructors, faculty, planners, and other individuals who are in a position to control the content of CME activities. All relevant conflicts of interest that are identified are thoroughly vetted by EOCME for fair balance, scientific objectivity, and patient care recommendations. EOCME is committed to providing its learners with CME activities that promote improvements or quality in healthcare and not a specific proprietary business or a commercial interest.

The planning committee, staff, authors and editors listed below have identified no financial relationships or relationships to products or devices they or their spouse/life partner have with commercial interest related to the content of this CME activity:

Nirav H. Amin, MD; Gary Calabrese, PT; Gilbert Chan, MD; Matthew W. Colman, MD; Sheila A. Conway, MD; Anthony Philip Cooper, MBChB, FRCS; Siddesh Nandi Doddabasappa, MBBS, MS, FRCS; Christopher C. Dodson, MD; Jennifer Flynn-Briggs; Kevin L. Garvin, MD; Stephen M. Gryzlo, MD; Angela L. Hewlett, MD, MS; Francis J. Hornicek, MD, PhD G. Russell Huffman, MD, MPH; Brynne Hunter; Asif M. Ilyas, MD; John D. Kelly IV, MD; Stuart D. Kinsella, BA, MD, MTR; Erik N. Kubiak, MD; Sandy Lavery; Kevin J. Little, MD; Santiago A. Lozano-Calderon, MD, PhD; T. Sean Lynch, MD; Jill McNair; Kishore Mulpuri, MBBS, MS, MHSc; Saravanaraja Muthusamy, MD; Shital N. Parikh, MD; Lindsay Parnell; Ronak M. Patel, MD; E. Scott Paxton, MD; Santha Priya; Kevin A. Raskin, MD; Raveesh Daniel Richard, MD; H. Thomas Temple, MD; Stephen J. Thomas, PhD, ATC.

The planning committee, staff, authors and editors listed below have identified financial relationships or relationships to products or devices they or their spouse/life partner have with commercial interest related to the content of this CME activity:

Antonia F. Chen, MD, MBA has royalties/patents with Slack Publishing.

Mark C. Gebhardt, MD has royalties/patents with Up To Date; and has an employment affiliation with Clinical Orthopaedics and Affiliated Research.

Curtis W. Hartman, MD is a consultant/advisor for Smith & Nephew, Inc. and Trak Surgical, Inc.; has a research grant from Smith & Nephew, Inc.; and has stock ownership with Trak Surgical, Inc.

Daniel Scott Horwitz, MD is a consultant/advisor for Biomet, Inc. and Cardinal Health; has royalties/patents with Biomet, Inc.; and has a research grant with Synthes, Inc.

William J. Hozack, MD is a consultant/advisor for Stryker; and has an employment affiliation with Journal of Arthroplasty, an Elsevier journal.

Beau S. Konigsberg, MD is a consultant/advisor for Trak Surgical, Inc.

Mark D. Lazarus, MD is on speakers bureau for Tornier, Inc. and Depuy Mitek, Inc.; also is a consultant/advisor, has stock ownership, a research grant and royalties/patents with Tornier, Inc.

Saqib Rehman, MD is a consultant/advisor for Depuy Synthes Companies; and has royalties/patents with Jaypee Brothers Medical Publishing Ltd.

Mark S. Schickendantz, MD is a consultant/advisor for Arthrex, Inc.

Giles R. Scuderi, MD is on speakers bureau for Zimmer, Inc., ConvaTec, Inc., and Medtronic, Inc.; is a consultant/ advisor for Zimmer, Inc., Pacira Pharmaceuticals and Medtronic, Inc.; has a research grant from Pacira Pharmaceuticals; and has royalties/patents from Zimmer, Inc.

Felasfa M. Wodajo, MD has royalties/patents with Stryker and Elsevier Inc.

UNAPPROVED/OFF-LABEL USE DISCLOSURE

The EOCME requires CME faculty to disclose to the participants:

1. When products or procedures being discussed are off-label, unlabelled, experimental, and/or investigational (not US Food and Drug Administration (FDA) approved); and

2. Any limitations on the information presented, such as data that are preliminary or that represent ongoing research, interim analyses, and/or unsupported opinions. Faculty may discuss information about pharmaceutical agents that is outside of FDA-approved labelling. This information is intended solely for CME and is not intended to promote off-label use of these medications. If you have any questions, contact the medical affairs department of the manufacturer for the most recent prescribing information.

TO ENROLL

To enroll in the *OrthopedicClinics of North America* Continuing Medical Education program, call customer service at 1-800-654-2452 or sign up online at http://www.theclinics.com/home/cme. The CME program is available to subscribers for an additional annual fee of USD $310.

METHOD OF PARTICIPATION

In order to claim credit, participants must complete the following:

1. Complete enrolment as indicated above.
2. Read the activity.
3. Complete the CME Test and Evaluation. Participants must achieve a score of 70% on the test. All CME Tests and Evaluations must be completed online.

CME INQUIRIES/SPECIAL NEEDS

For all CME inquiries or special needs, please contact elsevierCME@elsevier.com.

ORTHOPEDIC CLINICS OF NORTH AMERICA

FORTHCOMING ISSUES

Beginning with the July 2013 issue, *Orthopedic Clinics of North America* began to appear in this new format. Rather than focusing on a single topic, each issue contains articles on key areas in orthopedics—adult reconstruction, upper extremity, trauma, pediatrics and oncology. Articles on sports medicine and foot and ankle will also be included on a regular basis. As the practice of orthopedics has become more specialized, the format of one topic per issue is no longer fulfilling our readers' needs. The new format is intended to address these changing needs.

Orthopedic Clinics of North America continues to publish a print issue four times a year, in January, April, July, and October. However, this series also includes online-only articles that will be published on a rolling basis (not in accordance with our quarterly publication dates). These articles, along with articles from our print issues, are available on http://www.orthopedic.theclinics. com/.

DOWNLOAD
Free App!

Review Articles
THE CLINICS

YOUR iPhone and iPad

Contributors

EDITORS

ASIF M. ILYAS, MD - *Upper Extremity*
Program Fellowship Director of Hand and
Upper Extremity Surgery, Rothman Institute;
Associate Professor of Orthopaedic Sugery,
Thomas Jefferson University, Philadelphia,
Pennsylvania

SHITAL N. PARIKH, MD - *Pediatric Orthopedics*
Pediatric Orthopaedic Sports Medicine,
Associate Professor of Orthopaedic Sugery,
Cincinnati Children's Hospital Medical Center,
University of Cincinnati School of Medicine,
Philadelphia, Pennsylvania

SAQIB REHMAN, MD - *Trauma*
Orthopaedic Surgery, Temple University
Hospital, Philadelphia, Pennsylvania

GILES R. SCUDERI, MD - *Adult
Reconstruction*
Vice President, Orthopedic Service Line,
Northshore LIJ Health System New York,
ISK Institute, New York

FELASFA M. WODAJO, MD - *Oncology*
Musculoskeletal Tumor Surgery, Virginia
Hospital Center, Arlington, Virginia; Assistant
Professor of Orthopedic Surgery, Georgetown
University Hospital, Washington, DC; Assistant
Professor, Orthopaedic Sugery, VCU School of
Medicine, Inova Campus, Falls Church,
Arlington, Virginia

AUTHORS

NIRAV H. AMIN, MD
Sports Health, Department of Orthopaedic
Surgery, The Cleveland Clinic Foundation,
Cleveland, Ohio

GARY CALABRESE, PT
Sports Health, Department of Orthopaedic
Surgery, The Cleveland Clinic Foundation,
Cleveland, Ohio

GILBERT CHAN, MD
Pediatric Orthopedic Surgeon, Children's
Orthopedics of Louisville, Kosair Children's
Hospital; Clinical Instructor, Department of
Orthopedics, University of Louisville, Louisville,
Kentucky

ANTONIA F. CHEN, MD, MBA
Clinical Adult Reconstruction Fellow,
Rothman Institute, Philadelphia,
Pennsylvania

MATTHEW W. COLMAN, MD
Department of Orthopedic Surgery, Beth Israel
Deaconess Medical Center, Massachusetts
General Hospital, Boston Children's Hospital,
Boston, Massachusetts

SHEILA A. CONWAY, MD
Associate Professor, Department of
Orthopaedic Surgery, University of Miami Miller
School of Medicine, Miami, Florida

**ANTHONY PHILIP COOPER, BSc(Hons),
MBChB, FRCS (Tr&Orth)**
Department of Orthopaedics, BC Children's
Hospital, Vancouver, British Columbia,
Canada

**SIDDESH NANDI DODDABASAPPA, MBBS,
MS(Ortho), FRCS(Glasg)**
Department of Orthopaedics, BC Children's
Hospital, Vancouver, British Columbia,
Canada

CHRISTOPHER C. DODSON, MD
Department of Orthopedics, Rothman Institute, Thomas Jefferson University, Philadelphia, Pennsylvania

KEVIN L. GARVIN, MD
Professor and Chair, Department of Orthopaedic Surgery and Rehabilitation, University of Nebraska Medical Center, Omaha, Nebraska

MARK GEBHARDT, MD
Department of Orthopedic Surgery, Beth Israel Deaconess Medical Center, Boston Children's Hospital, Boston, Massachusetts

STEPHEN M. GRYZLO, MD
Department of Orthopaedic Surgery, Feinberg School of Medicine, Northwestern University, Chicago, Illinois

CURTIS W. HARTMAN, MD
Assistant Professor, Department of Orthopaedic Surgery and Rehabilitation, University of Nebraska Medical Center, Omaha, Nebraska

ANGELA L. HEWLETT, MD
Assistant Professor, Internal Medicine-Infectious Diseases, University of Nebraska Medical Center, Omaha, Nebraska

FRANCIS J. HORNICEK, MD, PhD
Department of Orthopedic Surgery, Massachusetts General Hospital, Boston, Massachusetts

DANIEL SCOTT HORWITZ, MD
Chief of Orthopaedic Trauma, Department of Orthopaedics, Geisinger Health System, Danville, Pennsylvania

WILLIAM J. HOZACK, MD
Professor of Orthopaedic Surgery, Rothman Institute, Jefferson Medical College of Thomas Jefferson University, Philadelphia, Pennsylvania

G. RUSSELL HUFFMAN, MD, MPH
Assistant Professor, Department of Orthopaedic Surgery, Hospital of the University of Pennsylvania, Philadelphia, Pennsylvania

JOHN D. KELLY IV, MD
Associate Professor, Department of Orthopaedic Surgery, Hospital of the University of Pennsylvania, Philadelphia, Pennsylvania

STUART D. KINSELLA, BA, MD, MTR
Orthopaedic Resident, Department of Orthopaedic Surgery, Massachusetts General Hospital, Boston, Massachusetts

BEAU S. KONIGSBERG, MD
Assistant Professor, Department of Orthopaedic Surgery and Rehabilitation, University of Nebraska Medical Center, Omaha, Nebraska

ERIK KUBIAK, MD
Department of Orthopaedics, University of Utah, Salt Lake, Utah

MARK D. LAZARUS, MD
Department of Orthopedics, Rothman Institute, Thomas Jefferson University, Philadelphia, Pennsylvania

KEVIN J. LITTLE, MD
Division of Pediatric Orthopaedics, Hand and Upper Extremity Surgery, Cincinnati Children's Hospital Medical Center; Assistant Professor, Department of Orthopaedic Surgery, University of Cincinnati College of Medicine, Cincinnati, Ohio

SANTIAGO A. LOZANO-CALDERON, MD, PhD
Department of Orthopedic Surgery, Beth Israel Deaconess Medical Center, Boston Children's Hospital; Massachusetts General Hospital, Boston, Massachusetts

T. SEAN LYNCH, MD
Sports Health, Department of Orthopaedic Surgery, The Cleveland Clinic Foundation, Cleveland, Ohio

FREEMAN MILLER, MD
Pediatric Orthopedic Surgeon, Alfred I. DuPont Hospital for Children; Director, Cerebral Palsy Program, Alfred I DuPont Hospital for Children, Wilmington, Delaware

KISHORE MULPURI, MBBS, MS(Ortho), MHSc(Epi)
Assistant Professor, Department of Orthopaedics, Centre for Hip Health and Mobility (CHHM), BC Children's Hospital; UBC Faculty of Medicine, Vancouver, British Columbia, Canada

SARAVANARAJA MUTHUSAMY, MD
Musculoskeletal Oncology Fellow, Department of Orthopaedic Surgery, University of Miami Miller School of Medicine, Miami, Florida

RONAK M. PATEL, MD
Sports Health, Department of Orthopaedic Surgery, The Cleveland Clinic Foundation, Cleveland, Ohio

E. SCOTT PAXTON, MD
Assistant Professor of Orthopaedic Surgery; Division of Shoulder and Elbow Surgery, Warren Alpert Medical School of Brown University, Providence, Rhode Island

KEVIN A. RASKIN, MD
Department of Orthopedic Surgery, Massachusetts General Hospital, Boston, Massachusetts

RAVEESH DANIEL RICHARD, MD
Department of Orthopaedics, Geisinger Health System, Danville, Pennsylvania

MARK S. SCHICKENDANTZ, MD
Sports Health, Department of Orthopaedic Surgery, The Cleveland Clinic Foundation, Cleveland, Ohio

H. THOMAS TEMPLE, MD
Professor, Department of Orthopaedic Surgery, University of Miami Miller School of Medicine, Miami, Florida

STEPHEN J. THOMAS, PhD, ATC
Assistant Professor, Division of Nursing and Health Sciences, Neumann University, Aston, Pennsylvania

Contents

dislocations in older patients often present with complex injury patterns, including rotator cuff tears, fractures, and neurovascular injuries. Glenohumeral instability in patients older than 40 years requires a different approach to treatment. An algorithmic approach aids the surgeon in the stepwise decision-making process necessary to treat this injury pattern.

Throwers, or athletes who engage in repetitive overhead motions, are a unique subset of athletes that experience distinct shoulder injuries. Athletes engaged in baseball comprise the majority of patients seeking orthopedic care for throwing related injuries. Injuries specific to throwers most commonly involve the labrum and the undersurface of the rotator cuff. In addition, tissue changes in both the anterior and posterior glenohumeral capsule are common with repetitive overhead motions. These capsular changes alter. This article will examine the pathomechanics of injuries to throwers, elaborate means of diagnoses of cuff and labral injury and discuss recent advances in both non-operative and operative interventions, including preventative principles.

Oncology

Bisphosphonates are medications known to decrease bone resorption by inhibiting osteoclastic activity. They are the first-line therapy for the treatment of osteoporosis because a significant body of literature has proved their efficacy in reducing the risk of fracture in the hip, spine and other nonvertebral osseous sites. In addition, the use of bisphosphonates has significantly decreased morbidity and increased survival, and they have also proved to be cost-effective. Unexpected adverse effects have been reported recently, but the benefit of bisphosphonates use outweighs the risks. This article reviews the current use of bisphosphonates in orthopedic surgery.

General orthopedic surgeons frequently encounter patients with conditions affecting multiple bones. It is important to recognize common polyostotic diseases. This article describes five polyostotic conditions: Multipe Enchondromatosis (Ollier Disease and Maffucci syndrome), Multiple Hereditary Exostosis (Diaphyseal Aclasis), Fibrous Dysplasia (McCune-Albright syndrome and Mazabraud syndrome), Paget's Disease of bone (Osteitis Deformans), and Skeletal Metastases. This is a survey of the clinical, pathologic and radiographic features that assist in diagnosing these conditions. Also, an overview of the laboratory findings, treatment, follow-up, and prognosis is presented. Recognizing these diseases will aid in prompt and accurate diagnosis and appropriate referral and therapy.

Adult Reconstruction

Preface
Adult Reconstruction

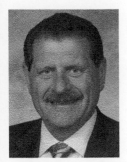

Giles R. Scuderi, MD
Editor

Total hip arthroplasty (THA) is one of the most common procedures performed in the United States and worldwide. Despite the high rate of success, there are reported complications that necessitate revision arthroplasty. These can be challenging cases, so in this current issue of *Orthopedic Clinics of North America*, we present two important topics: implant selection in revision THA and the management of the infected THA.

Critical to the success of revision THA is choosing the right implant. Component selection for revision THA is directed toward creating a stable hip, restoring appropriate leg lengths, and providing offset to optimize joint kinemanics. Multiple factors, described by Chen and Hozak, go into the decision-making process, including the mechanism of failure, the type of implant in situ, and femoral or acetabular bone loss. The utility of various implant choices should be clearly understood by those surgeons performing revision THA.

One of the more devastating complications is an infected THA. The appropriate diagnosis of a prosthetic hip infection is a critical first step to successful management and functional recovery of the patient. Konigsberg and coauthors report on the recent work by the Musculoskeletal Infection Society, which created a new uniform definition for both research and clinical use. It is imperative that orthopedic surgeons remain current in regard to recommendations for evaluation and diagnosis of prosthetic joint infection. Keeping up-to-date on the current evidence-based recommendations is an important part of the management of these complicated infections.

It is anticipated that the readers will find these two articles in the adult reconstruction section insightful and a resource for their clinical practice.

Giles R. Scuderi, MD
Vice President
Orthopedic Service Line
Northshore LIJ Health System
New York, NY, USA

ISK Institute
New York, NY, USA

E-mail address:
grscuderi@nshs.edu

Orthop Clin N Am 45 (2014) xv
http://dx.doi.org/10.1016/j.ocl.2014.04.009
0030-5898/14/$ – see front matter

Component Selection in Revision Total Hip Arthroplasty

Antonia F. Chen, MD, MBA*, William J. Hozack, MD

KEYWORDS

- Revision total hip arthroplasty • Fully porous coated stems • Modular components
- Trabecular metal • Acetabular augments • Cages

KEY POINTS

- Paprosky acetabular and femoral classification systems are important for diagnosis, prognosis, and treatment of bone loss when choosing revision total hip arthroplasty implants.
- Revision femoral stems provide diaphyseal fixation using either fully porous coated cylindrical stems or modular tapered stems for almost all bone deficiencies.
- For complete proximal bone loss, proximal femoral replacements may be used or an allograft-prosthetic composite can be grafted to existing host bone.
- Most acetabular defects can be addressed with second-generation porous coating hemispherical cups with or without the addition of metal augments.
- The preferred method for addressing severe acetabular defects is the cup-cage construct, in which a second-generation porous coating cup is held in place with a cage and secured with screws into the ischium and ilium. Bone loss rarely requires the use of a custom triflange implant.
- Acetabular liners can be used to change acetabular version, use effectively larger femoral heads through dual mobility liners, or constrain the femoral head.

INTRODUCTION

Component selection for revision total hip arthroplasty (THA) is dictated by choosing components that create a stable hip, restore appropriate leg lengths, and provide offset to maximize joint mechanics. Multiple factors go into the decision-making process for which components to use, including the amount of bone loss present and accounting for the components that are currently in place. For the femur, determining the geometry of the remaining bone helps to guide orthopedic surgeons to use fully porous coated stems for metaphyseal bone loss, modular stems that provide various stem versions, and proximal femoral replacements (PFRs) for reconstructions in which there is great proximal bone loss and no attachment for the abductors. Smaller acetabular defects can be contained by using hemispherical cups with second-generation porous coatings with or without metal augments or bone graft, whereas larger acetabular defects can be contained with cages or custom triflange implants. In addition, specific acetabular liners can be placed to alter the version of the cup by a set number of degrees, provide articulation through dual mobility liners, or constrain the femoral head. This article provides guidance as to which components to use in THA revisions.

Disclosures: A.F. Chen has no disclosures that are relevant to the topic discussed within this article. W.J. Hozack is a consultant and receives royalties from Stryker.
Department of Orthopaedic Surgery, Rothman Institute, 925 Chestnut Street, Philadelphia, PA 19107, USA
* Corresponding author.
E-mail address: antonia.chen@rothmaninstitute.com

Orthop Clin N Am 45 (2014) 275–286
http://dx.doi.org/10.1016/j.ocl.2014.03.001
0030-5898/14/$ – see front matter © 2014 Elsevier Inc. All rights reserved.

REVISION FEMORAL COMPONENTS

Choosing femoral components in revision THA depends on the type of fixation needed to stabilize a prosthesis within a femur with bone loss. Although metaphyseal fixation is often used in primary THA stems with wedge and taper stems, most stems used in revision THA are designed for diaphyseal fixation, because the metaphysis can be weakened or even absent in the revision setting. If too much proximal femoral bone is missing, then a PFR may need to be used. The options for femoral components in revision THA are described later.

Bone Loss Classification

The most useful classification system is the Paprosky classification,[1] which is both prognostic and helps to direct treatment options. For type I defects, there is minimal bone loss in the metaphyseal region and the diaphysis is intact. In this setting, a primary THA stem may be used. For type II defects, the femur has extensive metaphyseal cancellous bone loss, but the diaphysis is still intact. Type III defects are characterized by severe bone damage and are classified into 2 groups. Type IIIA defects have severe compromise of the metaphyseal bone, but have greater than 4 cm of bone remaining in the diaphysis. Type IIIB defects also have an unsupportive metaphysis, but have less than 4 cm of bone in the diaphysis to provide for fixation. In addition, type IV defects have extensive metaphyseal and diaphyseal bone loss with an unsupportive isthmus and a widened femoral canal.

Fully Porous Coated Cylindrical Stems

Fully porous coated stems require adequate diaphyseal bone present for fixation. These stems are cylindrical and achieve an interference fit in the diaphysis, and studies have shown the need for greater than 4 cm of intact diaphyseal bone for secure fixation.[2] The severity of the defect determines the long-term fixation and survivorship of these stems,[3,4] because Paprosky type I and II defects can be treated with fully porous coated stems[5] as long as the femoral canal is less than 19 mm in width.[6,7] Long-term results show that using fully porous coated stems leads to long survivorship and high rates of osseointegration determined by radiographic studies,[8] but one of the side effects is increased thigh pain and proximal stress shielding, because most of the stress transfer to bone occurs in the diaphysis.[9]

Modular Tapered Stems

Modular cementless stems are commonly used in revision THA (**Fig. 1**), because the proximal and distal femur are individually prepared to accommodate a prosthesis that fills bone defects. These implants can provide good diaphyseal fixation, limb length discrepancies can be restored,[10] and the version of the implant can be set to provide joint stability and maximize joint mechanics.[11] Although these modular stems can vary the distal stem configuration,[12] the tapered conical stem is now favored and has the best results. Studies show that modular tapered stems had lower failure rates, better osseointegration, and decreased revision rates compared with cylindrical stems.[13,14] These modular, tapered stems can be used to treat any level of bone damage, but are particularly effective (compared with cylindrical fully porous coated stems) for Paprosky type III femoral defects, with demonstrated 75% to 94% survivorship at 4.5 to 10 years.[15–20] Using proper technique, these implants have a low failure rate, but can subside if not fitted tightly, or can fracture at the interface between the neck and the stem of the prosthesis if that junction is not supported by bone.[21,22]

Allograft-Prosthetic Composite

Although modular stems can also be used to treat Paprosky type IV femoral defects, allograft-prosthetic composites (APCs) are another option for replacing bone loss by using a proximal femoral allograft and cementing or press fitting a stable implant into the allograft.[23] Distal fixation can be achieved by providing step cuts for fixation, or tunneling the graft bone into host bone (intussusception) for Paprosky type IV femurs. APCs were first used to reconstruct limbs in dogs with osteosarcoma who underwent limb-sparing surgery,[24] and they were subsequently used in revision THA to treat circumferential defects of greater than 3 cm from the calcar.[25] More current studies recommend using APCs in Paprosky type III and IV defects, with 69% survivorship at 10 years.[26] This method of fixation is beneficial because it restores bone stock, allows for load sharing of the revision construct with host bone, provides a biological anchor for abductor attachment, and improves the ease of reoperation if bone has incorporated by future revision surgery. However, implanting an APC is a technically demanding procedure, and because allograft is used there is a risk of fracture because the construct is not as strong as metal implants, there is a risk of disease transmission, and the graft may not incorporate and may lead to nonunion or resorption.

PFR

In the case of massive proximal bone loss in which treatment with the aforementioned implants

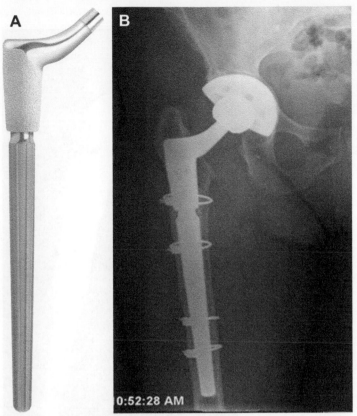

Fig. 1. Modular femoral stem. (*A*) Implant. (*B*) Radiograph. ([*A*] *Courtesy of* Howmedica Osteonics Corp, Mahwah (NJ); with permission.)

is not adequate for fixation, a PFR is an option that replaces the proximal femur with a metal prosthesis that allows for attachment of the abductors (**Fig. 2**).[27] These modular tumor megaprostheses can be used in patients with nonneoplastic conditions and are beneficial because they allow for version correction and leg length restoration.[28] The survivorship of these implants has been reported as 87% at 5 years[29] and 64% at 12 years.[30] After undergoing PFR, many patients report improvement in quality of life, as measured by Harris hip scores, Western Ontario and McMaster (WOMAC) Universities Arthritis Index, Oxford scores, and Short-form 12 mental component scores.[31] However, one study showed that, at a mean of 5 years' follow-up, all patients were still ambulating with assistive walking devices.[32] Complications after PFRs include dislocation and septic and aseptic loosening, which encourages the use of PFRs in low-demand, elderly patients who live sedentary lifestyles.[33] Additional PFRs using tantalum components have been described in the literature and may provide a better bone ingrowth surface for host bone to incorporate into the prosthesis.[34]

Custom Stems

In the revision THA setting, custom stems that have tantalum metal coatings can be used to improve fixation, especially in Paprosky type IV femurs with wide femoral canals.[35]

REVISION ACETABULAR COMPONENTS

Acetabular component selection is mostly based on the amount of bone loss present,[36,37] and the most useful classification system is another Paprosky classification, as described later. Determining the size of the existing implant is important for determining the minimum implant size that should be used in the revision setting. For implantation of the acetabular component, the options for components are listed later.

Bone Loss Classification

The Paprosky classification is the most commonly used, and it is also diagnostic, prognostic, and directs surgical management.[38] Type I Paprosky acetabular bone loss has the presence of a supportive rim of bone without bone lysis or migration.

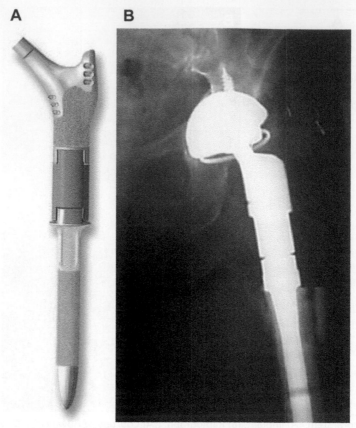

Fig. 2. Proximal femur replacement. (*A*) Implant. (*B*) Radiograph. ([*A*] *Courtesy of* Howmedica Osteonics Corp, Mahwah (NJ); with permission.)

Type II has a distorted acetabular hemisphere, but the anterior and posterior columns are intact and there is less than 2 cm of superomedial or superolateral migration. Type II is further divided into 3 groups: (1) type IIA, superomedial bone lysis with an intact superior rim; (2) type IIB, superolateral bone lysis with an absent superior rim; and (3) type IIC, medial wall bone lysis. Type III Paprosky acetabular bone loss is characterized by superior migration of greater than 2 cm and shows severe ischial and medial osteolysis. Type IIIA defects have bone loss between the 10 o'clock and 2 o'clock positions, and 30% to 60% of the bone is missing but the ilioischial line is intact. Type IIIB defects have bone loss between the 9 o'clock and 5 o'clock positions, and 60% of the bone is missing and the ilioischial line is not intact. This classification system has also been validated and is a reliable system, especially when individuals are taught about the classification system before looking at plain radiographs.[39]

Revision Acetabular Cups

Almost all revision acetabular cups are hemispherical with a second-generation porous coating to promote bone ingrowth (**Table 1**).[40,41] This second-generation coating promotes osseointegration by providing a porous surface that is seemingly biocompatible with osteoblasts,[42] and it also provides greater friction at the component-bone interface.[43] These cups have shown osseointegration with good long-term results when there is minimal bone loss in the revision setting.[44–46] Transacetabular screws can be used to augment fixation, whereas autograft or cancellous bone allograft can be used to fill acetabular defects.[47,48] These hemispherical cups can only be used if there is a contained defect with minimal migration of the failed cup, which requires that both the anterior and posterior columns are largely intact, so hemispherical revision cups work well in Paprosky I and most Paprosky II acetabular defects.

Acetabular Augments

To supplement acetabular fixation when there is segmental bone loss, acetabular augments can be used to fill specific defects.[49] In the past, structural allografts served this purpose. The problems with structural allografts are nonunion, infection,

Table 1
Revision acetabular cups

	Implant Name	Company	Composition	Surface
Hemispherical cups	Regenerex® Revision Acetabular Shells	Biomet	Titanium	Porous titanium
	Pinnacle® Revision Acetabular Cup System	DePuy	Titanium	3 options: 1. Titanium sintered metal beads (Porocoat®) 2. Super Textured Asperity Topography (Gription®) 3. Plasma sprayed hydroxyapatite (HA) or HA alone (DuoFix®)
	R3	Smith & Nephew	Titanium	STIKTITE porous coating
	Tritanium Acetabular Shell	Stryker	Titanium	Titanium matrix (Tritanium)
	Trabecular Metal™ Revision Shell	Zimmer	Titaniums	Trabecular metal
Acetabular augments	Regenerex® Acetabular Augments	Biomet	Titanium	Porous titanium
	Gription TF® Augments	DePuy	Titanium	Titanium foam
	Trabecular Metal™ Acetabular Augments	Zimmer	Titanium	Trabecular metal
	Restoration™ Acetabular Wedges	Stryker	Titanium	Titanium matrix (Tritanium)

aseptic loosening, graft resorption, immune reaction, disease transmission, and implant migration.[50,51] More recently, porous coated metal augments have become available with different shapes that can be used to fill specifically shaped defects. These augments have essentially replaced the need for structural allograft (**Fig. 3**). These augments can be used alone or in combination with other augments, and reamers are available to prepare the acetabular defect where augments will be placed. The augments are then impacted into the defect and secured with screws.

Once the augments are fixed with screws, a second-generation porous coated hemispherical cup can be press fitted into the acetabulum and cement placed at the augment-cup interface. Studies evaluating the use of acetabular augments have shown radiographically stable fixation at 2-year follow-up when used alone,[52–54] when combined with impaction grafting,[55,56] and when used with a cage-cup construct.[57] These augments extend the application of hemispherical revision cups to Paprosky type IIB and some type IIIA defects.[58]

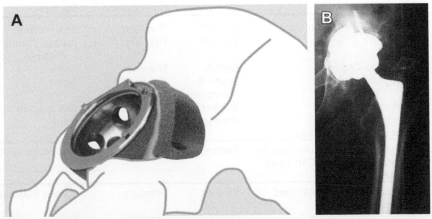

Fig. 3. Trabecular metal acetabular augments. (*A*) Implant. (*B*) Radiograph. ([*A*] *Courtesy of* Zimmer Holdings, Inc, Warsaw (IN); with permission.)

Cages

In Paprosky III acetabular defects in which there is substantial superior migration, bone loss, and/or pelvic discontinuity (type IIIB), these patients may be more appropriately treated with a cage construct. A cage is a prosthesis with multiple screw hole options, so that the prosthesis can be supported by the ilium and ischium instead of the acetabular dome alone (**Table 2**). This prosthesis is used to bridge bone loss as an antiprotrusio device,[59,60] and can be used to contain allograft placed within the acetabular defect to allow for integration of the graft with host bone.[61] Once adequate acetabular exposure is achieved, allograft can be reverse reamed and the cage can be fixed down through the dome screws first, then the superior flange, and then the inferior flange. An all-polyethylene cup or a polyethylene liner is then cemented into place to articulate with the femoral head. Although cages provide temporary fixation while bone graft incorporates into host bone, this method of treatment often lacks biological fixation and may lead to fatigue failure.[62,63]

The preferred option to provide acetabular fixation is to use a cup-cage construct. In this method, a second-generation porous cup is fixed in the pelvis. If there is minimal stability of the implant, an acetabular cage can be placed on top of the cup and secured with screw fixation into the ilium and ischium.[64] A polyethylene liner can then be cemented into the cup cage. This superior method of fixation allows the porous cup to achieve osseointegration, and one study showed that 88.5% of hips had no sign of clinical or radiographic loosening at 44.6 months.[65]

Custom Implants

An alternative treatment in the case of pelvic discontinuity (Paprosky IIIB), especially in situations of massive bone loss, is the use of a custom triflange cup. These components are beneficial because they supposedly match the patient's anatomy to try to minimize bone loss (**Fig. 4**). However, creating these triflange cups requires a computed tomography scan of the pelvis to evaluate the patient's anatomy and bone loss, and designing and manufacturing these implants is an expensive and time-consuming process.[66] When these custom triflange implants are used in selected patients, the radiographic results have shown bridging bone formation in pelvic discontinuity and patients have reported improved Harris hip scores.[67,68]

HEAD AND LINERS

Head and liners in revision THA must be selected to provide the most stable hip. Because soft tissues are more lax in the revision setting, using a larger head to reduce the likelihood of postoperative dislocation and liners that can change the version of the acetabulum provides a dual articulating surface, and provides constraint for the femoral head, which may be beneficial. The head and liner changes in revision THA are described later.

Table 2
Cage, cup-cage, and custom triflange implants

	Implant Name	Company	Composition	Surface
Cages	Recovery® Protrusio Cage	Biomet	Titanium	Grit blasted
	Par 5™	Biomet	Titanium Alloy	Porous Plasma Spray coating
	Protrusio Cage	DePuy	Titanium	None
	Contour	Smith & Nephew	Titanium	None
	Restoration Gap II	Stryker	Titanium	Grit blasted
	Burch-Schneider™ Reinforcement Cage	Zimmer	Titanium	None
Cup-cages	Trabecular Metal™ Acetabular Revision System Cup-Cage Construct	Zimmer	Titanium	Trabecular metal
Custom Triflange	BIOMET® Patient-Matched Implants (PMI®)	Biomet	Titanium	Porous Plasma Spray
	Pinnacle™ Triflange Acetabular System	DePuy	Titanium	Porous- and/or hydroxyapatite-coated

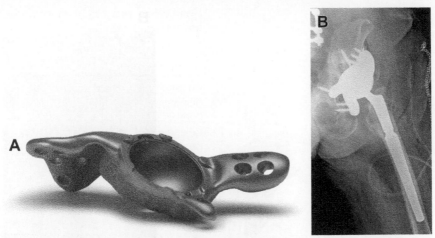

Fig. 4. Custom triflange prosthesis. (*A*) Implant. (*B*) Radiograph. ([*A*] *Courtesy of* Biomet Orthopedics, Inc, Warsaw (IN); with permission.)

Head Size Choice for Revision

The optimal head size for revision is dictated by the size of the acetabular cup and the need for a minimal amount of polyethylene. Studies have shown that the use of 32-mm, 38-mm, and 44-mm femoral heads can eliminate component-to-component impingement and increase range of motion, especially because a skirted neck does not need to be used with larger femoral heads.[69] As the head/neck ratio increases, greater translation is needed between the femoral head and the acetabulum before dislocation occurs, which is increased jump distance.[70] Thus, it is ideal to use larger femoral heads in the revision THA setting, because there is reduced impingement and greater jump distance, which reduces the likelihood of sustaining a dislocation.

Elevated Liners

Another liner option is to use an elevated liner, which is a liner that is elevated a certain number of degrees (often 10°). Elevated liners allow surgeons to change the angle or the face of the acetabular cup, especially in well-fixed components that are minimally malpositioned. In addition, if a cup needs to be placed in a less-than-ideal position to take advantage of available bone stock, an elevated liner may be used to provide appropriate version or inclination to the cup. Two early studies showed that the use of an elevated rim liner decreased hip dislocations compared with standard liners[71,72] and that the survivorship at 5 years was similar at 98.8%.[73] However, subsequent implant retrieval studies have shown that the use of these elevated implants can lead to greater impingement.[74,75]

Dual Mobility Liners

Dual articulation acetabular cups were first developed in France by Professor Gilles Bousquet in 1974, with which a small head is placed within a large polyethylene head that articulates with a metal acetabular component.[76] This construct then acts as a large femoral head, which has the benefit of increasing jump distance and improving range of motion before neck-socket impingement occurs (**Fig. 5**).[77,78] In the revision THA setting, one study showed that dual mobility cups can be used to treat recurrent dislocating hips, and these liners had a low rate of rerevision because of dislocation.[79] Another study even showed that cementing dual mobility liners into well-fixed metal shells, as in revision THA scenarios, was biomechanically stable.[80] As with all options, there are potential negatives for the dual mobility liners. One problem is intraprosthetic dislocation of the implant, or when the femoral head escapes from the thick polyethylene liner when there is polyethylene wear and loss of the retentive rim.[81]

Constrained Liners

To combat instability after revision THA, a constrained acetabular liner can be used, in which a locking mechanism from the liner captures the femoral head (**Fig. 6**). These liners are used when there is recurrent, multidirectional hip instability, when neurologic or neuromuscular diseases are present that can alter hip dynamics, or when there is proximal muscle weakness or soft tissue laxity that can increase the potential for dislocation.[82] However, constrained liners can fail and cause the acetabular component to loosen, or cause the acetabular liner and cup interface to fail.[83]

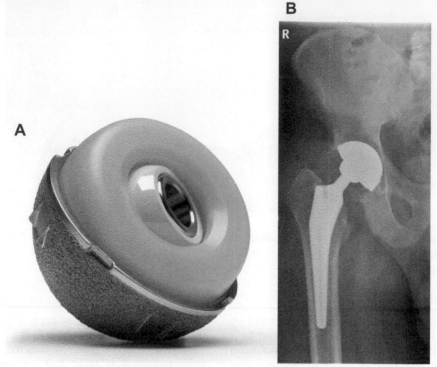

Fig. 5. Dual mobility liner. (*A*) Implant. (*B*) Radiograph. ([*A*] *Courtesy of* Biomet Orthopedics, Inc, Warsaw (IN); with permission.)

Because of the high failure rate, cementing constrained liners with cage constructs should be avoided if possible.[84,85] Because constrained acetabular liners have a significantly decreased primary arc, they are at higher risk for impingement. Thus, newer constrained liners have been designed from which the elevated rim is removed to allow for a greater arc of motion, while preserving the constrained liner benefit of minimizing dislocations.[86]

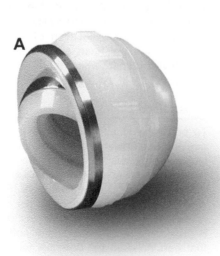

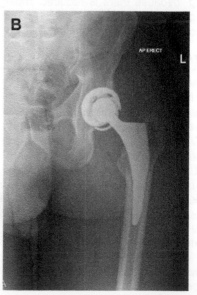

Fig. 6. Constrained liner. (*A*) Implant. (*B*) Radiograph. ([*A*] *Courtesy of* Howmedica Osteonics Corp, Mahwah (NJ); with permission.)

SUMMARY

Selecting appropriate components to perform revision THA is important for restoring hip stability, providing offset to optimize joint biomechanics, and restoring limb length if possible. There are different acetabular, femoral, liner, and head options to achieve stability and provide adequate fixation in the case of bone loss. Using the implant options described here should provide a template by which revision THA can successfully be performed.

REFERENCES

1. Valle CJ, Paprosky WG. Classification and an algorithmic approach to the reconstruction of femoral deficiency in revision total hip arthroplasty. J Bone Joint Surg Am 2003;85(Suppl 4):1–6.
2. Sheth NP, Nelson CL, Paprosky WG. Femoral bone loss in revision total hip arthroplasty: evaluation and management. J Am Acad Orthop Surg 2013; 21(10):601–12.
3. McAuley JP, Szuszczewicz ES, Young A, et al. Total hip arthroplasty in patients 50 years and younger. Clin Orthop Relat Res 2004;(418):119–25.
4. Weeden SH, Paprosky WG. Minimal 11-year follow-up of extensively porous-coated stems in femoral revision total hip arthroplasty. J Arthroplasty 2002;17(4 Suppl 1):134–7.
5. Chung LH, Wu PK, Chen CF, et al. Extensively porous-coated stems for femoral revision: reliable choice for stem revision in Paprosky femoral type III defects. Orthopedics 2012;35(7):e1017–21.
6. Sporer SM, Paprosky WG. Revision total hip arthroplasty: the limits of fully coated stems. Clin Orthop Relat Res 2003;(417):203–9.
7. Sporer SM, Paprosky WG. Extensively coated cementless femoral components in revision total hip arthoplasty: an update. Surg Technol Int 2005;14: 265–74.
8. Moon KH, Kang JS, Lee SH, et al. Revision total hip arthroplasty using an extensively porous coated femoral stem. Clin Orthop Surg 2009;1(2):105–9.
9. Garcia-Cimbrelo E, Garcia-Rey E, Cruz-Pardos A, et al. Stress-shielding of the proximal femur using an extensively porous-coated femoral component without allograft in revision surgery: a 5- to 17-year follow-up study. J Bone Joint Surg Br 2010;92(10):1363–9.
10. Restrepo C, Mashadi M, Parvizi J, et al. Modular femoral stems for revision total hip arthroplasty. Clin Orthop Relat Res 2011;469(2):476–82.
11. Kopec MA, Pemberton A, Milbrandt JC, et al. Component version in modular total hip revision. Iowa Orthop J 2009;29:5–10.
12. Jones RE. Modular revision stems in total hip arthroplasty. Clin Orthop Relat Res 2004;(420):142–7.
13. Revision Total Hip Arthroplasty Study Group. A comparison of modular tapered versus modular cylindrical stems for complex femoral revisions. J Arthroplasty 2013;28(8 Suppl):71–3.
14. Munro JT, Garbuz DS, Masri BA, et al. Role and results of tapered fluted modular titanium stems in revision total hip arthroplasty. J Bone Joint Surg Br 2012;94(11 Suppl A):58–60.
15. Palumbo BT, Morrison KL, Baumgarten AS, et al. Results of revision total hip arthroplasty with modular, titanium-tapered femoral stems in severe proximal metaphyseal and diaphyseal bone loss. J Arthroplasty 2013;28(4):690–4.
16. Wang L, Dai Z, Wen T, et al. Three to seven year follow-up of a tapered modular femoral prosthesis in revision total hip arthroplasty. Arch Orthop Trauma Surg 2013;133(2):275–81.
17. Jibodh SR, Schwarzkopf R, Anthony SG, et al. Revision hip arthroplasty with a modular cementless stem: mid-term follow up. J Arthroplasty 2013; 28(7):1167–72.
18. Klauser W, Bangert Y, Lubinus P, et al. Medium-term follow-up of a modular tapered noncemented titanium stem in revision total hip arthroplasty: a single-surgeon experience. J Arthroplasty 2013; 28(1):84–9.
19. Skytta ET, Eskelinen A, Remes V. Successful femoral reconstruction with a fluted and tapered modular distal fixation stem in revision total hip arthroplasty. Scand J Surg 2012;101(3):222–6.
20. Van Houwelingen AP, Duncan CP, Masri BA, et al. High survival of modular tapered stems for proximal femoral bone defects at 5 to 10 years followup. Clin Orthop Relat Res 2013;471(2):454–62.
21. Lakstein D, Eliaz N, Levi O, et al. Fracture of cementless femoral stems at the mid-stem junction in modular revision hip arthroplasty systems. J Bone Joint Surg Am 2011;93(1):57–65.
22. Efe T, Schmitt J. Analyses of prosthesis stem failures in noncemented modular hip revision prostheses. J Arthroplasty 2011;26(4):665.e7–12.
23. Mayle RE Jr, Paprosky WG. Massive bone loss: allograft-prosthetic composites and beyond. J Bone Joint Surg Br 2012;94(11 Suppl A):61–4.
24. Liptak JM, Pluhar GE, Dernell WS, et al. Limb-sparing surgery in a dog with osteosarcoma of the proximal femur. Vet Surg 2005;34(1):71–7.
25. Gross AE, Hutchison CR. Proximal femoral allografts for reconstruction of bone stock in revision hip arthroplasty. Orthopedics 1998;21(9): 999–1001.
26. Babis GC, Sakellariou VI, O'Connor MI, et al. Proximal femoral allograft-prosthesis composites in revision hip replacement: a 12-year follow-up study. J Bone Joint Surg Br 2010;92(3):349–55.
27. Maurer SG, Baitner AC, Di Cesare PE. Reconstruction of the failed femoral component and proximal

femoral bone loss in revision hip surgery. J Am Acad Orthop Surg 2000;8(6):354–63.

28. Parvizi J, Tarity TD, Slenker N, et al. Proximal femoral replacement in patients with non-neoplastic conditions. J Bone Joint Surg Am 2007;89(5):1036–43.

29. Sewell MD, Hanna SA, Carrington RW, et al. Modular proximal femoral replacement in salvage hip surgery for non-neoplastic conditions. Acta Orthop Belg 2010;76(4):493–502.

30. Malkani AL, Settecerri JJ, Sim FH, et al. Long-term results of proximal femoral replacement for non-neoplastic disorders. J Bone Joint Surg Br 1995; 77(3):351–6.

31. Al-Taki MM, Masri BA, Duncan CP, et al. Quality of life following proximal femoral replacement using a modular system in revision THA. Clin Orthop Relat Res 2011;469(2):470–5.

32. Haentjens P, De Boeck H, Opdecam P. Proximal femoral replacement prosthesis for salvage of failed hip arthroplasty: complications in a 2-11 year follow-up study in 19 elderly patients. Acta Orthop Scand 1996;67(1):37–42.

33. Parvizi J, Sim FH. Proximal femoral replacements with megaprostheses. Clin Orthop Relat Res 2004;(420):169–75.

34. Chalkin B, Minter J. Limb salvage and abductor re-attachment using a custom prosthesis with porous tantalum components. J Arthroplasty 2005;20(1): 127–30.

35. Levine B, Della Valle CJ, Jacobs JJ. Applications of porous tantalum in total hip arthroplasty. J Am Acad Orthop Surg 2006;14(12):646–55.

36. Sheth NP, Nelson CL, Springer BD, et al. Acetabular bone loss in revision total hip arthroplasty: evaluation and management. J Am Acad Orthop Surg 2013;21(3):128–39.

37. Deirmengian GK, Zmistowski B, O'Neil JT, et al. Management of acetabular bone loss in revision total hip arthroplasty. J Bone Joint Surg Am 2011; 93(19):1842–52.

38. Paprosky WG, Perona PG, Lawrence JM. Acetabular defect classification and surgical reconstruction in revision arthroplasty. A 6-year follow-up evaluation. J Arthroplasty 1994;9(1):33–44.

39. Yu R, Hofstaetter, Sullivan T, et al. Validity and reliability of the Paprosky acetabular defect classification. Clin Orthop Relat Res 2013;471(7): 2259–65.

40. Hanzlik JA, Day JS, Acknowledged Contributors: Ingrowth Retrieval Study Group. Bone ingrowth in well-fixed retrieved porous tantalum implants. J Arthroplasty 2013;28(6):922–7.

41. Jafari SM, Bender B, Coyle C, et al. Do tantalum and titanium cups show similar results in revision hip arthroplasty? Clin Orthop Relat Res 2010; 468(2):459–65.

42. Welldon KJ, Atkins GJ, Howie DW, et al. Primary human osteoblasts grow into porous tantalum and maintain an osteoblastic phenotype. J Biomed Mater Res A 2008;84(3):691–701.

43. Bobyn JD, Stackpool GJ, Hacking SA, et al. Characteristics of bone ingrowth and interface mechanics of a new porous tantalum biomaterial. J Bone Joint Surg Br 1999;81(5):907–14.

44. Della Valle CJ, Berger RA, Rosenberg AG, et al. Cementless acetabular reconstruction in revision total hip arthroplasty. Clin Orthop Relat Res 2004;(420):96–100.

45. Della Valle CJ, Shuaipaj T, Berger RA, et al. Revision of the acetabular component without cement after total hip arthroplasty. A concise follow-up, at fifteen to nineteen years, of a previous report. J Bone Joint Surg Am 2005;87(8):1795–800.

46. Hallstrom BR, Golladay GJ, Vittetoe DA, et al. Cementless acetabular revision with the Harris-Galante porous prosthesis. Results after a minimum of ten years of follow-up. J Bone Joint Surg Am 2004;86(5):1007–11.

47. Blom AW, Wylde V, Livesey C, et al. Impaction bone grafting of the acetabulum at hip revision using a mix of bone chips and a biphasic porous ceramic bone graft substitute. Acta Orthop 2009;80(2): 150–4.

48. Levai JP, Boisgard S. Acetabular reconstruction in total hip revision using a bone graft substitute. Early clinical and radiographic results. Clin Orthop Relat Res 1996;(330):108–14.

49. Nehme A, Lewallen DG, Hanssen AD. Modular porous metal augments for treatment of severe acetabular bone loss during revision hip arthroplasty. Clin Orthop Relat Res 2004;(429):201–8.

50. Bilgen OF, Bilgen MS, Oncan T, et al. Acetabular reconstruction by impacted cancellous allografts in cementless total hip arthroplasty revision. Acta Orthop Traumatol Turc 2012;46(2):120–5.

51. Lee PT, Clayton RA, Safir OA, et al. Structural allograft as an option for treating infected hip arthroplasty with massive bone loss. Clin Orthop Relat Res 2011;469(4):1016–23.

52. Van Kleunen JP, Lee GC, Lementowski PW, et al. Acetabular revisions using trabecular metal cups and augments. J Arthroplasty 2009;24(Suppl 6): 64–8.

53. Siegmeth A, Duncan CP, Masri BA, et al. Modular tantalum augments for acetabular defects in revision hip arthroplasty. Clin Orthop Relat Res 2009; 467(1):199–205.

54. Abolghasemian M, Tangsataporn S, Sternheim A, et al. Combined trabecular metal acetabular shell and augment for acetabular revision with substantial bone loss: a mid-term review. Bone Joint J Br 2013;95(2):166–72.

55. Borland WS, Bhattacharya R, Holland JP, et al. Use of porous trabecular metal augments with impaction bone grafting in management of acetabular bone loss. Acta Orthop 2012;83(4):347–52.

56. Gill K, Wilson MJ, Whitehouse SL, et al. Results using trabecular metal augments in combination with acetabular impaction bone grafting in deficient acetabula. Hip Int 2013;23:522–8.

57. Ballester Alfaro JJ, Sueiro Fernandez J. Trabecular metal buttress augment and the trabecular metal cup-cage construct in revision hip arthroplasty for severe acetabular bone loss and pelvic discontinuity. Hip Int 2010;20(Suppl 7):S119–27.

58. Gehrke T, Bangert Y, Schwantes B, et al. Acetabular revision in THA using tantalum augments combined with impaction bone grafting. Hip Int 2013; 23(4):359–65.

59. Berry DJ, Muller ME. Revision arthroplasty using an anti-protrusio cage for massive acetabular bone deficiency. J Bone Joint Surg Br 1992;74(5): 711–5.

60. Gill TJ, Sledge JB, Muller ME. The Burch-Schneider anti-protrusio cage in revision total hip arthroplasty: indications, principles and long-term results. J Bone Joint Surg Br 1998;80(6):946–53.

61. Hansen E, Shearer D, Ries MD. Does a cemented cage improve revision THA for severe acetabular defects? Clin Orthop Relat Res 2011;469(2): 494–502.

62. Paprosky WG, Sporer SS, Murphy BP. Addressing severe bone deficiency: what a cage will not do. J Arthroplasty 2007;22(4 Suppl 1):111–5.

63. Sembrano JN, Cheng EY. Acetabular cage survival and analysis of factors related to failure. Clin Orthop Relat Res 2008;466(7):1657–65.

64. Malhotra R, Kancherla R, Kumar V, et al. Trabecular metal acetabular revision system (cup-cage construct) to address the massive acetabular defects in revision arthroplasty. Indian J Orthop 2012; 46(4):483–6.

65. Kosashvili Y, Backstein D, Safir O, et al. Acetabular revision using an anti-protrusion (ilio-ischial) cage and trabecular metal acetabular component for severe acetabular bone loss associated with pelvic discontinuity. J Bone Joint Surg Br 2009;91(7): 870–6.

66. Taunton MJ, Fehring TK, Edwards P, et al. Pelvic discontinuity treated with custom triflange component: a reliable option. Clin Orthop Relat Res 2012;470(2):428–34.

67. DeBoer DK, Christie MJ, Brinson MF, et al. Revision total hip arthroplasty for pelvic discontinuity. J Bone Joint Surg Am 2007;89(4):835–40.

68. Joshi AB, Lee J, Christensen C. Results for a custom acetabular component for acetabular deficiency. J Arthroplasty 2002;17(5):643–8.

69. Burroughs BR, Hallstrom B, Golladay GJ, et al. Range of motion and stability in total hip arthroplasty with 28-, 32-, 38-, and 44-mm femoral head sizes. J Arthroplasty 2005;20(1):11–9.

70. Nevelos J, Johnson A, Heffernan C, et al. What factors affect posterior dislocation distance in THA? Clin Orthop Relat Res 2013;471(2):519–26.

71. Alberton GM, High WA, Morrey BF. Dislocation after revision total hip arthroplasty: an analysis of risk factors and treatment options. J Bone Joint Surg Am 2002;84(10):1788–92.

72. Cobb TK, Morrey BF, Ilstrup DM. The elevated-rim acetabular liner in total hip arthroplasty: relationship to postoperative dislocation. J Bone Joint Surg Am 1996;78(1):80–6.

73. Cobb TK, Morrey BF, Ilstrup DM. Effect of the elevated-rim acetabular liner on loosening after total hip arthroplasty. J Bone Joint Surg Am 1997; 79(9):1361–4.

74. Marchetti E, Krantz N, Berton C, et al. Component impingement in total hip arthroplasty: frequency and risk factors. A continuous retrieval analysis series of 416 cup. Orthop Traumatol Surg Res 2011; 97(2):127–33.

75. Shon WY, Baldini T, Peterson MG, et al. Impingement in total hip arthroplasty a study of retrieved acetabular components. J Arthroplasty 2005; 20(4):427–35.

76. Philippot R, Camilleri JP, Boyer B, et al. The use of a dual-articulation acetabular cup system to prevent dislocation after primary total hip arthroplasty: analysis of 384 cases at a mean follow-up of 15 years. Int Orthop 2009;33(4):927–32.

77. Lachiewicz PF, Watters TS. The use of dual-mobility components in total hip arthroplasty. J Am Acad Orthop Surg 2012;20(8):481–6.

78. Stulberg SD. Dual poly liner mobility optimizes wear and stability in THA: affirms. Orthopedics 2011;34(9):e445–8.

79. Hailer NP, Weiss RJ, Stark A, et al. Dual-mobility cups for revision due to instability are associated with a low rate of re-revisions due to dislocation: 228 patients from the Swedish hip arthroplasty register. Acta Orthop 2012;83(6):566–71.

80. Wegrzyn J, Thoreson AR, Guyen O, et al. Cementation of a dual-mobility acetabular component into a well-fixed metal shell during revision total hip arthroplasty: a biomechanical validation. J Orthop Res 2013;31(6):991–7.

81. Philippot R, Boyer B, Farizon F. Intraprosthetic dislocation: a specific complication of the dual-mobility system. Clin Orthop Relat Res 2013; 471(3):965–70.

82. Lombardi AV Jr. Constrained liners in revision: total hip arthroplasty an overuse syndrome: in opposition. J Arthroplasty 2006;21(4 Suppl 1):126–30.

83. Fricka KB, Marshall A, Paprosky WG. Constrained liners in revision total hip arthroplasty: an overuse syndrome: in the affirmative. J Arthroplasty 2006; 21(4 Suppl 1):121–5.

84. Khoury JI, Malkani AL, Adler EM, et al. Constrained acetabular liners cemented into cages during total hip revision arthroplasty. J Arthroplasty 2010;25(6): 901–5.

85. Klein GR, Rapuri V, Hozack WJ, et al. Caution on the use of combined constrained liners and cages in revision total hip arthroplasty. Orthopedics 2007; 30(11):970–1.

86. Munro JT, Vioreanu MH, Masri BA, et al. Acetabular liner with focal constraint to prevent dislocation afterk THA. Clin Orthop Relat Res 2013;471(12): 3883–90.

Current and Future Trends in the Diagnosis of Periprosthetic Hip Infection

Beau S. Konigsberg, MD[a], Curtis W. Hartman, MD[a],
Angela L. Hewlett, MD[b], Kevin L. Garvin, MD[a],*

KEYWORDS

- Hip arthroplasty • Revision arthroplasty • Periprosthetic infection
- Diagnosis of prosthetic hip infection

KEY POINTS

- The diagnosis of prosthetic hip infection involves multiple modalities, including an initial clinical evaluation, appropriate laboratory studies, and intraoperative assessment.
- Arthrocentesis should be performed in all patients with suspected prosthetic joint.
- A minimum of three, optimally up to six cultures of the periprosthetic tissue should be obtained to aid in the diagnosis of prosthetic joint infection.
- Although ESR and CRP remain the standard of care in serum laboratory diagnosis of prosthetic joint infection, other biomarkers are under investigation.
- Newer diagnostic techniques, such as sonication and molecular analysis, may be helpful in the diagnosis of prosthetic joint infection.

INTRODUCTION

The appropriate diagnosis of a prosthetic hip infection is a critical first step to successful management and functional recovery of the patient. The challenge of confirming the diagnosis is two-fold. First, the presentation of the patient with a prosthetic hip infection often has limited or few subjective complaints and physical findings, nonconfirmatory inflammatory laboratory markers, and negative culture results. Secondly, there has not been consistent agreement of the definition of prosthetic join infection. Different authors and institutions have used many combinations of blood tests, histologic analysis, synovial fluid,

and tissue culture results and clinical findings to define the presence of infection. Recent work by the Musculoskeletal Infection Society has created a new uniform definition for research and clinical use.[1] This may improve the ability to accurately diagnose prosthetic hip infections individually and share data among different sites for research collaboration. The incidence of prosthetic hip infection has remained at approximately 2% for the last past several years.[2] By following consistent diagnosis criteria established for hip and knee infections, we may actually see an increase in the number of identified prosthetic hip infections (**Figs. 1** and **2**).

Conflict of Interest: TRAK Surgical, Omaha, NE (B.S. Konigsberg, and C.W. Hartman); Smith and Nephew, Memphis, TN (C.W. Hartman); None (A.L. Hewlett); Biomet, Warsaw, IN (K.L. Garvin).
[a] Department of Orthopaedic Surgery and Rehabilitation, University of Nebraska Medical Center, 981080 Nebraska Medical Center, Omaha, NE 68198–1080, USA; [b] University of Nebraska Medical Center, 985400 Nebraska Medical Center, Omaha, NE 68198-5400, USA
* Corresponding author.
E-mail address: kgarvin@unmc.edu

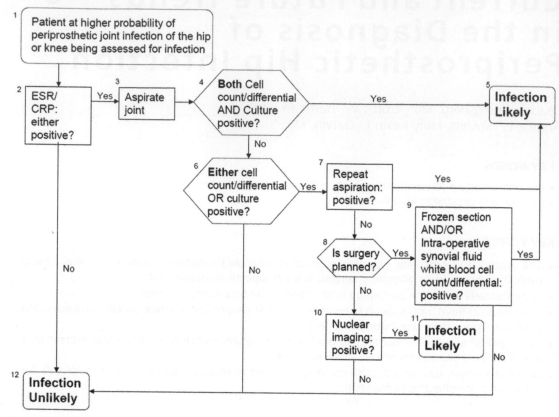

Fig. 1. Algorithm for patients with a higher probability of periprosthetic joint infection of the hip or knee being assessed for infection. CRP, C-reactive protein; ESR, erythrocyte sedimentation rate. (© 2010 American Academy of Orthopaedic Surgeons. *Reprinted from* Della Valle C, Parvizi J, Bauer TW, et al. AAOS clinical practical guideline summary: diagnosis of periprosthetic joint infections of the hip and knee. J Am Acad Orthop Surg 2010;18:762; with permission.)

CLINICAL EXAMINATION

The clinician evaluating a patient with a possible prosthetic hip infection must be aware of the vast array of signs and symptoms that may be present. The most common complaint is pain in the hip area (buttock, lateral hip, groin, or thigh). The symptom of pain associated with this inflammatory process is usually present at all times, but may be most noticeable while the patient is inactive or at rest. Activity usually has little effect on the pain, but may distract the patient from its presence and intensity for brief periods of time. A complete clinical history including questions about the presence of comorbid conditions, history of previous infections and subsequent management, history of poor wound healing, and information about any current symptoms should be obtained. While the clinician is obtaining history from the patient, it is important to ask about the history of the surgical procedure. Specifically, surgical records that can inform the clinician about the length of surgery, type of implant that was used, and if there

were intraoperative challenges that resulted in prolonged surgical time. Any history of perioperative infections (such as urinary tract or pneumonia, wound infections, or others that may have caused transient bacteremia) should also be noted. All pertinent medical records should be obtained and reviewed, including prior history and physical assessments, operative reports, and any relevant diagnostic studies including previous culture results.

A thorough physical examination should be performed, paying close attention to the surgical incision, including evaluation of drainage or the presence of a sinus tract. Areas of tenderness about the hip reflecting sites of inflammation or abscesses should also be evaluated. Range-of-motion of the hip may or may not be affected; however, stiffness of the joint is a common finding for those patients with an infection.

Radiographs of the prosthetic joint are routinely ordered to evaluate for the presence of findings consistent with infection (progressive radiolucent lines, osteolysis, or periosteal new bone formation).

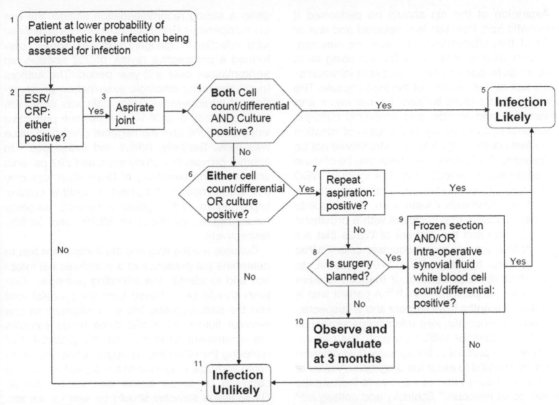

Fig. 2. Algorithm for patients at lower probability of periprosthetic knee Infection being assessed for infection. CRP, C-reactive protein; ESR, erythrocyte sedimentation rate. (© 2010 American Academy of Orthopaedic Surgeons. *Reprinted from* Della Valle C, Parvizi J, Bauer TW, et al. AAOS clinical practical guideline summary: diagnosis of periprosthetic joint infections of the hip and knee. J Am Acad Orthop Surg 2010;18:763; with permission.)

The use of additional radiographs is of limited value. Specifically, nuclear imaging (labeled-leukocyte imaging combined with bone or bone marrow imaging, F-18 fluorodeoxyglucose-positron emission tomography [FDG-PET] imaging, or gallium imaging) may be of benefit but limited information supports their routine use.[3] Furthermore, with variability in imaging studies special expertise may be required for these particular images. Magnetic resonance imaging is another diagnostic test that has the potential to be helpful, but this has not been definitively established.[4]

Inflammatory markers, such as erythrocyte sedimentation rate (ESR) and C-reactive protein (CRP), are essential laboratory tests to be included in the diagnostic evaluation of a patient suspected of having a prosthetic joint infection. Greidanus and colleagues[5] performed a prospective study on patients being evaluated before revision surgery. Schinsky and colleagues[6] performed preoperative evaluation in 235 painful total hip arthroplasties. The studies performed in the work-up of this population included ESR, CRP, fluid aspiration for white blood cell (WBC) count, intraoperative frozen

section analysis of patients from the joint tissue, and permanent histopathologic examination of this tissue. When the CRP and ESR were both elevated above their normal ranges, the sensitivity and specificity were 91% and 95%, respectively, and the positive predictive value and negative predictive value were 83% and 91%, respectively. In contrast, if the ESR was less than 30 mm/h and the CRP less than 10 mg/dL, the specificity for asepsis was 100%. The value of the ESR and CRP has been reported by other investigators.[7,8] Alternative biomarkers for diagnosis of prosthetic joint infection are under investigation, including interleukin-6, synovial CRP, and synovial alpha-defensin.

Blood cultures (two sets) should be performed in patients with systemic symptoms including fever, acute onset of symptoms, or if a concomitant infection is present that would make the presence of a bloodstream infection more likely.[9] The presence of bacteremia can aid in the identification of the offending pathogen to tailor antibiotic therapy, and may also change the clinical management of the patient.

Aspiration of the hip should be performed if prosthetic joint infection is suspected and one or both of the inflammatory markers are elevated. The aspiration should be performed using strict aseptic technique in a clinic setting or intraoperatively just before incision of the joint capsule. The synovial fluid should be sent for cell count and differential, and aerobic and anaerobic cultures. Additional cultures for atypical causes of infection (acid-fast bacilli, fungi, and so forth) should not be obtained routinely; however, these may be of value in certain patient populations. The synovial WBC count should be interpreted in reference to the time from prosthesis implantation. The absolute number of WBCs that correlate with a prosthetic joint infection and the percent of WBCs that are present that are polymorphonuclear cells (PMNs) are reported to range from 1700 cells/mL to approximately 4200 cells/mL if the joint is more than 6 months postoperative.[6,10] A patient who is less than 6 months from surgery and is suspected of having a prosthetic joint infection generally has a higher number of WBCs present. The percent of PMN cells present in the synovial fluid differential is also helpful to aid in the diagnosis. A value of greater than 80% has been shown to indicate the presence of infection.[6] Schinsky and colleagues[6] also demonstrated that in the presence of elevated ESR and CRP, the optimal cut-point for prosthetic hip infection was a synovial fluid WBC count of greater than 3000 cells/mL. Synovial fluid WBC counts have been shown to be variable in failed metal-on-metal hip implants, making interpretation of synovial fluid analysis difficult in this patient population.[11]

INTRAOPERATIVE EVALUATION FOR A PROSTHETIC JOINT INFECTION

Intraoperative assessment of the prosthetic hip is a critical next step in the evaluation for the presence of infection. If synovial fluid was not obtained preoperatively, then it should be obtained intraoperatively. Tissue specimens obtained from the interface tissue adjacent or juxtaposed to the implant or the interior surface of the capsule should be sent for histopathology by frozen section analysis. A minimum of three specimens should be obtained. Mirra and colleagues[12] defined acute inflammation, consistent with infection, if more than five PMNs were seen on at least 10 high-powered fields at ×400 magnification. The American Academy of Orthopaedic Surgeons (AAOS) Evidence Based Guideline included a meta-analysis also supporting five PMNs per high-powered field with excellent specificity.[3] The AAOS Evidence Based Guideline has also

given a strong recommendation against the use of intraoperative Gram stain to rule out a prosthetic joint infection.[3] Spangehl and colleagues[7] performed a prospective review of 202 revision hip arthroplasties over a 2-year period. The authors found the histopathologic examination on sensitivity of intraoperative Gram stain was only 19% and specificity was 98%. The positive predictive value was 63% and the negative predictive value was 89%. Similarly, Atkins and colleagues[13] in another prospective study evaluated 297 patients and found the sensitivity of Gram stain was only 6% when measured against a positive culture, improving to 12% against a positive histology result and a specificity of 99.7% and 98.8%, respectively.

Cultures are the final and most important test to determine the presence of a prosthetic hip infection and to identify the offending pathogen. Cultures should be obtained from the synovial fluid and the periprosthetic tissue. A minimum of one synovial fluid sample and three tissue samples are recommended to increase the probability of retrieving the offending pathogen. Obtaining additional samples may increase the yield further, so obtaining up to six tissue samples is optimal. These tissue samples should be sent for aerobic and anaerobic cultures. Similarly to the synovial fluid analysis, additional cultures for atypical organisms should not be routinely obtained, but may be necessary in certain patient populations. Although there is no defined standard for incubation time of periprosthetic tissue specimens, it is reasonable to pursue a longer incubation time (up to 14 days) because some organisms may require a prolonged period of time to grow. This is especially important when *Propionibacterium* sp is suspected.[14,15]

Other modalities have been shown to enhance the yield of traditional cultures. The process of sonication (subjecting the explanted prosthetic material to ultrasound waves, and culturing the remaining ultrasonicate fluid) was demonstrated to improve the sensitivity of traditional cultures.[16] However, the use of this procedure should be considered relative to the sensitivity of the clinical microbiology laboratory to detect positive cultures in patients with prosthetic joint infection. Sonication may not be necessary in centers with clinical microbiology laboratories that achieve high sensitivities using standard microbiologic techniques.[17]

The use of preoperative antibiotics in this setting, including routine prophylaxis, should be avoided to maximize the yield of the intraoperative cultures. Berbari and colleagues[18] reviewed the experience of culture-negative prosthetic joint infection. Of 897 episodes of prosthetic joint infection, 60 (7%) were initial episodes of culture-negative infection. Antibiotics had been used in 32 (53%) of the 60 episodes during the 3 months before the diagnosis of the culture-negative prosthetic joint infection.

Given the complexity of management of culture-negative prosthetic joint infections, the challenge of pathogen identification is always present. One additional modality to assist with pathogen identification is the use of molecular diagnostic techniques. Advantages of molecular diagnostic techniques include a short time until results are available and accurate detection of the infectious agent, even if it is present at low levels. It is also possible to identify genetic determinants of virulence of some organisms and the presence of antibiotic resistance, which can aid in the management of these infections.[19-26] A recent investigation by Gomez and colleagues[27] compared PCR (16S rRNA gene real-time PCR sequences) of the fluid obtained after sonication of removed implants to culture of synovial fluid, tissue and sonicate fluid, tissue, and sonicate fluid. One hundred thirty-five samples from prosthetic joint infections in 231 from aseptic failure were studied. The authors concluded that broad-range PCR and culture of sonicate fluid have equivalent performance in the diagnosis of a prosthetic joint infection.[27] The advantages include a high sensitivity because only a small number of bacteria need to be present for identification. The disadvantages of the routine use of PCR are the additional cost and the high number of false-positive results, because it is possible that commensal pathogens can be amplified and thought to be responsible for an infection when either there is not an infection present or the infection is not caused by the commensal that has been identified. Nonetheless, because of the number of false-negative culture results that are present with prosthetic hip infection, molecular diagnostic tests continue to be an option for the diagnosis of prosthetic hip infection. It is hoped that future work in this area will result in important information to aid in the identification of the pathogens associated with prosthetic hip infection.

SUMMARY

The tests and the sequence of performing appropriate tests while evaluating a patient suspected of having a prosthetic hip infection have been described in this article. One short-coming in the evaluation process is that there is not a single test to confirm the diagnosis of prosthetic hip infection for all patients. Because of this, definitions for diagnosing infection have been established to aid clinicians with this diagnostic dilemma. The Work Group for the Musculoskeletal Infection Society convened to analyze the evidence and propose a new definition for prosthetic joint infection (**Box 1**).[28] The authors acknowledge that the diagnosis includes current tests but numerous other tests are under evaluation. This dynamic process will allow upgrading of the diagnostic criteria as necessary.

In summary, the diagnosis of a prosthetic hip infection requires clinician awareness of various patient presentations. There are many factors that contribute to the patient presentation, including patient-related factors like comorbid conditions including immunosuppression, proximity of the surgical procedure, and the virulence of the offending pathogen. Early infections are likely to cause severe pain, and be associated with poor wound healing and drainage, and even systemic symptoms of fever, night sweats, or malaise. Patients with a chronic infection require the

---

Box 1
Definition of periprosthetic joint infection

Based on the proposed criteria, definite prosthetic joint infection exists when:

1. There is a sinus tract communicating with the prosthesis; or

2. A pathogen is isolated by culture from at least two separate tissue or fluid samples obtained from the affected prosthetic joint; or

3. Four of the following six criteria exist:

   a. Elevated serum erythrocyte sedimentation rate and serum C-reactive protein concentration

   b. Elevated synovial leukocyte count

   c. Elevated synovial neutrophil percentage (polymorphonuclear cell %)

   d. Presence of purulence in the affected joint

   e. Isolation of a microorganism in one culture of periprosthetic tissue or fluid, or

   f. Greater than five neutrophils per high-power field in five high-power fields observed from histologic analysis of periprosthetic tissue at ×400 magnification.

Prosthetic joint infection may be present if fewer than four of these criteria are met.

Adapted from Parvizi J, Zmistowski B, Berbari EF, et al. The workgroup convened by the Musculoskeletal Infection Society: brief communication: new definition for periprosthetic joint infection. J Arthroplasty 2011;26(8):1136–8; with permission.

clinician's vigilance because of the possibility of less acute symptoms and physical findings. A painful loose implant 2 years after surgery may reflect a low-grade infection and therefore a thorough evaluation as described in this article is necessary to establish the diagnosis.

The evaluation of a patient with suspected prosthetic joint infection consists of a history and physical examination and appropriate diagnostic tests. A multidisciplinary approach is optimal, and obtaining the opinion of an infectious diseases specialist may aid in the appropriate management of patients with prosthetic joint infections.

It is imperative that providers remain current in regards to recommendations for evaluation and diagnosis of prosthetic joint infection. Interest in newer diagnostic techniques and assays is apparent, and keeping up-to-date on the current evidence-based recommendations is an important part of the management of these complicated infections.

REFERENCES

1. Workgroup Convened by the Musculoskeletal Infection Society. New definition for periprosthetic joint infection. J Arthroplasty 2011;26(8):1136–8. http://dx.doi.org/10.1016/j.arth.2011.09.026.

2. Kurtz SM, Lau E, Watson H, et al. Economic burden of periprosthetic joint infection in the United States. J Arthroplasty 2012;27(Suppl 8):61–5.e1.

3. Della Valle C, Parvizi J, Bauer TW, et al. Diagnosis of periprosthetic joint infections of the hip and knee. J Am Acad Orthop Surg 2010;18(12):760–70.

4. Hayter CL, Koff MF, Potter HG. Magnetic resonance imaging of the postoperative hip. J Magn Reson Imaging 2012;35(5):1013–25.

5. Greidanus NV, Masri BA, Garbuz DS, et al. Use of erythrocyte sedimentation rate and C-reactive protein level to diagnose infection before revision total knee arthroplasty. A prospective evaluation. J Bone Joint Surg Am 2007;89(7):1409–16. http://dx.doi.org/10.2106/JBJS.D.02602.

6. Schinsky MF, Della Valle CJ, Sporer SM, et al. Perioperative testing for joint infection in patients undergoing revision total hip arthroplasty. J Bone Joint Surg Am 2008;90(9):1869–75. http://dx.doi.org/10.2106/JBJS.G.01255.

7. Spangehl MJ, Masri BA, O'Connell JX, et al. Prospective analysis of preoperative and intraoperative investigations for the diagnosis of infection at the sites of two hundred and two revision total hip arthroplasties. J Bone Joint Surg Am 1999;81(5):672–83.

8. Levitsky KA, Hozack WJ, Balderston RA, et al. Evaluation of the painful prosthetic joint. Relative value of bone scan, sedimentation rate, and joint aspiration. J Arthroplasty 1991;6(3):237–44.

9. Osmon DR, Berbari EF, Berendt AR, et al. Diagnosis and management of prosthetic joint infection: clinical practice guidelines by the Infectious Diseases Society of America. Clin Infect Dis 2013;56(1):e1–25. http://dx.doi.org/10.1093/cid/cis803.

10. Trampuz A, Hanssen AD, Osmon DR, et al. Synovial fluid leukocyte count and differential for the diagnosis of prosthetic knee infection. Am J Med 2004; 117(8):556–62. http://dx.doi.org/10.1016/j.amjmed.2004.06.022.

11. Wyles C, Larson D, Houdek M, et al. Diagnosing infection in failed metal-on-metal hip arthroplasty: are synovial fluid aspirations helpful?: Philadelphia; Musculoskeletal Infection Society meeting, August 2-3, 2013.

12. Mirra JM, Amstutz HC, Matos M, et al. The pathology of the joint tissues and its clinical relevance in prosthesis failure. Clin Orthop Relat Res 1976;(117): 221–40.

13. Atkins BL, Athanasou N, Deeks JJ, et al. Prospective evaluation of criteria for microbiological diagnosis of prosthetic-joint infection at revision arthroplasty. J Clin Microbiol 1998;36(10):2932–9.

14. Butler-Wu SM, Burns EM, Pottinger PS, et al. Optimization of periprosthetic culture for diagnosis of Propionibacterium acnes prosthetic joint infection. J Clin Microbiol 2011;49(7):2490–5.

15. Schäfer P, Fink B, Sandow D, et al. Prolonged bacterial culture to identify late periprosthetic joint infection: a promising strategy. Clin Infect Dis 2008; 47(11):1403–9.

16. Trampuz A, Piper KE, Jacobson MJ, et al. Sonication of removed hip and knee prostheses for diagnosis of infection. N Engl J Med 2007;357(7):654–63.

17. Hartman CW, Kildow BJ, Antoniak D, et al. Sonication for enhanced diagnosis of prosthetic joint infection. 2013 annual meeting of the Musculoskeletal Infection Society.

18. Berbari EF, Marculescu C, Sia I, et al. Culture-negative prosthetic joint infection. Clin Infect Dis 2007; 45(9):1113–9. http://dx.doi.org/10.1086/522184.

19. Kim HB, Lee B, Jang HC, et al. A high frequency of macrolide-lincosamide-streptogramin resistance determinants in Staphylococcus aureus isolated in South Korea. Microb Drug Resist 2004;10(3):248–54. http://dx.doi.org/10.1089/mdr.2004.10.248.

20. Jorgensen JH, Crawford SA, McElmeel ML, et al. Detection of inducible clindamycin resistance of staphylococci in conjunction with performance of automated broth susceptibility testing. J Clin Microbiol 2004;42(4):1800–2.

21. Lapierre P, Huletsky A, Fortin V, et al. Real-time PCR assay for detection of fluoroquinolone resistance associated with grlA mutations in Staphylococcus aureus. J Clin Microbiol 2003;41(7):3246–51.

22. Ramos-Trujillo E, Perez-Roth E, Mendez-Alvarez S, et al. Multiplex PCR for simultaneous detection of

enterococcal genes vanA and vanB and staphylococcal genes mecA, ileS-2 and femB. Int Microbiol 2003;6(2):113–5. http://dx.doi.org/10.1007/s10123-003-0118-z.

23. Spiliopoulou I, Petinaki E, Papandreou P, et al. Erm(C) is the predominant genetic determinant for the expression of resistance to macrolides among methicillin-resistant *Staphylococcus aureus* clinical isolates in Greece. J Antimicrob Chemother 2004; 53(5):814–7. http://dx.doi.org/10.1093/jac/dkh197.

24. Strommenger B, Kettlitz C, Werner G, et al. Multiplex PCR assay for simultaneous detection of nine clinically relevant antibiotic resistance genes in *Staphylococcus aureus*. J Clin Microbiol 2003; 41(9):4089–94.

25. Verdier I, Reverdy ME, Etienne J, et al. *Staphylococcus aureus* isolates with reduced susceptibility to glycopeptides belong to accessory gene regulator group I or II. Antimicrob Agents Chemother 2004;48(3):1024–7.

26. Morsczeck C, Langendorfer D, Schierholz JM. A quantitative real-time PCR assay for the detection of tetR of Tn10 in *Escherichia coli* using SYBR green and the opticon. J Biochem Biophys Methods 2004; 59(3):217–27. http://dx.doi.org/10.1016/j.jbbm.2004.02.003.

27. Gomez E, Cazanave C, Cunningham SA, et al. Prosthetic joint infection diagnosis using broad-range PCR of biofilms dislodged from knee and hip arthroplasty surfaces using sonication. J Clin Microbiol 2012;50(11):3501–8.

28. Parvizi J, Zmistowski B, Berbari EF, et al. New definition for periprosthetic joint infection: from the workgroup of the Musculoskeletal Infection Society. Clin Orthop Relat Res 2011;469(11):2992–4. http://dx.doi.org/10.1007/s11999-011-2102-9.

Trauma

Preface
Trauma

 CrossMark

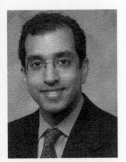

Saqib Rehman, MD
Editor

Distal tibia fractures continue to be challenging injuries to treat, even for those surgeons with extensive experience. Complications with wound and bone healing can be humbling, and controversy exists regarding the appropriate surgical timing of these injuries. Especially with the advent of locked plates and minimally invasive methods (including nailing of extremely distal extra-articular distal tibia fractures), indirect reduction methods and critical evaluation of fracture reduction and alignment are extremely important. Drs Richard, Kubiak, and Horwitz review many of the surgical techniques that can be used to properly manage these difficult injuries. I hope you find these techniques and this article useful in your practice.

Saqib Rehman, MD
Orthopaedic Surgery
Temple University Hospital
3401 North Broad Street
Philadelphia, PA 19140, USA

E-mail address:
Saqib.rehman@tuhs.temple.edu

http://dx.doi.org/10.1016/j.ocl.2014.04.007
0030-5898/14/$ – see front matter

orthopedic.theclinics.com

Techniques for the Surgical Treatment of Distal Tibia Fractures

Raveesh Daniel Richard, MD[a], Erik Kubiak, MD[b],
Daniel Scott Horwitz, MD[a],*

KEYWORDS

- Distal tibia fractures • Surgical treatment • Open reduction • Internal fixation

KEY POINTS

- Surgical management of extra-articular distal tibia fractures has evolved because of the high rate of complications with conventional techniques and the technically challenging aspects of the surgery.
- Open reduction and internal fixation with plating or nailing remain the gold standards of treatment, and minimally invasive techniques have reduced wound complications and increased healing.
- Adequate reduction and stabilization as well as appropriate soft tissue management are imperative to achieving good outcomes in these fractures.

ANATOMY

Distal tibial metaphyseal fractures are those that extend within approximately 4 cm of the tibial plafond.[1] The Orthopedic Trauma Association's (OTA) fracture classification, similar to Muller's definition, defines these fractures as those contained within a square with a side length equal to the widest portion of the epiphysis; extra-articular fractures are those with no or with simple extension of a nondisplaced fracture line into the plafond.[2]

In an axial cross section of the tibia, moving distally from the diaphysis to the metaphysis, the shape of the tibia transitions from that of a triangle with an anterior apex to a more circular shape.[3] Compared with that of the diaphysis, metaphyseal cortical bone is thinner and the central cortex is replaced by secondary spongiosa and cancellous bone, making screw fixation more challenging. However, the material properties of this cancellous bone vary based on the age and activity level of patients and can be quite dense in patients less than 50 years old, which allows for stronger screw purchase. The medullary canal of the tibia has an hourglass shape, with a narrow diaphyseal region

and wider metaphyseal regions. This flaring out of the metaphyseal region poses a challenge for intramedullary (IM) fixation, as a tight endosteal fit with the nail is achieved only in the middle few centimeters of the diaphysis.

The fibula is situated posterolateral to the tibia and distally joins with the lateral surface of the distal tibial metaphysis at the inferior tibiofibular articulation. This articulation is composed of the lateral syndesmotic ligaments and the distal interosseous membrane and is the reason why the fibula is often injured in higher-energy fracture patterns. Conversely, the inferior tibiofibular articulation is important because an intact or repaired fibula may help maintain tibial alignment during fracture healing. The lateral malleolus and the lateral ligamentous complex are critical to maintaining stability at the ankle joint.

Blood supply to the distal tibia is derived from 2 sources. Perfusion to the outer one-tenth to one-third of the tibial cortex is extraosseous and arises from a network of periosteal vessels on the medial surface that are branches of the anterior and posterior tibial arteries. The inner two-thirds of the distal tibia are supplied by intraosseous nutrient arteries, which are branches of the posterior tibial

[a] Department of Orthopaedics, Geisinger Health System, 100 North Academy, Danville, PA 17821, USA;
[b] Department of Orthopaedics, University of Utah, 590 Wakara Way, Salt Lake, UT 84108, USA
* Corresponding author.
E-mail address: dshorwitz@geisinger.edu

Orthop Clin N Am 45 (2014) 295–312
http://dx.doi.org/10.1016/j.ocl.2014.04.001

artery. Segmental fractures can potentially obliterate this intraosseous supply, leaving only the extraosseous supply intact. As a result, significant periosteal stripping during fixation may destroy the remaining blood supply and cause avascular necrosis of the bone, with consequent complications in bone healing.

At the level of the distal tibia, the structures most at risk during medial fixation are the great saphenous vein and the saphenous nerve. This vein and the major branch of the saphenous nerve intersect at the posterior cortex of the tibia at an average of 10 cm from the tip of the medial malleolus and then pass the anterior cortex approximately 3 cm from the tip of the medial malleolus.

CLASSIFICATION

Multiple classification systems have been developed to describe distal tibia fractures. Soft tissue injury can be evaluated with the Gustilo-Anderson or Tscherne-Gotzen classification systems for open or closed fractures, respectively. Robinson and colleagues[4] developed a classification system after studying distal tibia metaphyseal fractures treated with IM nailing (IMN). Two distinct injuries were noted: type I fractures resulted from a direct bending force producing a transverse fracture pattern, and type II fractures resulted from a torsional force producing a spiral/helical fracture pattern of the tibia with an associated oblique fibular fracture at the same or different level. The Association for Osteosynthesis/Association for the Study of Internal Fixation (AO/ASIF) system was also developed primarily for use in research and describes all fractures in the form of an alphanumeric code. Distal tibial extra-articular metaphyseal fractures are 43-A (4 = tibia, 3 = distal metaphysis, A = extra-articular). Based on the degree of comminution of the fracture, 43-A1 are noncomminuted extra-articular fractures, 43-A2 are wedge fractures, and 43-A3 are comminuted extra-articular fractures. Simple extension of the fracture line into the tibiotalar joint without depression of the joint surface is classified as 43-B1 and can often be treated in the same manner as extra-articular (43-A) fractures.

PRESENTATION AND INITIAL MANAGEMENT

Distal tibia fractures are frequently caused by high-energy trauma and are often associated with life-threatening injuries. Management of these injuries should be initiated according to Advanced Trauma Life Support principles.

A thorough medical history should be obtained identifying patient factors associated with the risk of soft tissue complications, poor fracture healing, and fixation failure. Preexisting peripheral vascular disease, smoking, diabetes mellitus and associated neuropathy, alcoholism, malnutrition, and osteoporosis have all been associated with an increased risk of infection and nonunion and may affect the choice of fixation.

A complete physical examination should be performed, and it is critical to evaluate for neurovascular compromise of the lower extremity. In the event of vascular compromise, immediate fracture reduction should be attempted. A full evaluation for possible compartment syndrome is mandatory, especially in closed injuries; urgent 4-compartment fasciotomy should be performed if suspected.

The soft tissue envelope of the involved lower extremity should be closely examined. Early recognition of impending skin compromise and urgent fracture reduction reduces the risk of conversion to an open fracture and a compromised surgical approach. Soft tissue injury signs include edema, ecchymosis, fracture blisters, and open fracture wounds; injury is often greater with distal metaphyseal fractures than with diaphyseal fractures. Open distal tibia fractures occur with an approximate incidence of 20%; the medial surface of the tibia, covered by thin subcutaneous tissue, is the most common site of open injury. Prompt administration of antibiotics, tetanus vaccination, and urgent debridement and irrigation should be performed. The limb should always be splinted pending definitive management.

RADIOGRAPHY/IMAGING

Radiographic imaging is necessary for injury classification and determining surgical technique and approach. Imaging of the fracture should include orthogonal views of the distal tibia and ankle mortise. Full-length radiographs of the tibia and fibula and orthogonal views of the knee are routinely obtained. Computed tomography (CT) is also useful for preoperative planning as it has been shown to add information in 82% of patients and change the surgical plan in 64%.[5,6] It is especially recommended if there is concern for intra-articular extension of the fracture.

It is important to define similar standards of radiographic outcomes that can be used by all studies, but this has not always been the case. Union can be defined as healing of at least 3 of 4 cortices on anteroposterior and lateral radiographs. Nonunion can be defined as a lack of healing within 6 months. Malunion is typically defined as fracture healing of greater than 5° of angular deformity in any plane or shortening greater than 10 mm.[7–9]

NONOPERATIVE MANAGEMENT

Nonoperative management of distal tibia metaphyseal fractures involves the use of casting cast bracing and avoids the risks of surgery and postoperative complications. There are, however, few published studies examining nonoperative management of distal tibia fractures.

Sarmiento and Latta[7] reviewed 450 cases of closed fractures of the distal tibia. Nonoperative management was chosen for fractures that were closed, with initial shortening less than 15 mm and angulation after manipulation less than 5° in any plane. A long leg cast was applied for these fractures, with the knee in 7° of flexion and the ankle in 90° of dorsiflexion. Patients were allowed to bear weight as tolerated and mobilize using walking aids. Early functional bracing demonstrated a longer healing time, with a mean time to union of 16.6 weeks and malunion of 13.1%. Of note, malunion was defined as greater than 7° angulation or 12 mm shortening, which is more forgiving than the accepted 5° angulation or 10 mm shortening.

Similarly, Böstman and colleagues[10] reviewed 103 patients managed initially with a long leg cast and subsequent IMN if there was loss of reduction. A malunion rate of 26.4% was observed in the nonoperatively managed group. Approximately 4% of the patients developed nonunion and required bone grafting. The time to union was faster in those who underwent subsequent IMN than those who were managed by functional bracing alone.

Although surgical complications are minimized with nonoperative management, significant complications have been reported with its use. For axially unstable fractures, the risk of shortening is substantial. Loss of reduction with angular malunion is also an issue, with approximately 33% of patients healing with a deformity of greater than 5° in any plane. The increased occurrence of malunion leads to increased tibiotalar contact pressures, which can cause significant hindfoot and ankle stiffness in these patients. In fact, joint stiffness caused by conservative treatment has been reported to be as high as 40% in these cases.[11-13] Because of these high rates of shortening, angulation, and malunion, nonoperative management should be used only for a select few patients with relatively stable fractures and the opportunity for close monitoring.

OPERATIVE MANAGEMENT

Most distal tibial metaphyseal fractures necessitate operative management because of the potential for displacement and malunion with conservative treatment. After the initial reduction and stabilization in the emergency setting, patients should be medically optimized for definitive fixation. Classically, these fractures are treated with the use of IMN or plating, although the use of external fixation as the definitive management has also been described.

For open fractures, surgical debridement has historically been recommended within 6 hours of presentation; but the evidence for this time frame is weak, and multiple studies have failed to show any impact in infection rate with debridement occurring after 6 hours.[9] Evidence does support the early administration of intravenous broad-spectrum antibiotics, and the Tscherne-Gotzen classification system can be used to guide surgical management in open wounds. Grade 0 and I fractures are amenable to definitive fixation within 24 hours, and grade II and III fractures are initially stabilized with external fixation until the soft tissue injury allows definitive fixation at a later date. With delays of 7 to 24 days for definitive treatment of the higher-grade injuries, a significant reduction in complication rates has been observed.[8,14,15]

IMN

IM devices for diaphyseal tibia fractures have been implemented since the 1940s, allowing for sufficient movement at the fracture site to induce callus formation while minimizing the risk of pseudoarthrosis and malunion. In distal tibia fractures, IMN is associated with high union rates and minimally interferes with the soft tissue envelope at the time of surgery. Historically, this technique was reserved for fractures greater than 5 cm proximal to the ankle joint; but with newer nail designs, this limitation no longer exists.

Biomechanics

The fixation of distal tibial fractures with IM nails has been limited by the fact that there is reduced bone-to-implant contact at the distal metaphysis. The cortical flare of the metaphysis allows a windscreen-wiper action of the distal fragment in relation to the IM nail, minimizing the intrinsic stability of the construct when compared with plate fixation. When cortical contact distal to the fracture site is poor, a higher proportion of the mechanical load is borne by the nail and is transmitted to the distal screws. This results in inferior load sharing between the distal screws and the metaphysis, which can result in 4-point bending of the screws and failure of the construct. Multiple techniques exist to add stability to these constructs, including fibular fixation, multiplane distal locking screws, and blocking (Poller) screws.

Indications

Although multiple innovations in IM nail design have increased the indications for nailing in distal metaphyseal tibial fractures, challenges with reduction, distal propagation of the fracture line, inadequate distal fixation, and potential articular involvement still limit its applicability. Some researchers have concluded that IMN is both effective and safe to use for distal tibia fractures without significant articular involvement.[4,16] Im and Tae[17] demonstrated shorter operative times with improved function in the nailing group compared with plate fixation. Others disagree citing the potential for malalignment and reduced stability as reasons for increased fracture propagation, hardware failure, malunion, nonunion, and delayed healing.[9,18] Indications for IMN in these fractures are older patients with thin skin, compromised soft tissue, patients with diabetes with compromised wound healing, and fractures with limited distal extension allowing the use of at least 2 distal interlocking screws.

Operative Technique

In comparison with plate fixation, IMN can be performed acutely without the need to wait for soft tissue stabilization. Initial reduction of the fracture may be achieved with gentle manipulation and traction by an assistant or with the use of percutaneously placed pointed reduction forceps (**Fig. 1**). The use of gravity while flexing the knee over a support, such as a radiolucent foam wedge, may also assist reduction. Alternatively, a femoral distractor can provide length and alignment during traction and fracture reduction (**Fig. 2**A). Pins are placed proximally in the posterior metaphysis of the tibia and distally in the tibia (see **Fig. 2**B), serving as an additional check to anatomic reduction (ie, the nail should be perpendicular to the pin and plafond; see **Fig. 2**C). The use of a femoral distractor avoids the need for conventional fracture tables and provides complete control over the involved extremity. The importance of achieving and maintaining reduction of the fracture cannot be understated, as this is often the most difficult aspect of nailing distal tibial metaphyseal fractures.

The starting point of the IM nail is similar to that of diaphyseal tibial nails; however, the end point of the guidewire must be center-center to prevent deformity (**Fig. 3**). The use of a guidewire with a minimal bend at the tip is helpful, and the wire should be kept perpendicular to the tibiotalar joint line during reaming to minimize deformity in the coronal plane. If intra-articular extension of the fracture line exists, lag screws should be placed before reaming and nailing to stabilize the fracture at the metaphysis and prevent propagation or displacement; but care must be taken to avoid blocking the passage of the subsequent nail.

Unlike diaphyseal fractures, the insertion of the nail in distal metaphyseal fractures does not result in fracture reduction; consequently, careful control of the distal fragment is critical to allow the nail to advance centrally into the distal fragment in both anteroposterior and lateral planes. Eccentric reaming or failure to control the distal fragment can lead to significant malalignment and deformity (**Fig. 4**). Percutaneous bone reduction clamps are particularly helpful in spiral/oblique fractures in facilitating reduction. In the case of open fractures, the application of small fragment plates for provisional reduction has been described in combination with nailing. Distal locking of the nail with multiple distal fixation points and the use of at least 3 locking screws are recommended to facilitate reduction to healing (**Fig. 5**).

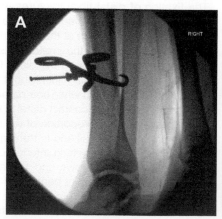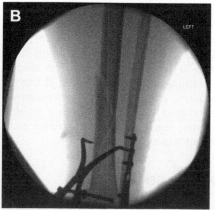

Fig. 1. AP (*A*) and lateral (*B*) fluoroscopic images showing percutaneous application of pointed reduction clamps. The near anatomic alignment achieved simplifies ball-tipped wire passage and initial reaming.

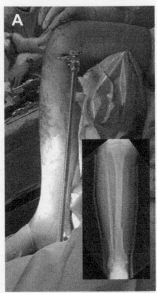

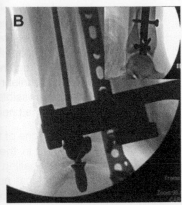

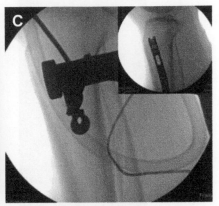

Fig. 2. (*A*) Clinical image of the tibia in preparation for nailing with femoral distractor in place ready for nail insertion. (*Inset*) Radiograph of typical fracture where this is of greatest utility; comminuted distal third fracture of tibia with associated fibula fracture at the same level. (*B*) Radiograph of proximal tibia with distractor pin in place. (*C*) Radiograph of the distal tibia with the distractor pin in place. Again the pin should be placed distal and posterior to the nail path, doing so will aid in confirming that restoration of alignment has been achieved. The distal pin, like the proximal pin, should be in line with the posterior cortex of the tibia. Note in the inset that the pin is posterior to the nail path and in line with the posterior cortex of the tibia.

Approach

There are multiple surgical approaches to the proximal tibia for nailing, and these include the following:

1. *Medial parapatellar tendon*: This approach is the most common starting point but is prone to valgus malalignment when used to treat proximal tibial fractures.
2. *Lateral parapatellar tendon*: This approach aids in maintaining the reduction of proximal metaphyseal fractures but makes it more difficult to reach the correct starting point.
3. *Patellar tendon splitting*: This approach gives direct access to the starting point but can

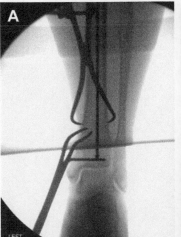

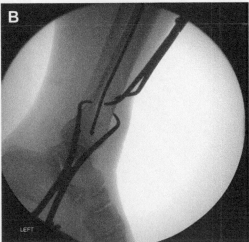

Fig. 3. Placement of the guidewire center-center and fully seated in the distal metaphysis is essential to avoiding final deformity. It is imperative that a true anteroposterior view (*A*) as well as a true lateral view (*B*) be obtained. Note the slight anterior bend at the terminal aspect of the wire allowing for precise positioning as well as matching the slight anterior bend of many commonly used nails.

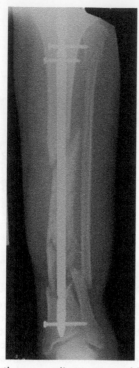

Fig. 4. Note the poor alignment established before reaming results in eccentric distal nail placement and significant malreduction. It is imperative that the alignment is confirmed on both anteroposterior and lateral views before reaming. In this case, reduction would have been facilitated by initial reduction and plating of the fibula.

inadvertently damage the patellar tendon or lead to patella baja.

4. *Semiextended medial or lateral parapatellar*: The advantages include ease of positioning and imaging and aiding in the reduction of proximal and distal fractures. Inadvertent injury to femoral cartilage is possible as well as anterior nail migration during reaming.

5. *Suprapatellar (trans quadriceps tendon)*: This approach is similar to the semiextended technique but requires special instruments. Inadvertent trochlear damage to the patella and femur is possible, and deposition of reaming debris in the knee is a concern.

The use of one of the semiextended techniques, as described in the literature, can be extremely helpful when nailing distal shaft fractures, as it allows for surgical approach to the fibula as well as more intuitive control of the tibia and ease of fluoroscopic viewing (**Fig. 6**).[19,20]

Choice of Implant

The length of the nail must be closely matched to the length of the tibia because the placement of distal locking screws depends on this. Preoperative assessment is helpful in determining appropriate implant length; using the contralateral limb as a template is essential in highly comminuted fractures, but exact measurements made on radiographs should be carefully scrutinized because magnification can affect the perceived length.

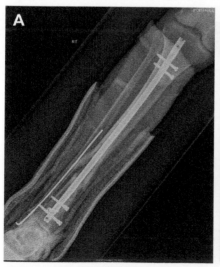
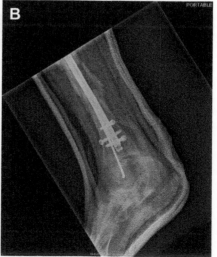

Fig. 5. This highly unstable distal tibia fracture has been stabilized with an IM fibular implant as well as multiple fixed-angle screws in 2 planes. In this case, the fixed-angle screws were chosen because of the extremely poor bone and concern for backing out of the interlock. Acceptable alignment has been achieved on both the anteroposterior (*A*) and lateral (*B*) views.

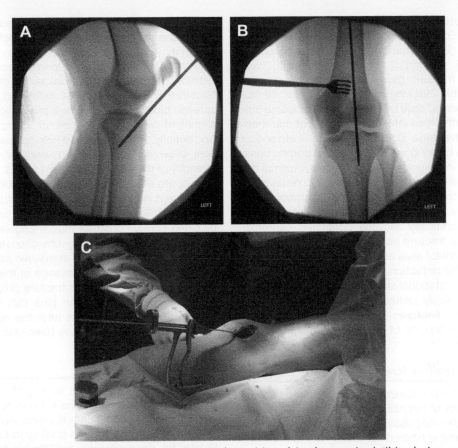

Fig. 6. (*A*) The lateral view of an entry wire properly positioned in the proximal tibia during parapatellar extended nailing. Note the wire penetrates the proximal tibia behind the anterior cortex. (*B*) The anteroposterior view of the same entry site, showing the wire properly positioned and aligning with the lateral aspect of the tibial spine. (*C*) An intraoperative view showing a guidewire in place with the knee in the semiextended position.

Distal Locking Screws

Distal locking screws are used in IM nail designs to provide stability in the coronal and sagittal planes in addition to controlling length and rotation. Early generations of IM nails did not allow adequate fixation of shorter distal tibial fracture fragments because the distal interlocks were several centimeters from the nail tip and, as a result, surgeons began modifying the implants by sawing off the tip distal to the interlocks to achieve more distal fixation. This technique was shown to be a reliable treatment of distal tibial metaphyseal fractures without extension into the ankle joint.[4,16] Newer generations of IM nails have since been developed and allow the insertion of more locking screws within the distal 15 mm in multiple planes. Three distal interlocking holes at 5, 15, and 25 mm, respectively, from the nail tip are common in current tibial nails. A laboratory study demonstrated that the insertion of 2 distal interlocking screws reduced the rate of hardware failure and increased

fatigue strength compared with the use of a single interlocking screw, and Kneifel and Buckley[21] reported a failure rate of 59% with one distal screw versus 5% with 2 distal screws when nailing tibial shaft fractures. Furthermore, the use of a single screw has been reported to increase the rate of nonunion when compared with 2 locking screws in distal tibia fractures.

In theory, the placement of screws in multiple planes increases the stability of the distal segment. To date, however, biomechanical studies have not demonstrated the superiority of any one screw configuration. In a cadaveric model, no significant difference in fixation strength was observed between parallel and orthogonally oriented distal interlocks. Most surgeons aim for the maximum possible but at least 2 distal locking screws to hold reduction.

Angle-stable locking screws have been used to address angular and rotational instability. Multiple designs exist, and a construct that uses these angle-stable screws draws increased stability from greater cortical purchase and is less reliant on the endosteal fit between the nail and the distal fragment. Biomechanical studies have confirmed improved construct stability, stiffness, and reduced fracture gap motion with the use of angle-stable locking screws.[22,23] No clinical studies exist to date that show better or worse outcomes with these interlock screws, but one theoretical advantage is the decreased likelihood of the screw backing out from the osteoporotic bone.

Nailing in a dynamic mode, with a proximal dynamic interlocking screw and 2 static distal interlocking screws, provides excellent rotational and angulatory stability in simple fracture patterns while theoretically allowing controlled compression at the fracture site. Attaining at least a 50% cortical contact area across the fracture site via intraoperative reduction techniques significantly improves the rotational stability after dynamic nailing, but dynamically locked nailing of distal metaphyseal tibia fractures is strongly discouraged because of reports of unacceptably high rates of shortening.[24–26]

Blocking (Poller) Screws

The use of Poller screws may be required to allow the passage of the nail into the desired location by blocking the nail passage into an undesirable location, and this is often done initially with a medium-sized Kirschner wire (K wire) (**Fig. 7**). These wires can be inserted percutaneously in the sagittal or coronal plane adjacent to the nail along the concave side of an observed deformity to decrease the diameter of the medullary canal.

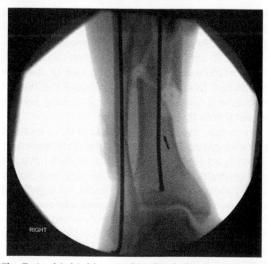

Fig. 7. In this highly unstable distal tibia fracture, the fibula has been stabilized; the resulting likely deformity is, therefore, varus. Placement of a blocking pin in the proximal-medial aspect of the distal fracture fragment helps minimize this varus deformity.

Anteroposterior blocking screws placed medially in the distal fragment will help correct a varus deformity, whereas anteroposterior blocking screws placed laterally will help to correct a valgus deformity (**Fig. 8**). In a clinical series of 21 tibial fractures managed with IM nails and blocking screws, blocking screws were shown to improve alignment with minimal risk or complications. Additionally, blocking screws help facilitate reduction, prevent nail translation, and increase the strength of the fixation construct.[27] Still, blocking screws are more helpful in holding reduction than achieving it initially because the distal fragment is often short (ie, 3–4 cm) and the lever arm of the blocking screw construct makes angular correction challenging. Some surgeons choose to place smaller-diameter 2.0- to 2.5-mm wires as blocking pins as they allow easier passage of the reamers and the nail with the risk of fracture propagation, as discussed earlier. These pins can be easily changed to 3.5-mm screws after the nail is fully seated and all interlocks have been placed.

Fibular Fixation

Fixation of the fibula in the setting of distal tibia fractures adds stability to the ankle joint and aids in tibial fracture reduction and union. An absolute indication for fibular fixation is injury to the inferior tibiofibular syndesmosis, but fibular fixation is often necessary to avoid valgus deformity when medial plating of the distal tibia is performed. Usually, if normal length, axis, and rotation of the tibial fracture are not easily achieved with standard reduction, the fibula is plated first using a flexible tubular plate to provide lateral stability while permitting fine tuning of the tibial length and alignment.

Care must be taken to avoid overdistraction at the tibial fracture site while plating the fibula, as evidence demonstrates that there is an increased risk of nonunion as a result of reduced strain across the tibial fracture site caused by overdistraction with fibular plating.[1] Although anatomic reduction of the tibia is facilitated, the potential for delayed healing is increased. In a study of 113 distal tibia fractures located 4 to 11 cm from the plafond, Vallier and colleagues[28] found a higher rate of nonunion in fractures managed with tibial and fibular fixation than tibial fixation alone (14.0% vs 2.6%, $P = .04$). More recently, similar findings were observed between the two groups with an increased rate of nonunion in those who underwent fibular fixation, although this was not significant (12.0% vs 4.1%, $P = .09$).[9] It is essential that any plate used be flexible to allow adjustments during reduction. Fibula fractures

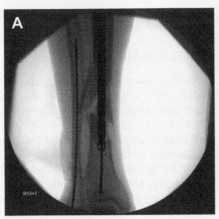
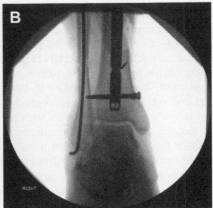

Fig. 8. (*A*) The anteroposterior view of a comminuted distal tibia fracture. The fibula has been stabilized with an IM device, and the tendency is for the tibia to drift into varus. This tendency is prevented by centering the tip of the guidewire distally and using a blocking pin, or Poller screw, on the concave side of the distal fragment. (*B*) In this case, the blocking wire is left in place until distal interlocks are placed. If necessary, the wire can be replaced with a small fragment screw; or if the construct is stable, it can simply be removed. Note the intimate contact of the blocking device with the nail.

can also be stabilized with an IM implant, such as a rush rod, flexible nail, or guidewire (see **Fig. 5**A; **Fig. 9**).

Studies have also reported on the use of fibular plating with plating and external fixation. Investigations by Williams and colleagues[29] and Pugh and colleagues[30] demonstrated that fibular fixation does not reduce the incidence of malunion in externally fixated fractures. In open plating, fibular fixation is helpful in reducing the risk of malreduction by correcting angular or rotational deformity and correcting length. Strauss and colleagues[31] demonstrated that fixation of a concomitant fracture of the fibula increased construct stiffness in the setting of open plating or IMN. An "en peigne" fixation, in which a fibular plate and long screws gain both fibular and tibial purchase, has been described in nonarticular distal tibia fractures with extensive medial soft tissue injury and healthy lateral soft tissues.[32]

In IMN, fibular fixation is useful, especially in extensively comminuted fractures in which rotational and sagittal alignment are difficult to maintain with nail fixation alone.[14] For fractures with significant valgus angulation, fibular plating can be used as an adjunct for reduction before IMN. A biomechanical study has confirmed that fibular fixation in the setting of IMN reduces malunion and angular displacement.[33] Egol and colleagues[14] reported on 72 distal fractures of the distal tibia and fibula managed with IMN with or without plating of the fibula. Those managed with fibular plating in addition to nailing had a reduced incidence of late malalignment versus those who were managed with nailing only (4%

vs 13%, respectively), although Dogra and colleagues[16] observed an incidence of malunion of 20% following fibular fixation and IMN in a case series.

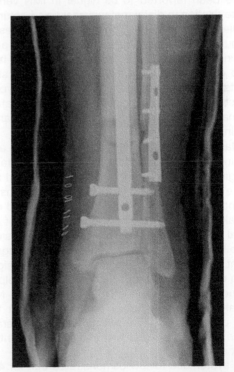

Fig. 9. Note this distal tibial nailing has been simplified by initial open reduction internal fixation of the fibula using a flexible tubular plate. This technique helps restore rotational alignment and prevents collapse into excessive valgus.

Complications

IMN of distal tibia fractures has been reported to cause an increased risk of anterior knee pain.[9] The cause of knee pain following tibial IMN is unclear but seems to be related to the extent of soft tissue injury and, in particular, injury to the patellar tendon and retropatellar fat pad. A study in which patients underwent reamed IMN with a parapatellar approach and meticulous dissection of the retropatellar fat pad demonstrated a relatively low incidence of knee pain (19%).[34] This incidence is significantly less than the reported average of 50% of all patients undergoing IMN of distal tibial fractures.[4,32] A meta-analysis that included 20 studies evaluating knee pain after tibial nailing reported the that incidence of knee pain ranged from 10% to 86% in all studies, and approximately 51% of patients still reported knee pain after the removal of the IM nail.[35]

Angular malunion is frequently observed with IMN in comminuted distal metaphyseal tibia fractures, with reports demonstrating a malunion rate ranging from 0% to 29%.[36] Often, malunion can be attributed to intraoperative technical error and inadequate fracture reduction before reaming and nailing. Similarly, delayed union or nonunion have been reported to be higher in IMN versus plate fixation in distal metaphyseal tibia fractures. Vallier and colleagues[9] observed higher rates of nonunion and primary angular malalignment after nailing compared with open plating. The high rate of delayed union after unreamed IMN supports routine reaming in these fracture types. Most cases of nonunion can be successfully managed with bone grafting and/or exchange nailing.

Nail and distal locking screw breakage are also frequently reported complications. Breakage rates ranging from 5% to 59% have been reported but were mainly attributable to older generations of IM nails.[21,36] Hahn and colleagues[37] reported nail breakage in 5 cases of fixation within 7 cm of the tibial plafond where the proximal interlock was unable to bypass the fracture line, generating significant stress on the construct. Newer nail designs with more distal locking screw holes have helped reduce the incidence of this complication. Nail breakage is also another argument against the use of unreamed tibial nails, which are generally 9 mm or smaller in diameter and use smaller interlock screws.

A systematic review demonstrated that for 489 patients treated with IMN, the nonunion rate was 5.5%; the infection rate was 4.3%; the malunion rate was 16.2%; and 16.4% of patients required secondary surgical procedures.[18] Infection, cortical necrosis, and increased risk of compartment syndrome are less frequent complications.

PLATE FIXATION: OPEN

The main advantage of open reduction internal fixation with a plate construct is near anatomic reduction ensuring accurate alignment of the fracture fragments under direct visualization. There are minimal limits to the length of the distal fragment as needed for distal locking of IM nails. The biomechanics of plate fixation have shown that plate constructs are approximately twice as stiff as IM nails under an axial load.[1,31] Additionally, multiple studies have demonstrated high rates of union and low incidences of infection, malunion, nonunion, and malalignment with plate fixation.[18] Although malunion after plating has been reported to be as high as 35%, most of the literature cites rates less than 10%.[9,17,28,38,39] In a study of distal metaphyseal tibia fractures treated with IMN or open plating, Im and Tae[17] found that mean angulation was approximately 1.9° less in the plate fixation group. Vallier and colleagues[9] reported that approximately 8% of patients treated with conventional open plate fixation had an unacceptable angulation greater than 4° versus more than 23% of patients treated with IMN.

Indications

Open plate fixation may be indicated for fractures at risk for malalignment because direct exposure is used to achieve reduction, which may be difficult to achieve with a nail alone. Fractures with a simple articular split are prime candidates for open plating, as small fragment screws can be used to achieve articular reduction. Fractures with extensive soft tissue damage but not amenable to IMN (ie, too distal) can be treated with plating in a staged fashion after initial external fixation. Patients who are less likely to benefit from open plating include patients with diabetes, those with open fractures, or those with hemorrhagic fracture blisters overlying the desired incision site.

Operative Technique

Multiple surgical approaches have been developed for operative plating of distal tibia fractures and include anteromedial, anterolateral, posterolateral, and direct lateral approaches.[1,8,40–48] Generally, preoperative planning including the assessment of soft tissue injury, degree of comminution, and type of fracture pattern are important in deciding the prime location of the implant. Reduction techniques include the use of bone clamps and external fixators. Similar to nailing, intra-articular reduction is essential and should be achieved before meta-diaphyseal realignment and fixation. The availability of precontoured plates facilitates reduction of the meta-diaphyseal region to the plate, and the use of locking screws in the metaphysis may be useful in improving stability but are not generally necessary proximally. In fact, overuse of locked screws, especially in the diaphysis, can easily create a construct that is too stiff in the setting of an imperfect reduction (as little as a 0.5-mm gap) and may result in nonunion (**Fig. 10**). Fracture reduction and plate position should be satisfactory before insertion of locking screws. Fixation should include at least 3 to 4 screws distally (if feasible) and balanced fixation proximally to optimize bony stability.

Anteromedial Approach

The most common approach to open plating of the distal tibia is anterior, as it offers excellent exposure. The medial soft tissue envelope is very thin and provides easy access to the medial aspect of the distal tibia with minimal dissection. For the same reason, however, the medial surface is at an increased risk for postoperative complications. The initial injury often causes contusions or lacerations to the medial soft tissue envelope, increasing

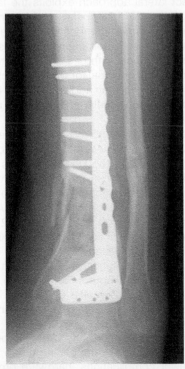

Fig. 10. The excessive use of locked screws in the diaphysis has resulted in nonunion in this complex, comminuted fracture.

the risk of wound sloughing. Furthermore, medial plating increases skin tension on the anteromedial aspect of the tibia and can lead to infection and nonunion.

Cheng and colleagues[41] described the use of an AO locking compression plate (LCP) for fixation of these fractures. The researchers emphasized the need for premolding of the plates, although precontoured plates have simplified this step. The distal end of the plate should be externally rotated approximately 15 degrees in order to match the anatomy of the tibia. One additional option considered for open medial plating involves a more posteriorly based incision, creating an anterior flap that covers the hardware. This technique preserves the blood supply to the anterior-medial skin and avoids placing the incision directly over the prominent plate. Alternatively, a percutaneous technique can be used that similarly minimizes the risk of soft tissue compromise and infection (**Fig. 11**).

Anterolateral Approach

The anterolateral approach requires more dissection than the anteromedial approach, which can compromise the blood supply and lead to subsequent delayed healing or nonunion. In a cadaver study, Wolinksy and Lee[48] observed that the dorsalis pedis and deep peroneal arteries, as well as the terminal branches of the peroneal nerve, are at an increased risk of injury during the anterolateral approach. An advantage of the anterolateral approach is that the anterior compartment musculature lies adjacent to the anterolateral surface of the tibia, and so there is less concern for soft tissue complications. Anterolateral plating provides mechanical benefits for fixation of valgus distal tibia fractures in that it allows the hardware to be placed in a buttress fashion, thereby directly resisting the drift into valgus through the stable fixation in the diaphysis.

Posterolateral Approach

Harmon described the posterolateral approach to the tibia in 1945 for the treatment of tibial nonunion, and this approach has been used when soft tissue concerns preclude an anterior approach.[42,47,49] Reduction and fixation of both the tibia and fibula can be performed with the use of a single incision. Moreover, the flexor hallucis longus muscle belly is directly above the posterior tibia and can act as a cushion between the tibia and the skin. This approach decreases the incidence of hardware irritation and wound complications compared with the traditional anterior approaches. This approach also allows bone graft

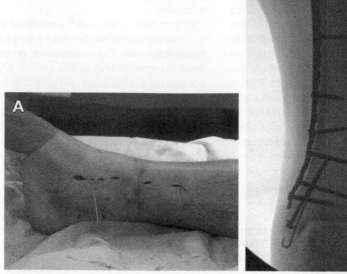

Fig. 11. (A) The distal tibia fracture in this case is treated with a percutaneous medially based plate. The technique allows for clamp reduction and soft tissue preservation. (B) A medial plate used to treat a nonunion in a patient with significant soft tissue compromise. Similar to an acute fracture, extensive fixation is achieved with minimal incisions.

to be placed through soft tissues that have not been or are minimally traumatized.

Disadvantages to the posterolateral approach include limited visualization of the articular surface and an increased learning curve of operating with patients in the prone position. For fractures with anterior comminution, the posterolateral approach should be avoided, as anatomic reduction is difficult to achieve. Additionally, some researchers have noted the proximity of the sural nerve and lesser saphenous vein to the distal surgical incision. The sural nerve in particular poses considerable variations in anatomy and is at greatest risk of injury during this approach. For the proximal incision, injury to the posterior tibial artery and tibial nerve are potential risks. To reduce the risk of neurovascular injury, dissection in the correct intermuscular plane is crucial.

The use of a 4.5-mm cannulated blade plate via a posterolateral approach has also been described. All patients included sustained distal tibia fractures deemed unsuitable for IMN because of the distal extent of the fracture line or the degree of soft tissue injury. All patients achieved fracture union at an average of 21 weeks and had acceptable American Orthopaedic Foot and Ankle Society's ankle-hindfoot scores.[47] Currently, no anatomic plate exists for plating the posterior aspect of the tibia necessitating precontouring of the plate before fixation.

Direct Lateral Approach

The direct lateral approach exploits the fact that fixation of both the distal fibula and tibia can be approached via a single lateral incision while avoiding severe soft tissue complications. The most distal fractures of the tibia with or without anterolateral joint involvement are ideal for this approach. Fixation of the fibula using an additional lateral incision compromises the vascular supply of the anterior soft tissues.

Studies that have reported on using the lateral approach using a single incision have typically reported good results, although sample sizes tend to be small.[43,45] Manninen and colleagues[45] reported on 20 patients who underwent a single lateral approach for fractures of the distal tibia. All fractures healed; malunion was found in 2 cases (10%); and 4 superficial infections (20%) were noted. Lee and colleagues[44] compared medial plating using an anterior approach with lateral plating using a lateral approach. The mean healing time was 16.1 ± 3.1 weeks. Union rate, healing time, reduction rate, malunion, infection, functional outcome scores, ankle dorsiflexion, and plantar flexion were not significantly different between the two groups. The lateral plating group experienced fewer complications, hardware problems, and elective hardware removals than the medial plating group.

Previous studies have reported that lateral plating using a lateral approach can be technically challenging. The most distal medially comminuted fractures and pilon fractures are difficult to reduce from the lateral approach. However, Lee and colleagues[44] demonstrated that operative time and surgeon experience were no different among those who performed the lateral approach versus the anterior approach.

Complications

Open reduction internal fixation with plating has been associated with a high risk of soft tissue complications. Soft tissue breakdown, delayed wound healing, superficial infection, and deep infection are all cited complications, particularly with the anteromedial approach whereby the soft tissue coverage is minimal. High rates of infection (range 8.3%–20.0%) and nonunion (range 8.3%–35.0%) have been reported, especially when acute plating is performed; Im and Tae[17] reported a significantly higher incidence of wound complications in an open plating group compared with an IM nail group (7 of 30 vs 1 of 34, $P = .03$).[32] However, these findings have not been consistent throughout studies because several researchers have cited minimal soft tissue complications following plate fixation.[50] Some researchers suggest that wound problems are often attributable to patient-related factors, including diabetes, smoking, and the degree of initial trauma.[9]

Lee and colleagues[44] compared medial and lateral open plating and found that symptomatic hardware was a more common issue in the medial plating group (42.9%) than the lateral plating group (5.1%), likely due to placement of the plate beneath the anterior compartment musculature with thick soft-tissue coverage in the lateral plating group. Symptomatic patients often require hardware removal, and Mauffrey and colleagues[51] found that more secondary procedures occurred in open plating than IM nailing.

MINIMALLY INVASIVE PLATE OSTEOSYNTHESIS

Because of the high risk of infection and wound complications associated with open plating techniques, minimally invasive plate osteosynthesis (MIPO) was developed for the treatment of distal tibia fractures.[27] Percutaneous plating using minimal incisions minimizes the compromise to circulation at wound edges after closure and has greatly reduced soft tissue disturbance and the rate of infection. Small incisions are advantageous in restoring mechanical axes, decreasing iatrogenic soft tissue injury, and preserving the fracture

hematoma. This technique has proven especially useful for comminuted fracture patterns. Multiple researchers have claimed that the advantages of IMN (ie, minimal soft tissue exposure and dissection) are comparable with those of MIPO.

Excellent healing and union rates have been observed with the use of this technique.[52,53] A cadaver study by Borrelli and colleagues[54] demonstrated substantially less injury to the medial extraosseous blood supply of the distal tibia with percutaneous plating versus conventional open plating. A large prospective study of 142 acute tibia fractures (including distal metaphyseal injuries) demonstrated 100% union, satisfactory clinical outcomes, and a low rate of complications with the use of minimally invasive plating.[55] Studies by Helfet and colleagues[52] and Oh and colleagues[53] demonstrated 100% union and no complications in a small series of patients with nonarticular distal tibia fractures treated with MIPO. No angular deformities greater than 5° or shortening greater than 1 cm were observed. In addition, Ahmad and colleagues[11] demonstrated that MIPO takes approximately 4.7 weeks less to union than open plating.[56]

Indications

Because MIPO preserves the soft tissues and blood supply to the distal tibia, comminuted extra-articular fracture patterns are ideal candidates for this technique, primarily because smaller incisions are advantageous in restoring mechanical axes, decreasing iatrogenic soft tissue injury, and preserving the fracture hematoma. Remote fractures, active infection, articular surface involvement, and compartment syndrome are contraindications to minimally invasive procedures.

Operative Technique

MIPO requires initial closed reduction of the fracture, which can be obtained directly via percutaneous reduction forceps or indirectly via manual traction, a femoral distractor, or spanning external fixator (see Fig. 1). Additionally, concurrent fibular fixation, as previously discussed, may significantly aid in initial reduction. Reduction should be performed cautiously because of the potential for sagittal plane malreduction.[57] Typically, a 3-cm curvilinear incision is made over the medial malleolus, avoiding the great saphenous vein and saphenous nerve, and a subcutaneous plane developed. Lag screws should be used to address intra-articular extension before definitive fixation. A plate is anatomically contoured to restore supramalleolar anatomy, help reduce its prominence, and decrease the likelihood of varus/valgus or rotational deformity.[32] It is then inserted in a distal-to-proximal direction through the subcutaneous tunnel over the medial border of the tibia. A suture passed through a proximal hole of the plate can be used to assist with this retrograde insertion. With the aid of fluoroscopy, K wires are used to temporary stabilize the construct while the plate position is confirmed on orthogonal views. Screws can then be inserted through stab incisions to fix the construct, ensuring that distal screws do not violate the inferior tibiofibular articulation. At least 3 screws at each end and engagement of 4 to 6 cortices of fixation of each side of the fracture is generally considered adequate, and care must be taken to avoid fixation with distraction at the fracture site.[41] Closure is performed in a standard fashion; postoperatively, patients' weight bearing is limited until callus has formed, at which point full weight bearing can commence. Failure to achieve acceptable alignment or congruity with MIPO necessitates open plating; the use of overlocked constructs with an imperfect reduction, as previously noted, is likely to result in nonunion and eventual plate breakage.

Types of Plates Used in MIPO

Multiple types of plates have been used for MIPO, including dynamic compression plates (DCP), limited-contact DCP (LC-DCP), and the anatomically contoured LCP.

Compared with conventional plates, locking plates, via a rigid interface between the plate and the screw, impart a higher degree of construct stability and reduction while minimizing bone contact. Rather than relying on the frictional force between the plate and bone, stability is obtained from the screw-plate interface as locked plates function as fixed-angle devices, which eliminates screw toggling, ensures angular and axial stability, and reduces the risk of losing reduction. This system functions as a locked internal fixator and stimulates callus formation because of the flexible elastic fixation. This type of construct is especially useful for maintaining alignment during the healing of short-segment periarticular fractures. Decreased trauma to soft tissues with the use of locking plates has also been observed. Osteoporotic patients and those with multi-fragmentary fractures particularly benefit from these advantages.[58] The LC-DCP has been noted to have high fatigue resistance compared with earlier plates, although a limitation is the low number of screws that can be placed in a short distal fragment.[59]

The LCP is a popular plate as the locked fixed-angle construct helps the plate sit off the bone, preserving the periosteal blood supply and fracture hematoma. A conventional screw can be used close to the fracture site to draw the bone and plate close together, reducing the prominence of the plate and increasing construct stability. The trajectories of the LCP interfragmentary screws are nearly perpendicular to the major fracture lines. The anatomic shape of the LCP prevents primary displacement of the fracture and allows a better load distribution around the plate compared with improperly contoured conventional plates. Additionally, lower-profile LCPs have been developed for improved cosmesis and to decrease the chance of articular impingement. For extremely distal fractures, within 11 mm of the tibial plafond, polyaxial locking plates have been used to disperse multidirectional locking screws in a larger volume of periarticular fragments, providing potential better pullout strength than monoaxial locking plates.

Outcomes

Studies of MIPO have generally demonstrated favorable results with low infection rates (<8%), even in the setting of extensive soft tissue injury.[55] Lau and colleagues[39] noted a delayed union rate of 10%, deep infection in 8%, and hardware removal in 48% in a series of 48 patients treated with medial locked plating, although prolonged healing times were observed in simple fracture patterns. Similarly, a study by Ahmad and colleagues[11] demonstrated an average time to union of 23.1 weeks in 16 of 18 patients treated with the MIPO technique. Bahari and colleagues[60] reported one hardware failure, 2 superficial infections, one deep infection, and appropriate alignment in all 42 patients managed with medial locking plates. Collinge and colleagues[38] found a high infection rate of 19%, although these were all high-energy fractures; higher complication rates were expected.

A prospective randomized study of 85 distal tibia fractures managed with either IMN or MIPO by Guo and colleagues[50] demonstrated no significant difference in union rates or functional outcomes. No patients had greater than 10° of coronal or sagittal malalignment. Cheng and colleagues[41] compared MIPO with open plating and found no malunion or loosening in either group and concluded that there was no significant difference between the 2 methods of fixation. Studies by Bahari and colleagues[60] and Collinge and colleagues[38] showed that functional outcome scores for patients treated with MIPO were comparable with that of the general population by 6 months postoperatively.

Complications

Many of the complications seen in open plating can also be found with minimally invasive techniques, although often to a lesser degree. There is a surprising potential for increased hardware prominence and irritation associated with the MIPO technique. A retrospective comparison of MIPO with open plating by Cheng and colleagues[41] found more soft tissue irritation in the MIPO group, and Lau and colleagues[39] encountered an implant removal rate of 52% of patients managed with MIPO caused by hardware irritation. Monoaxial locking plates have been associated with skin irritation from wearing tall boots and pain over the medial malleolus. Lower-profile and anatomically contoured plates have been designed to address this issue, although residual malreduction also contributes to the imprecision of plate and bone contouring.

Residual malreduction caused by inaccurate precontouring of the plate or overdistraction at the fracture site can result in malunion or nonunion. When fragments are not tightly compressed across the main fracture lines, delayed healing occurs, especially in simple fracture patterns. Reported delayed union and nonunion rates have ranged from 5% to 17% in previous studies involving the MIPO technique, and angular deformities greater than 7° (range 7.1%–35.0%) and hardware failure (range 0%–10%) have been reported.[36] Maffulli and colleagues[61] noted that 7 out of 20 patients treated with MIPO of distal tibia fractures had 7° to 10° of angular deformity postoperatively. Sagittal plane malreduction is also a noted risk.[57] The risk of malreduction can be attributed to the lack of direct visualization and reduction in percutaneous plating, which makes it challenging to obtain optimal alignment and compression. Contouring of the plate to restore supramalleolar anatomy is essential and prevents pushing the distal fragment into angular or rotational malalignment, particularly valgus and external rotation. Judicious use of an image intensifier can help prevent unacceptable deformity.

Risks such as injury to the saphenous nerve and long saphenous vein have been reported and call for careful dissection during percutaneous plating. Additionally, for those surgeons who are unfamiliar with the technique, an increased infection risk is present because of the repeated insertion and removal of the plate from the subcutaneous tunnel.

EXTERNAL FIXATION

External fixation can be used for either temporary stabilization or definitive fixation of distal tibia fractures. Spanning external fixation can be used for temporary fixation of open nonarticular or extensively comminuted fractures with significant soft tissue injury. Consisting of a unilateral or delta frame spanning the ankle joint, these devices allow for restoration of length and alignment while allowing swelling to reduce and the soft tissues to heal until definitive management (**Fig. 12**).

Definitive fixation with the use of an external fixator can be used for fractures with extensive intra-articular and extra-articular comminution and open fractures with extensive soft tissue damage. Hybrid or Ilizarov fixation is an alternative to nail or plate fixation of periarticular fractures. These devices involved the passage of pins directly into the distal fragment; this has the potential advantage of early weight bearing and ankle range-of-motion exercises, allowing for simultaneous soft tissue and bone healing over time.

Complications caused by external fixation are predominantly pin tract infection, ankle stiffness, loosening, and delayed union. Hybrid external fixation can result in inaccurate reduction, with reported rates of malunion (range 5%–25%), nonunion (range 2.0%–17.6%), and pin tract infection (range 10%–100%) in some studies. Pin tract infection and secondary loosening can result in deep infection and osteomyelitis, and septic arthritis has been documented with wires placed within 1 cm of subchondral bone.[62] When used

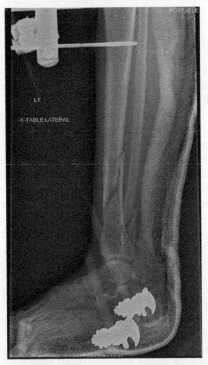

Fig. 12. An external fixator has been used temporarily in this open, distal tibia fracture in order to allow full evaluation with CT scan and staged definitive fixation. Ultimate choice of IM or plate fixation is determined based on surgeon comfort and degree of intra-articular involvement.

for temporary stabilization, there is an increased risk of subsequent infection of the IM nail used for definitive management, resulting in the current recommendation that conversion to an IM nail takes place within 2 weeks of fixator application.

Studies reporting on the outcomes of hybrid external fixation are few. Tornetta and colleagues[63] prospectively managed 26 distal tibia fractures with limited articular surface internal fixation and hybrid external fixation, observing 80% good to excellent clinical outcomes at the long-term follow-up. Demiralp and colleagues[64] looked at 27 distal tibia fractures and reported no malunion, 5 pin tract infections, and 3 cases of ankle stiffness. Most recently, a series by Ristiniemi and colleagues[65] reported on 47 fractures treated with hybrid external fixation, with 25.5% of fractures needing additional procedures because of a delayed union.

POSTOPERATIVE MANAGEMENT

Postoperative care must be individualized to the patients, mechanism of injury, implant selection, and quality of fixation. In general, most patients should be restricted from early weight bearing, as biomechanical studies have clearly shown early failure of plates and nails with only moderate loads.[32,66] Early ankle mobilization, however, is important and should be encouraged to prevent ankle stiffness. Once callus formation has occurred, typically at 6 to 8 weeks, weight bearing can be advanced, generally under the supervision of trained physical therapists.

For patients with extensive soft tissue complications, negative-pressure wound therapy (NPWT) can be a useful adjunct. Although historically used for open wounds, recently it has been used over closed surgical incisions to decrease edema and drainage after plating.[67] A prospective randomized trial compared the Vacuum-Assisted Closure (VAC) system (Kinetic Concepts, San Antonio, TX) with standard dressings for wound management, and decreased drainage time was found in the NPWT group ($P<.03$, hematoma study; $P<.02$, fracture study).

In active infection, protocols tend to be institution specific. For those with cellulitis, recommended coverage is with penicillin group antibiotics for 1 week. For abscesses, surgical incision and drainage combined with intravenous antibiotics is essential. In some cases of deep infection, hardware may be preserved in order to provide needed stability; but recurrent or persistent infection generally necessitates the removal of deep hardware and conversion to external fixation if the fracture has not yet healed.

SUMMARY

Surgical management of extra-articular distal tibia fractures has evolved because of the high rate of complications with conventional techniques and the technically challenging aspects of the surgery. Open reduction and internal fixation with plating or nailing remain the gold standards of treatment, and minimally invasive techniques have reduced wound complications and increased healing. Adequate reduction and stabilization as well as appropriate soft tissue management are imperative to achieving good outcomes in these fractures.

REFERENCES

1. Casstevens C, Le T, Archdeacon MT, et al. Management of extra-articular fractures of the distal tibia: intramedullary nailing versus plate fixation. J Am Acad Orthop Surg 2012;20(11):675–83.
2. Marsh JL, Slongo TF, Agel J, et al. Fracture and dislocation classification compendium - 2007: Orthopaedic Trauma Association classification, database and outcomes committee. J Orthop Trauma 2007;21(Suppl 10):S1–133.
3. Trafton P. Skeletal trauma. Philadelphia: WB Saunders; 2009. p. 2319–451. Tibial shaft fractures.
4. Robinson CM, McLauchlan GJ, McLean IP, et al. Distal metaphyseal fractures of the tibia with minimal involvement of the ankle. Classification and treatment by locked intramedullary nailing. J Bone Joint Surg Br 1995;77(5):781–7.
5. Crist BD, Khazzam M, Murtha YM, et al. Pilon fractures: advances in surgical management. J Am Acad Orthop Surg 2011;19(10):612–22.
6. Topliss CJ, Jackson M, Atkins RM. Anatomy of pilon fractures of the distal tibia. J Bone Joint Surg Br 2005;87(5):692–7.
7. Sarmiento A, Latta LL. 450 closed fractures of the distal third of the tibia treated with a functional brace. Clin Orthop Relat Res 2004;(428):261–71.
8. Newman SD, Mauffrey CP, Krikler S. Distal metadiaphyseal tibial fractures. Injury 2011;42(10):975–84.
9. Vallier HA, Cureton BA, Patterson BM. Randomized, prospective comparison of plate versus intramedullary nail fixation for distal tibia shaft fractures. J Orthop Trauma 2011;25(12):736–41.
10. Böstman O, Vainionpää S, Saikku K. Infra-isthmal longitudinal fractures of the tibial diaphysis: results of treatment using closed intramedullary compression nailing. J Trauma 1984;24(11):964–9.
11. Ahmad MA, Sivaraman A, Zia A, et al. Percutaneous locking plates for fractures of the distal tibia: our experience and a review of the literature. J Trauma Acute Care Surg 2012;72(2):E81–7.

12. Rüedi TP, Allgöwer M. The operative treatment of intra-articular fractures of the lower end of the tibia. Clin Orthop Relat Res 1979;(138):105–10.

13. Oni OO, Stafford H, Gregg PJ. A study of diaphyseal fracture repair using tissue isolation techniques. Injury 1992;23(7):467–70.

14. Egol KA, Weisz R, Hiebert R, et al. Does fibular plating improve alignment after intramedullary nailing of distal metaphyseal tibia fractures? J Orthop Trauma 2006;20(2):94–103.

15. Fulkerson EW, Egol KA. Timing issues in fracture management: a review of current concepts. Bull NYU Hosp Jt Dis 2009;67(1):58–67.

16. Dogra AS, Ruiz AL, Thompson NS, et al. Dia-metaphyseal distal tibial fractures–treatment with a shortened intramedullary nail: a review of 15 cases. Injury 2000;31(10):799–804.

17. Im GI, Tae SK. Distal metaphyseal fractures of tibia: a prospective randomized trial of closed reduction and intramedullary nail versus open reduction and plate and screws fixation. J Trauma 2005;59(5):1219–23.

18. Zelle BA, Bhandari M, Espiritu M, et al, Evidence-Based Orthopaedic Trauma Working Group. Treatment of distal tibia fractures without articular involvement: a systematic review of 1125 fractures. J Orthop Trauma 2006;20(1):76–9.

19. Tornetta P 3rd, Riina J, Geller J, et al. Intraarticular anatomic risks of tibial nailing. J Orthop Trauma 1999;13(4):247–51.

20. Kubiak EN, Widmer BJ, Horwitz DS. Extra-articular technique for semiextended tibial nailing. J Orthop Trauma 2010;24(11):704–8.

21. Kneifel T, Buckley R. A comparison of one versus two distal locking screws in tibial fractures treated with unreamed tibial nails: a prospective randomized clinical trial. Injury 1996;27(4):271–3.

22. Horn J, Linke B, Höntzsch D, et al. Angle stable interlocking screws improve construct stability of intramedullary nailing of distal tibia fractures: a biomechanical study. Injury 2009;40(7):767–71.

23. Gueorguiev B, Wähnert D, Albrecht D, et al. Effect on dynamic mechanical stability and interfragmentary movement of angle-stable locking of intramedullary nails in unstable distal tibia fractures: a biomechanical study. J Trauma 2011;70(2):358–65.

24. Henley MB, Meier M, Tencer AF. Influences of some design parameters on the biomechanics of the unreamed tibial intramedullary nail. J Orthop Trauma 1993;7(4):311–9.

25. Tornetta P 3rd. Technical considerations in the surgical management of tibial fractures. Instr Course Lect 1997;46:271–80.

26. Tornetta P 3rd, Collins E. Semiextended position of intramedullary nailing of the proximal tibia. Clin Orthop Relat Res 1996;(328):185–9.

27. Krettek C, Miclau T, Schandelmaier P, et al. The mechanical effect of blocking screws ("Poller screws") in stabilizing tibia fractures with short proximal or distal fragments after insertion of small-diameter intramedullary nails. J Orthop Trauma 1999;13(8):550–3.

28. Vallier HA, Le TT, Bedi A. Radiographic and clinical comparisons of distal tibia shaft fractures (4 to 11 cm proximal to the plafond): plating versus intramedullary nailing. J Orthop Trauma 2008;22(5):307–11.

29. Williams TM, Marsh JL, Nepola JV, et al. External fixation of tibial plafond fractures: is routine plating of the fibula necessary? J Orthop Trauma 1998;12(1):16–20.

30. Pugh KJ, Wolinsky PR, McAndrew MP, et al. Tibial pilon fractures: a comparison of treatment methods. J Trauma 1999;47(5):937–41.

31. Strauss EJ, Alfonso D, Kummer FJ, et al. The effect of concurrent fibular fracture on the fixation of distal tibia fractures: a laboratory comparison of intramedullary nails with locked plates. J Orthop Trauma 2007;21(3):172–7.

32. Bedi A, Le TT, Karunakar MA. Surgical treatment of nonarticular distal tibia fractures. J Am Acad Orthop Surg 2006;14(7):406–16.

33. Kumar A, Charlebois SJ, Cain EL, et al. Effect of fibular plate fixation on rotational stability of simulated distal tibial fractures treated with intramedullary nailing. J Bone Joint Surg Am 2003;85A(4):604–8.

34. Weil YA, Gardner MJ, Boraiah S, et al. Anterior knee pain following the lateral parapatellar approach for tibial nailing. Arch Orthop Trauma Surg 2009;129(6):773–7.

35. Katsoulis E, Court-Brown C, Giannoudis PV. Incidence and aetiology of anterior knee pain after intramedullary nailing of the femur and tibia. J Bone Joint Surg Br 2006;88(5):576–80.

36. Ronga M, Longo UG, Maffulli N. Minimally invasive locked plating of distal tibia fractures is safe and effective. Clin Orthop Relat Res 2010;468(4):975–82.

37. Hahn D, Bradbury N, Hartley R, et al. Intramedullary nail breakage in distal fractures of the tibia. Injury 1996;27(5):323–7.

38. Collinge C, Kuper M, Larson K, et al. Minimally invasive plating of high-energy metaphyseal distal tibia fractures. J Orthop Trauma 2007;21(6):355–61.

39. Lau TW, Leung F, Chan CF, et al. Wound complication of minimally invasive plate osteosynthesis in distal tibia fractures. Int Orthop 2008;32(5):697–703.

40. Clifford RP, Beauchamp CG, Kellam JF, et al. Plate fixation of open fractures of the tibia. J Bone Joint Surg Br 1988;70(4):644–8.

41. Cheng W, Li Y, Manyi W. Comparison study of two surgical options for distal tibia fracture-minimally invasive plate osteosynthesis vs. open reduction and internal fixation. Int Orthop 2011;35(5):737–42.

42. Kritsaneephaiboon A, Vaseenon T, Tangtrakulwanich B. Minimally invasive plate osteosynthesis of distal tibial fracture using a posterolateral approach: a cadaveric study and preliminary report. Int Orthop 2013;37(1):105–11.

43. Femino JE, Vaseenon T. The direct lateral approach to the distal tibia and fibula: a single incision technique for distal tibial and pilon fractures. Iowa Orthop J 2009;29:143–8.

44. Lee YS, Chen SH, Lin JC, et al. Surgical treatment of distal tibia fractures: a comparison of medial and lateral plating. Orthopedics 2009;32(3):163.

45. Manninen MJ, Lindahl J, Kankare J, et al. Lateral approach for fixation of the fractures of the distal tibia. Outcome of 20 patients. Technical note. Arch Orthop Trauma Surg 2007;127(5):349–53.

46. Shantharam SS, Naeni F, Wilson EP. Single-incision technique for internal fixation of distal tibia and fibula fractures. Orthopedics 2000;23(5):429–31.

47. Sheerin DV, Turen CH, Nascone JW. Reconstruction of distal tibia fractures using a posterolateral approach and a blade plate. J Orthop Trauma 2006;20(4):247–52.

48. Wolinsky P, Lee M. The distal approach for anterolateral plate fixation of the tibia: an anatomic study. J Orthop Trauma 2008;22(6):404–7.

49. Bhattacharyya T, Crichlow R, Gobezie R, et al. Complications associated with the posterolateral approach for pilon fractures. J Orthop Trauma 2006;20(2):104–7.

50. Guo JJ, Tang N, Yang HL, et al. A prospective, randomised trial comparing closed intramedullary nailing with percutaneous plating in the treatment of distal metaphyseal fractures of the tibia. J Bone Joint Surg Br 2010;92(7):984–8.

51. Mauffrey C, McGuinness K, Parsons N, et al. A randomised pilot trial of "locking plate" fixation versus intramedullary nailing for extra-articular fractures of the distal tibia. J Bone Joint Surg Br 2012;94(5):704–8.

52. Helfet DL, Shonnard PY, Levine D, et al. Minimally invasive plate osteosynthesis of distal fractures of the tibia. Injury 1997;28(Suppl 1):A42–7.

53. Oh CW, Kyung HS, Park IH, et al. Distal tibia metaphyseal fractures treated by percutaneous plate osteosynthesis. Clin Orthop Relat Res 2003;(408):286–91.

54. Borrelli J Jr, Prickett W, Song E, et al. Extraosseous blood supply of the tibia and the effects of different plating techniques: a human cadaveric study. J Orthop Trauma 2002;16(10):691–5.

55. Batten RL, Donaldson LJ, Aldridge MJ. Experience with the AO method in the treatment of 142 cases of fresh fracture of the tibial shaft treated in the UK. Injury 1978;10(2):108–14.

56. Yang SW, Tzeng HM, Chou YJ, et al. Treatment of distal tibial metaphyseal fractures: plating versus shortened intramedullary nailing. Injury 2006; 37(6):531–5.

57. Khoury A, Liebergall M, London E, et al. Percutaneous plating of distal tibial fractures. Foot Ankle Int 2002;23(9):818–24.

58. Hoenig M, Gao F, Kinder J, et al. Extra-articular distal tibia fractures: a mechanical evaluation of 4 different treatment methods. J Orthop Trauma 2010;24(1):30–5.

59. Borg T, Larsson S, Lindsjö U. Percutaneous plating of distal tibial fractures. Preliminary results in 21 patients. Injury 2004;35(6):608–14.

60. Bahari S, Lenehan B, Khan H, et al. Minimally invasive percutaneous plate fixation of distal tibia fractures. Acta Orthop Belg 2007;73(5):635–40.

61. Maffulli N, Toms AD, McMurtie A, et al. Percutaneous plating of distal tibial fractures. Int Orthop 2004;28(3):159–62.

62. Hutson JJ Jr, Zych GA. Infections in periarticular fractures of the lower extremity treated with tensioned wire hybrid fixators. J Orthop Trauma 1998;12(3):214–8.

63. Tornetta P 3rd, Weiner L, Bergman M, et al. Pilon fractures: treatment with combined internal and external fixation. J Orthop Trauma 1993;7(6): 489–96.

64. Demiralp B, Atesalp AS, Bozkurt M, et al. Spiral and oblique fractures of distal one-third of tibia-fibula: treatment results with circular external fixator. Ann Acad Med Singapore 2007;36(4): 267–71.

65. Ristiniemi J, Flinkkilä T, Hyvönen P, et al. Two-ring hybrid external fixation of distal tibial fractures: a review of 47 cases. J Trauma 2007;62(1):174–83.

66. Gorczyca JT, McKale J, Pugh K, et al. Modified tibial nails for treating distal tibia fractures. J Orthop Trauma 2002;16(1):18–22.

67. Stannard JP, Robinson JT, Anderson ER, et al. Negative pressure wound therapy to treat hematomas and surgical incisions following high-energy trauma. J Trauma 2006;60(6):1301–6.

Pediatric Orthopedics

Preface
Pediatrics Orthopedics

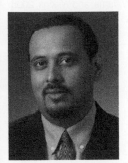

Shital N. Parikh, MD
Editor

William John Little (1810–1894) first described the deformities related to spastic rigidity, traceable to causes operative at birth, based on his personal encounter with about two hundred patients with "Little's disease."[1] The deformities have not changed since then; the condition is now known as cerebral palsy. Although there is no cure for cerebral palsy, advances have been made in its medical management including the use of Botulinum toxin, intrathecal baclofen therapy, and/or selective dorsal rhizotomy. The orthopedic management includes assessment of the patient's functional level based on gross motor functional classification system, functional mobility scale, and/or gait analysis. The current surgical treatment strategy has evolved and focuses on single-event–multilevel surgery and an interdisciplinary team approach. The current article by Chan and Miller provides a comprehensive review of the current orthopedic assessment and management of deformities of the lower extremity and spine in patients with cerebral palsy.

The treatment of developmental dysplasia of hip continues to be challenging. Screening strategies, diagnostic ultrasound, and Pavlik harness are routinely used for the newborn. Closed reduction and cast or brace is used in infants who fail initial treatment or present late. Open hip reduction, once considered "bloody reposition of congenital hip joint dislocation" due to massive loss of blood and perioperative deaths,[2] is now considered to be the treatment of choice for hips irreducible by closed methods. Cooper and colleagues provide evidence-based guidelines for the management of developmental dysplasia of hip, including the role of pelvic osteotomies.

The change in the approach to management of pediatric elbow fractures and dislocations can be summarized by the introductory remarks on elbow fractures in the first and third editions of *Children's Fractures* by Mercer Rang.[3] The first-edition phrase, "Pity the young surgeon whose first case is a fracture around the elbow," emphasized the difficulties in diagnosis, vascular and neurological problems, malunion, and stiffness of elbow due to traumatic injuries. The revised statement in the third edition, "It is no longer necessary to pity the young surgeon—save the pity for the old surgeon unacquainted with the advances in diagnosis and treatment of elbow fractures," summarizes the advancement in knowledge in treatment of pediatric elbow injuries. The review article by Little is an update on treatment of supracondylar humerus fractures, intra-articular humerus fractures, apophyseal injuries, elbow dislocation, and proximal radius and ulna fractures, including Monteggia fracture-dislocations.

I hope the readers enjoy these articles, which provide improved understanding of complex pediatric conditions.

Shital N. Parikh, MD
Pediatric Orthopaedic Sports Medicine
Cincinnati Children's Hospital Medical Center
University of Cincinnati School of Medicine
530 Walnut Street, Philadelphia
PA 19106, USA

E-mail address:
Shital.Parikh@cchmc.org

Orthop Clin N Am 45 (2014) xix–xx
http://dx.doi.org/10.1016/j.ocl.2014.04.006
0030-5898/14/$ – see front matter © 2014 Published by Elsevier Inc.

orthopedic.theclinics.com

REFERENCES

1. Little WJ. Hospital for the cure of deformities: course of lectures in the deformities of the human frame. Lancet 1843;41:350–4.

2. Warbasse JP. Lorenz on the bloody reposition of congenital hip-joint dislocation. Ann Surg 1895; 21(6):727–44.

3. Wenger DR, Pring ME, editors. Rang's children's fractures. 3rd edition. Lippincott, Williams, and Wilkins; 2005.

Assessment and Treatment of Children with Cerebral Palsy

Gilbert Chan, MD[a],*, Freeman Miller, MD[b]

KEYWORDS

- Orthopedics • Cerebral palsy • Hips • Spine • Spasticity • Neuromuscular • Feet

KEY POINTS

- Children with cerebral palsy are prone to development of musculoskeletal deformities.
- The underlying neurologic insult may results in a loss of selective motor control, an increase in underlying muscle tone, and muscle imbalance, which lead to abnormal deforming forces acting on the immature skeleton.
- The severely involved child is one who is at increased risk for developing progressive musculoskeletal deformities.
- Close surveillance and evaluation are key to addressing the underlying deformity and improving and maintaining overall function.

INTRODUCTION

Orthopedic management of children with cerebral palsy is a challenging task. The presentation is highly variable, ranging from those with mild clinical manifestations to those who are severely involved. The critical part in the initial assessment of children with cerebral palsy is the identification of risk factors for development of deformities so that attempts can be made to circumvent these events. This, in turn, maintains or improves a child's overall function.

Cerebral palsy is characterized by an injury or insult to the immature brain. This may occur before, during, or up to 5 years after birth. The pathology in the brain is permanent and nonprogressive. It results in a wide variety of postural and movement disorders. Clinical manifestations are determined by the timing of the injury and whether they occur in the preterm (immature) or term (mature) infant. The underlying pathology can

point to probable patterns of involvement. An immature or preterm infant with periventricular leukomalacia typically presents with spastic diplegia, whereas a child with periventricular hemorrhage is more likely to present with hemiplegia. Cerebellar involvement may present with hypotonia and ataxia. Occasionally, more than one lesion exists in the brain, resulting in a mixed presentation. A full-term child with watershed ischemia between the anterior and middle cerebral artery presents with quadriparesis whereas a focal ischemic injury in a full-term child presents with hemiparesis. Although the brain lesion is static, its manifestations are progressive. The primary manifestations of the neurologic insult include loss of selective motor control alteration in muscular balance and muscle tone abnormalities. This results in secondary manifestations of abnormal growth and development of the musculoskeletal system. It significantly affects a child's function, including

The authors have nothing to disclose.
a Children's Orthopedics of Louisville, Kosair Children's Hospital, 3999 Dutchman's Lane, Plaza 1, 6th Floor, Louisville, KY 40207, USA; b Alfred I. DuPont Hospital for Children, 1600 Rockland Road, Wilmington, DE 19803, USA
* Corresponding author.
E-mail address: Gilbert.Chan@nortonhealthcare.org

Orthop Clin N Am 45 (2014) 313–325
http://dx.doi.org/10.1016/j.ocl.2014.03.003
0030-5898/14/$ – see front matter © 2014 Elsevier Inc. All rights reserved.

abnormalities in gait and ambulation. The compensations that children undertake to overcome or adapt to these secondary manifestations are termed, *tertiary manifestations*.[1] It is in addressing the secondary and tertiary manifestations where orthopedists take a lead role, with the goal of correcting lever arm dysfunction, preventing progression of deformity, and optimizing overall function. In a sense, the role of orthopedic surgeons is to maintain, improve, or optimize a child's function and alter the natural history of the condition.

CLASSIFICATION

Classification systems help define and quantify the underlying pathology. They help determine and guide clinicians toward the most appropriate treatment and aid in communication between clinicians. Several classification systems have been proposed, dating as far back as the 1800s. The most comprehensive of these is the classification proposed by Minear in 1956,[2] which takes into consideration every aspect of a child, including physiologic, topographic, etiologic, traumatic, neuroanatomic, functional, and therapeutic involvement. Bax and colleagues[3] proposed a simpler classification system based on motor abnormalities, associated impairments, anatomic and radiographic findings, and causation and timing. Functional classification schemes are also commonly used and these are based on a child's overall functional capability. The Gross Motor Functional Classification System (GMFCS) is the most widely used functional scheme. It divides children into 5 groups based on the overall functional capability (**Table 1**).[4] The Functional Mobility Scale (FMS) describes motor function into 6 levels in 3 domains based on typical walking distance of 5, 50, or 500 m. This system is used to monitor change in motor function over time.[5]

Table 1
Gross motor function classification system

GMFCS Level	Description
I	No functional impairment
II	Functional limitation, may need assistive device
III	Assistive device needed for ambulation
IV	Limited self-mobility, wheelchair often required
V	Wheelchair bound

ASSESSMENT

Assessment of children with cerebral palsy centers on a complete history and physical evaluation. The history must include birth history and associated underlying medical conditions. The clinical evaluation should consist of a clinical evaluation of gait, both barefoot and with the use of orthotics, if any. Rotational profile should be checked to evaluate underlying torsional malalignment. Range of motion should be checked for the presence of any contractures. The specific underlying muscle tone is evaluated and recorded. A more detailed evaluation may include strength testing and an evaluation for selective motor control. Orthotics, assistive devices, and wheelchairs are evaluated to ensure that they fit properly.

Radiographs should be taken on the first orthopedic visit to establish a baseline; this is particularly true of the hips and pelvis. The severity of involvement and amount of deformity present dictate the frequency and need for sequential imaging studies on follow-up visits. Other advanced imaging techniques may be required prior to planning of reconstructive procedures.

A comprehensive gait analysis can be performed to obtain an objective assessment of the gait pattern that could be measured and quantified. This information can be further assessed to help in preoperative planning. It also provides a permanent record to compare the outcome of surgery. Studies have shown that gait analysis may aid and improve in surgical decision making in children with cerebral palsy.

HIPS

The hips in children with cerebral palsy are normal at birth. The deformity occurs from loss of selective motor control and abnormalities in muscle tone and balance. Such deformities include coxa valga, femoral anteversion, and acetabular dysplasia. The muscular imbalance is typically due to strong hip flexors and adductors overpowering the hip extensors and abductors. The rate of hip subluxation in cerebral palsy has been reported as high as 75%.[6–15] It is related to a child's level of function. Lonstein and Beck[7] found the rate of hip subluxation 11% in ambulators and 57% in nonambulators. Root[8] reported the incidence of dislocation to be 8% and subluxation 38%. Soo and colleagues[16] found no displacement in children who were GMFCS 1% and found 90% displacement in children who were GMFCS V. Increased femoral anteversion and coxa valga were also noted to be related to children's GMFCS level; Robin and colleagues[17] found femoral anteversion and neck shaft angles 30° and 135.9°, respectively, in those who were GMFCS I and 40° and 163°, respectively, in those who were GMFCS V.

Close surveillance of the hip joint is necessary. Identifying the hip at risk can lead to early and appropriate intervention to prevent the long-term sequelae of an untreated hip. Initial evaluation should include the hip range of motion; the presence or absence of contractures; pelvic obliquity; spinal deformity, if any; and femoral anteversion. Radiographic evaluation of the hip should quantify the amount of subluxation, if any. This is best assessed by the Reimer migration index (migration percentage) (**Fig. 1**), which is the measurement of the width of the uncovered femoral head relative to the total width of the femoral head. In children with cerebral palsy, the migration index is believed within acceptable limits if it is below 30. An increasing migration index has been correlated to the increased risk for hip dislocation. Hagglund and colleagues[9] reported that hips with a migration index greater than 40 had a high risk for dislocation and require treatment. Miller and Bagg[18] reported that children with a migration index below 30 were at low risk for dislocation and those with a migration index of greater than 60% had complete dislocation. The acetabular index is used to evaluate and quantify acetabular dysplasia (see **Fig. 1**). Acetabular index of less than 20° is considered normal in adulthood. In children below 5 years

of age, 25° is considered normal. An increased angle may denote the need to address the pelvic component of the deformity during surgical reconstruction. Radiographically, the amount of coxa valga may be assessed by measuring the neck shaft angle, which is typically increased. The radiographs must be taken with the hips in internal rotation to get an accurate measurement of the proximal femur.[19] In more complex deformities, a CT scan may be useful in preoperative planning.

A severely involved child who is at an increased risk for the development of hip dysplasia and subsequent dislocation should be observed closely, with radiographs taken at regular intervals (approximately 6 months). In more functional ambulatory children, a baseline radiograph should be obtained and the need for follow-up radiographs should be at the discretion of the physician based on a child's clinical evaluation. This may depend on whether there are initial concerns on the radiographs or if there are changes in the range of motion of the hip during regular evaluations. Nonoperative modalities should focus on maintaining hip range of motion, with or without formal physical therapy. Hip abduction bracing maybe attempted, but it may be difficult to maintain in the presence of a child's underlying tone. Focal spasticity management may be performed to improve range of motion and allow children to tolerate bracing better. Short-term studies have shown initial benefit with the use of botulinum toxin, particularly in younger children. These findings have not been substantiated, however, by other studies. In a randomized study, Graham and colleagues[20] reported a 1.4% decrease in the rate of hip displacement and they did not recommend botulinum toxin. In a long-term study, Willoughby and colleagues[21] showed that botulinum toxin injection combined with abduction bracing did not significantly reduce the rate of hip reconstructive surgery or influence the development of the hips at skeletal maturity. The current recommendation is to get one anteroposterior pelvis radiograph between 2 to 4 years of age for GMFCS I and II (independent ambulators) and one radiograph every year until age 8 and then every 2 years until skeletal maturity for GMFCS III, IV, and V as long as the migration index is less than 30. If the migration index is more than 30, more frequent radiographs and possible intervention should be planned.

Operative modalities are intended to prevent progression of deformity or to address an established deformity, subluxation, and/or dislocation. Soft tissue procedures may be carried out to maintain and improve hip range of motion. Miller and colleagues[22] performed iliopsoas and adductor lengthening in children with hip abduction of less

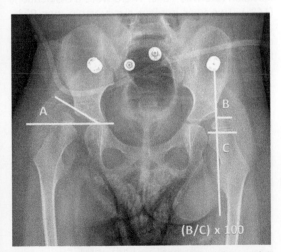

Fig. 1. Anteroposterior radiograph taken of the pelvis exhibiting measures of both the acetabular index (A) and Reimer migration index; (B and C) the angle subtended by Hilgenreiner line and the acetabular roof forms the acetabular index (A). The amount of the femoral head extruded (B) divided by the entire width of the femoral head (C) multiplied by 100 equates to the Reimer migration index.

than or equal to 30° and migration percentages of greater than or equal to 25%. At a mean follow-up of 39 months, 54% had good and 34% had fair outcome. The investigators concluded that early detection and intervention can lead to satisfactory outcome in 80% of children with spastic hips. This study, however, did not answer the question as to how many children would eventually require bony reconstruction. In a later long-term follow-up study, Presedo and colleagues[23] reported that soft tissue releases were effective for prevention of hip dislocation. The best predictors of good outcome in their study were ambulatory status and migration percentage. In those children who develop progressive subluxation or dislocation, hip reconstruction may be required (**Fig. 2**). During surgery, the deformity of the proximal femur and the acetabulum are assessed and addressed. In children with progressive subluxation or dislocation without significant acetabular dysplasia, a femoral varus derotation osteotomy combined with appropriate soft tissue procedures is often sufficient. In those with significant acetabular involvement, a pelvic osteotomy may be required. The osteotomy is performed to address the deficiency, which, in children with cerebral palsy, is more commonly posterior.[24,25] Outcomes after operative intervention have been favorable. McNerney and colleagues[26] reviewed 104 hips with a mean follow-up of 6.9 years. A total of 95% of the hips remained well reduced and there were no redislocations. Similarly, Miller and colleagues,[27] in a review of 49 subluxated and 21 dislocated hips, reported 2 hip redislocations at a mean follow-up of 34 months; 82% of cases had complete pain relief. The current recommendations are as follows: children under the age of 8 years and with migration index between 30%

and 60% should undergo adductor and iliopsoas lengthening, and children over the age of 8 years with migration percentage greater than 40% and all children with migration index greater than 60% should be recommended for hip reconstruction with femoral varus shortening osteotomy, pelvic osteotomy, and adductor lengthening.

In the skeletally mature hip, treatment is more challenging. Pelvic osteotomies, such as the Dega osteotomy or the Bernese periacetabular osteotomy, could be performed[28–32] but the results might not be as optimal. Often the severity of deformity dictates the most appropriate course. The results of primary reconstruction in hips with chronic degenerative changes and significant deformity (**Fig. 3**) may be dismal because pain may persist despite reconstruction. A fixed, painful, subluxated, or dislocated hip in a more mature patient with cerebral palsy often presents with a treatment conundrum. Typically, the hip shows denudation and loss of cartilage. Hip replacement can be performed and has the advantage of preserving hip motion. There are, however, substantial risks of hip dislocation, infection, and implant-related complications. Raphael and colleagues[33] reported on 56 patients (59 hips) who underwent total hip arthroplasty. Patients were routinely placed in a unilateral hip spica postoperatively for 3 weeks. All patients had a minimum follow-up of 2 years (mean 9.7 years). There was complete pain relief in 48/59 (81%) hips and 52/59 (88%) returned to their prepain GMFCS level. Revision rate was 15%. There were 8 dislocations (14%). Two-year implant survivorship was 95%, and the10-year survivorship was 85%. Alternatively, Gabos and colleagues[34] performed interpositional arthroplasty in 11 GMFCS V (non–weight-bearing) patients (14 hips) and achieved

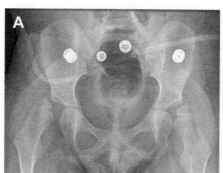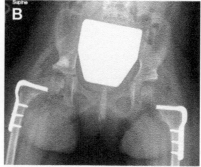

Fig. 2. (*A*) A 7-year-old child with quadriplegic cerebral palsy, exhibiting progressive subluxation of both hips with significant coxa valga and acetabular dysplasia; a decision was made to undergo surgical intervention. (*B*) Patient underwent correction of both hips. Soft tissue releases were done followed by bilateral varus derotation osteotomies and bilateral pelvic osteotomies to correct the acetabular component of the deformity. Postoperative radiographs taken show excellent correction of deformity.

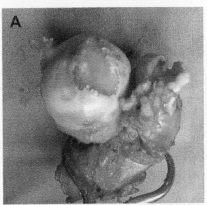
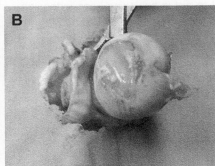

Fig. 3. (*A*, *B*) Photographs of a resected hip from an 15-year-old child with quadriplegic cerebral palsy. He had presented with significant hip pain and a windswept deformity and a decision was made to perform a resection of the hip. Resected specimen shows denudation of the superolateral portion of the hip with complete loss of cartilage.

improvement in pain in 10 of 11 cases. Proximal femoral resection and interpositional arthroplasty were initially introduced by Castle and Schneider.[35] McCarthy and colleagues[36] revised the technique to perform the resection at the level of the ischial tuberosity; in their series, all but 1 patient achieved improvement in seating. The concerns related to proximal femoral resection are heterotopic ossification, increased time to pain relief, prolonged hospital stay, and migration of the proximal femur. To address the issue of heterotopic ossification, Egermann and colleagues[37] used femoral head to cap the proximal femur and showed a decreased rate of heterotopic ossification. Another option in lieu of proximal femoral resection is a valgus osteotomy (McHale procedure). The goal of this procedure is to aim the femoral head away from the acetabulum while allowing for an indirect transfer of load. Several studies have shown an improvement in seating and pain relief.[38,39] Leet and colleagues[40] compared the results of proximal femoral resection with a valgus osteotomy with a mean follow-up of 3.4 years. Those treated with the McHale procedure had a shorter hospital stay and decreased proximal femoral migration. Both groups achieved improved seating and caretaker satisfaction.

KNEES

Anterior knee pain may present as a significant issue in children with cerebral palsy. It is often related to the patellofemoral joint. The common causes of anterior knee pain include patella alta, patellar subluxation or dislocation, quadriceps weakness, angular deformity, and rotational malalignment. Senaran and colleagues[41] looked at patients with anterior knee pain secondary to

patellafemoral symptoms; in their study, the patients were classified based on patella alta, fracture of the inferior pole of the patella, and patellar subluxation or dislocation. The investigators advocated aggressive treatment to prevent future deterioration.

Knee flexion contractures frequently occur in children with cerebral palsy. It is more severe in nonambulatory children. In younger children (age <12 years) with less severe deformity (contractures <15°), serial casting has shown effective at achieving and maintain correction for at least 1 year.[42] In more severe cases, hamstring release may be required to achieve adequate range of motion. In younger children with severe knee flexion deformity, guided growth in the form of an anterior hemiepiphysiodesis of the distal femur may be attempted.[43] In ambulatory children with knee flexion contractures, treatment should be aimed at correction of the contracture and improvement in the gait pattern. Typically, these patients have a crouch gait pattern. Children with crouch gait ambulate with the hip, knee, and ankle in flexion. This gait pattern has been described as increased knee flexion in stance phase in spastic diplegics.[44–46] The development of crouch gait has often been attributed to the natural progression of gait in ambulatory children with cerebral palsy.[47] Muscle weakness has also been implicated in the development of progressive crouch gait after lengthening of the triceps surae.[48–50] The cause of crouch is probably multifactorial and cannot be totally attributed to any single factor. In children with crouch gait, there is a failure of the plantar flexion–knee extension couple; hence, the knee maintains a flexed position with the ground reaction force falling behind the knee.

Several options exist to correct crouch gait. Initially, a ground reaction ankle foot orthosis may be used to aid in achieving knee extension. Surgical intervention for correction of crouch includes lengthening of the contracted muscle tendon units. Rethlefsen and colleagues[51] showed, however, that repetitive hamstring lengthening does not result in long-term correction of crouch. A complete evaluation of children needs to be undertaken prior to surgical intervention. Correction of all underlying deformities and restoration of the knee extensor mechanism are essential in correction of crouch gait. Stout and colleagues[52] showed that adequate correction can be achieved by addressing the knee flexion contracture through a distal femoral extension osteotomy (DFEO) and the patella alta with an advancement and transfer of the patellar tendon. In their series, children who underwent a combined DFEO with patellar tendon advancement did better than children who underwent DFEO alone or patellar tendon advancement alone.[53] In a majority of cases of undergoing a DFEO, hamstring lengthening does not seem required.[54] Correction of the other aspects of lower extremity malalignment, such as rotational malalignment (tibial torsion or femoral anteversion), planovalgus feet and muscle imbalance should be undertaken to restore and improve overall function. In a smaller series, Rodda and colleagues[55] showed that the use of multilevel orthopedic surgery was effective in improving the knee extensor mechanism, relieving knee pain, and achieving improved function in children with crouch gait. Children should not be allowed to develop severe crouch to the point where they lose function and ambulatory potential and become wheelchair bound. Correction is indicated when the crouch increases or a child's functional ability decreases.

Stiff knee gait results from increase spasticity of the rectus femoris muscle and is one of the common gait patterns seen in cerebral palsy. It interferes with the swing phase of gait by keeping the knee in extension, hence interfering with foot clearance. During the normal gait cycle, the rectus femoris is active during toe-off and inactive during midswing; it then reactivates during terminal swing and early stance to allow and prepare the limb for load acceptance. In stiff knee gait, the rectus femoris seems active during the entire swing phase of gait.[56,57] Stiff knee gait is defined as decreased magnitude of peak knee flexion of less than 45°, decreased range of knee flexion, and delay in peak knee flexion.[58] This may cause frequent tripping and falling. Other contributors to stiff knee gait include femoral torsional malalignment, poor push-off from the ankle, and weak hip flexor power.

Indications for treatment of stiff knee gait include decreased peak knee flexion, delay in time to peak knee flexion, and rectus femoris activity during swing phase of the gait. Transfer of the rectus femoris is the treatment of choice for stiff knee gait. The area or the site to where the rectus femoris is transferred does not seem to show any difference in the outcome of treatment when the area of the transfer is evaluated.[59,60] It seems that the improvement in peak knee flexion is maintained long term.[61] Although the results of simple release of rectus femoris in the treatment of stiff knee gait have not been good, there have been good results with a rectus femoris tendon resection of 4 to 6 cm[62]; rectus femoris transfer still seems superior to a release of the muscle in treatment of stiff knee gait.[63,64] It seems that when the rectus femoris is firing out of phase, when it fires predominantly during swing as documented by electromyography, is when maximal benefit can be achieved with a rectus femoris transfer.[65]

FEET

The feet are an essential part of gait providing a stable base of support to allow for standing and ambulation. The foot consists of 2 columns—the lateral and the medial columns, and 3 parts—forefoot, midfoot, and the hindfoot. It is essential that all these segments be assessed to correct the underlying deformity. The underlying muscular imbalance in cerebral palsy plays a large role in the development and progression of deformity. The necessity of correcting the foot in ambulatory children relies on restoring the lever arm to allow for appropriate push off, especially in children with a crouch gait pattern. In nonambulatory children, correction of deformity is centered on achieving a corrected foot that allows for shoe wear, bracing, standing, and pain relief. If the deformity is flexible, it may be amenable to bracing or soft tissue procedures. Radiographs may be used to document malalignment in various foot segments. Gait analysis with an electromyogram may be performed to assess and evaluate dynamic muscle imbalance. Dynamic pedobarographs may be used to assess plantar pressure distribution.

Planovalgus and equinovarus are the common deformities seen in cerebral palsy. In achieving appropriate correction of the foot, the role of the gastrocnemius cannot be stressed enough. The tightness of the Achilles tendon exacerbates the deformity, preventing the calcaneus from coming down to achieve an appropriate correction; most of this contracture tends to occur in the gastrocnemius and not the soleus. Lengthening of the gastrocsoleus mechanism should be undertaken with great caution in diplegic children, because overlengthening may lead to exacerbation or worsening of crouch gait from weakening of the plantar flexors.[48] Correction of the planovalgus foot begins with correction of segmental malalignment. This is best achieved by lengthening of the lateral column.[66–68] Once the hindfoot and lateral column are lengthened and the forefoot is brought over, the medial side of the foot should be assessed. If full correction of the foot is achieved, then the initial lengthening of the lateral column may be all that is needed. If residual deformity in the forefoot is still present and the first ray remains in supination, a plantar flexion osteotomy of the first ray may be performed either through the cuneiform or the first metatarsal. In more severe cases, a talonavicular arthrodesis may be required.[69] The specific method of correction is dependent on the severity of the deformity and a child's age. Seldom should surgery be considered for children younger than 8 years of age, because the deformity can usually be managed with orthotics. In children up to 4 years of age, significant correction can occur as part of the natural history of the disease, with no treatment required. Most surgery for planovalgus deformity correction should be done after age 10 years, because correction is much better maintained. The specific correction for lateral column lengthening can be done through lengthening of the calcaneus. This procedure works well for children with excellent functional gait, usually in those who ambulate without any assistive device. For children with hypotonia, poor muscle control, and more severe gait problems requiring walkers or doing standing transfers, lateral lengthening is best done with correct reduction of the calcaneus to the talus followed by a subtalar fusion. Medial column correction must correct the forefoot supination; in mild cases, this correction may be achieved with excision of the navicular tuberosity and advancement of the tibialis posterior. In more severe cases, an osteotomy and correction at the apex of the deformity can be done, which is usually at the cuneiform to bring the first ray down; a fusion at the talonavicular joint can also be performed. Usually, a fusion of the joint at the apex has the best long-term results in the authors' experience. Often the gastrocnemius is contracted with large differences between foot dorsiflexion with the knee flexed and with the knee extended. Usually, a lengthening of the gastrocnemius is required, but lengthening at the level of the Achilles tendon should be avoided, if possible, because this only further lengthens the soleus unnecessarily.

The equinovarus foot is more common in hemiplegic children. The treatment relies on balancing or removing the deforming force and addressing the bony deformities. In mild cases, soft tissue correction may suffice; this may take the form of split tendon transfers.[70,71] Complete tendon transfers are not advocated. In the more severe cases, soft tissue procedures in combination with bony procedures, such as a sliding calcaneal osteotomy or a closing wedge osteotomy for residual varus is required. In the most severe cases, an arthrodesis may be required.[72] Posterior tibialis tendon surgery prior to age 8 years should be avoided because of a high rate of overcorrection. In hemiplegia and children over age 8 years, the tibialis posterior is the most common overactive tendon and a split transfer to the peroneus brevis is a reliable procedure. When the varus is accentuated during the swing phase of gait or if varus seems mainly from the forefoot, then a split transfer of the tibialis anterior is a good option. Dynamic electromyogram is helpful to sort out these 2 options. Almost all varus deformities are associated with equinus and need to have a lengthening of the gastrocnemius or tendo-Achilles depending on the source of contracture. An open Z-lengthening of the tendo-Achilles is safer then blind percutaneous approaches.

Forefoot deformities also occur often in combination with other deformities. Hallux valgus can be managed with toe straps in the brace. Surgical correction is reserved for recalcitrant deformities. Dorsal bunions may be secondary to an underlying muscle imbalance or from an iatrogenic injury. Surgery is reserved for recalcitrant cases that interfere with shoe wear or bracing.

SPINE

The development of spinal deformity has been well described in children with cerebral palsy. Spine involvement, as with the development of any other deformity in cerebral palsy, is related to the functional level of the child. Scoliosis is the most common form of spinal deformity in cerebral palsy; its incidence has been reported as high as 77% in some studies.[73–76] A majority of these studies agree that the incidence of scoliosis increases with the severity of involvement of a child. Koop[73] found a higher incidence of scoliosis in patients with quadriplegic involvement. Their study showed that 30% of quadriplegic children developed scoliosis of greater than 40° at skeletal maturity compared with only 2% in children with hemiplegia. In a more recent study, Persson-Bunke and colleagues[77] analyzed the relationship of the development of scoliosis with children's

GMFCS level. In their series, only children with GMFCS level IV and V developed significant scoliosis of greater than 40°.

A majority of children with cerebral palsy manifest with a long C-shaped curve that often involves the pelvis. This curve pattern is more typical in those who are severely involved, in particular quadriplegics. Other curve types, similar to the types seen in idiopathic scoliosis, do occur in the more functional individuals. The natural history of scoliosis in cerebral palsy is well described. Severely involved children who develop scoliosis at a younger age (<15 years of age) have a higher risk for progression, and progression can be seen even after skeletal maturity.[75] Thometz and Simon[76] showed that after skeletal maturity, curves under 50° progressed at a rate of 0.8° per year, whereas those above 50° progressed at a rate of 1.4° per year. When taking into account the ambulatory status, curves progress at a rate of 0.9° per year in ambulatory children and at a rate of 2.4° per year in nonambulatory children. Tone-reducing modalities have also been evaluated to assess whether they influence progression or induce the development of spinal deformity. Selective dorsal rhizotomy has been implicated in the development of spinal deformity. Turi and Kalen[78] showed a 36% rate of developing significant deformity and 6% rate of requiring surgical stabilization at an average of 4.9 years after the index procedure. Johnson and colleagues[79] likewise showed an increased rate of developing spinal deformity in patients who had undergone a laminectomy or laminoplasty. In their study, they showed no difference in the development of deformity in patients who had undergone either procedure. The role of intrathecal baclofen in the progression of scoliosis remains unclear. Ginsburg and Lauder[80] showed increased progression of scoliotic deformity after placement of intrathecal baclofen pump. They showed that progression increased to 11° per year after pump placement. On the other hand, Senaran and colleagues[81] and Shilt and colleagues[82] showed no difference in the rate of progression in patients with and without the baclofen pump. Curve progression typically results in significant functional impairment and may interfere with activities of daily living. These curves may result in significant pelvic obliquity and cause seating difficulty. The contact pressures resulting from seating in an unbalanced position may result in pain and pressure ulceration. The loss of upright sitting ability may also cause a decrease in pulmonary function and interfere with feeding and exacerbate gastroesophageal reflux. The goals for treatment differ depending on the curve type and a child's level of function. In more

functional individuals, treatment centers on prevention of curve progression and maintaining spinal balance. In ambulatory children, spinal curvature may be treated much in the same way as in children with idiopathic scoliosis; however, these scenarios are less common. The more common case is a quadriplegic child with severe neuromuscular scoliosis and significant pelvic obliquity, resulting in pain, discomfort, and loss of seating balance. In these instances, the treatment should be centered on correcting spinal balance, relieving pain, and maintaining spinal stability in the safest way possible. The restoration of sitting ability and overall functional improvement should be achieved after treatment.

Nonoperative treatment is usually achieved through either seating modifications or brace treatment. There is little to no evidence in the literature that nonoperative measures may halt the progression of spinal curvature. Nonoperative measures may be instituted to allow for seating comfort. Bracing may also be used to slow curve progression until such time as a definitive procedure may be undertaken. Care must be taken when instituting rigid bracing in children with pulmonary compromise because this may induce chest cage deformity and further compromise pulmonary function.

Surgical management depends on several factors, which include a patients' age, functional capacity, comorbid factors, and curve pattern. In more functional children without significant pelvic obliquity, fusion of the curve without extending to the sacropelvis has been advocated to preserve ambulatory capacity. When fusion to the sacropelvis is not avoidable, ambulatory capacity has been shown maintained at a mean follow-up of 2 years.[81] In younger children, nonoperative treatment may be initially instituted to allow for growth until children are amenable for definitive treatment. In young children with large progressive curves, techniques for the management of early-onset scoliosis, such as growing rods, serial casting, and vertical expandable prosthetic titanium rib may be used until children have achieved adequate growth to allow for definitive fusion.[82–84] Young children with cerebral palsy and scoliosis, however, usually have severe disability, do not tolerate casting, and have high complication rates with growing rod techniques. In most children with limited ambulatory capacity, fusion to the sacropelvis is the treatment of choice (**Fig. 4**). The proximal level extends to T3 or higher. Proximal fusion levels below T3 are not advisable given the kyphotic posture of the thoracic spine, because lower fusion levels are at risk for developing proximal junctional kyphosis. Fusion to the pelvis is

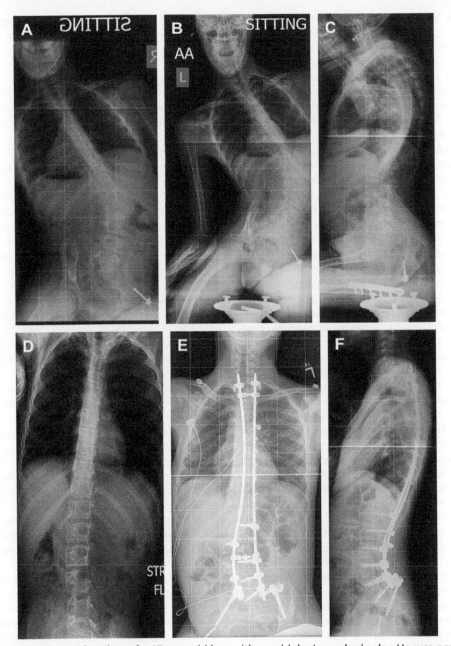

Fig. 4. (*A*) Initial radiographs taken of a 15-year-old boy with quadriplegic cerebral palsy. He was noted to have an XX degree curve; continued observation was advised. (*B, C*) On follow-up PA and lateral radiographs taken XX months later, he was noted to have progression of his curvature to XX degrees. (*D*) Traction films taken show excellent correction of his curvature with improvement of pelvic obliquity. (*E, F*) Postoperative films after a posterior spinal fusion was performed, which shows excellent correction of the curvature and pelvic obliquity. The child is sitting comfortably with a well-balanced spine.

often required to control and correct pelvic obliquity.[85] In most cases, the goals of surgery can be achieved through a posterior only approach, although occasionally, for a large, rigid curve, an anterior and posterior approach may be required. The necessity to go anterior can be determined by both clinical methods and radiographic methods. Clinically, the deformity and pelvis can be assessed for flexibility by applying traction or by using the side bending test.[86] Radiographically, flexibility films can be used to determine spinal flexibility.[87,88] Traction films are particularly useful in evaluating pelvic flexibility. Inability to correct the pelvis often necessitates an anterior release to provide additional flexibility to the spine.[89] In addition to adding flexibility, an anterior approach may be required in addressing the spine in younger children to prevent crankshaft phenomenon of the spine. Performing an anterior surgery is not without its risks. Significant postoperative complications may occur after an anterior approach. Pulmonary complications can occur especially if the thoracic cage is entered. The surgery may be performed either on the same day or in a staged fashion. Increased blood loss, prolonged operative time, and higher complication rates have been noted with sequential (single-stage) procedure.[90] Given the increased risk and morbidity associated with an anterior procedure, proper patient selection, patient preparation, and preoperative planning are required prior to surgery. Ideally, if surgery can be performed early with the spine maintaining adequate flexibility, then an anterior procedure can be obviated.

The choice of instrumentation is surgeon dependent. Several instrumentation techniques have been used successfully to address the deformity; these include the unit rod, Luque construct, Galveston technique, Cotrel-Dubousset instrumentation, third-generation instrumentation, and combinations thereof, which have been used successfully in the treatment of neuromuscular scoliosis.[91–96] The results after treatment with the various instrumentation systems have been comparable. When choosing instrumentation systems, surgeons must be reminded that the goal is not to achieve a straight spine but to correct the pelvic obliquity, achieve a balanced spine, restore seating ability, and relieve pain. The significant economic cost of newer-generation instrumentation must also be considered. Another factor for consideration is implant prominence, because soft tissue coverage may prove an issue in some of these children and, because most of these children are severely involved, osteopenia and poor bone quality in the areas of fixation may be a key issue during surgery. At the end of the day, the choice of instrumentation system relies on surgeon familiarity and preference.

SUMMARY

The orthopedic manifestations of children with cerebral palsy are wide and varied, with the clinical presentation directly correlating with the severity of a child's involvement. Although the underlying injury is static, its effects on a child's musculoskeletal system are progressive throughout the growing years. Close clinical surveillance and observation are needed to address these deformities as they develop and progress. The goal of treatment should not focus on the specific deformity but on the child as a whole, in an attempt to improve overall function.

REFERENCES

1. Gage JR, Schwarz MH, Koop SE, et al, editors. The identification and treatment of gait problems in cerebral palsy. Second edition. London: Mac Keith Press; 2009.
2. Minear WL. A classification of cerebral palsy. Pediatrics 1956;18(5):841–52.
3. Bax M, Goldstein M, Rosenbaum P, et al. Proposed definition and classification of cerebral palsy, April 2005. Dev Med Child Neurol 2005;47(8):571–6.
4. Palisano R, Rosenbaum P, Walter S, et al. Development and reliability of a system to classify gross motor function in children with cerebral palsy. Dev Med Child Neurol 1997;39(4):214–23.
5. Graham HK, Harvey A, Rodda J, et al. The Functional Mobility Scale (FMS). J Pediatr Orthop 2004;24(5):514–20.
6. Terjesen T. The natural history of hip development in cerebral palsy. Dev Med Child Neurol 2012; 54(10):951–7.
7. Lonstein JE, Beck K. Hip dislocation and subluxation in cerebral palsy. J Pediatr Orthop 1986;6(5):521–6.
8. Root L. Surgical treatment for hip pain in the adult cerebral palsy patient. Dev Med Child Neurol 2009;51(Suppl 4):84–91.
9. Hagglund G, Lauge-Pedersen H, Wagner P. Characteristics of children with hip displacement in cerebral palsy. BMC Musculoskelet Disord 2007;8:101.
10. Morton RE, Scott B, McClelland V, et al. Dislocation of the hips in children with bilateral spastic cerebral palsy, 1985-2000. Dev Med Child Neurol 2006; 48(7):555–8.
11. Howard CB, McKibbin B, Williams LA, et al. Factors affecting the incidence of hip dislocation in cerebral palsy. J Bone Joint Surg Br 1985;67(4):530–2.
12. Carr C, Gage JR. The fate of the nonoperated hip in cerebral palsy. J Pediatr Orthop 1987;7(3):262–7.
13. Gamble JG, Rinsky LA, Bleck EE. Established hip dislocations in children with cerebral palsy. Clin Orthop Relat Res 1990;(253):90–9.
14. Cooperman DR, Bartucci E, Dietrick E, et al. Hip dislocation in spastic cerebral palsy: long-term consequences. J Pediatr Orthop 1987;7(3):268–76.
15. Sherk HH, Pasquariello PD, Doherty J. Hip dislocation in cerebral palsy: selection for treatment. Dev Med Child Neurol 1983;25(6):738–46.
16. Soo B, Howard JJ, Boyd RN, et al. Hip displacement in cerebral palsy. J Bone Joint Surg Am 2006;88(1):121–9.
17. Robin J, Graham HK, Selber P, et al. Proximal femoral geometry in cerebral palsy: a

population-based cross-sectional study. J Bone Joint Surg Br 2008;90(10):1372–9.

18. Miller F, Bagg MR. Age and migration percentage as risk factors for progression in spastic hip disease. Dev Med Child Neurol 1995;37(5):449–55.

19. Kay RM, Jaki KA, Skaggs DL. The effect of femoral rotation on the projected femoral neck-shaft angle. J Pediatr Orthop 2000;20(6):736–9.

20. Graham HK, Boyd R, Carlin JB, et al. Does botulinum toxin a combined with bracing prevent hip displacement in children with cerebral palsy and "hips at risk"? A randomized, controlled trial. J Bone Joint Surg Am 2008;90(1):23–33.

21. Willoughby K, Ang SG, Thomason P, et al. The impact of botulinum toxin A and abduction bracing on long-term hip development in children with cerebral palsy. Dev Med Child Neurol 2012;54(8):743–7.

22. Miller F, Cardoso Dias R, Dabney KW, et al. Soft-tissue release for spastic hip subluxation in cerebral palsy. J Pediatr Orthop 1997;17(5):571–84.

23. Presedo A, Oh CW, Dabney KW, et al. Soft-tissue releases to treat spastic hip subluxation in children with cerebral palsy. J Bone Joint Surg Am 2005;87(4):832–41.

24. Buckley SL, Sponseller PD, Magid D. The acetabulum in congenital and neuromuscular hip instability. J Pediatr Orthop 1991;11(4):498–501.

25. Kim HT, Wenger DR. Location of acetabular deficiency and associated hip dislocation in neuromuscular hip dysplasia: three-dimensional computed tomographic analysis. J Pediatr Orthop 1997;17(2):143–51.

26. McNerney NP, Mubarak SJ, Wenger DR. One-stage correction of the dysplastic hip in cerebral palsy with the San Diego acetabuloplasty: results and complications in 104 hips. J Pediatr Orthop 2000;20(1):93–103.

27. Miller F, Girardi H, Lipton G, et al. Reconstruction of the dysplastic spastic hip with peri-ilial pelvic and femoral osteotomy followed by immediate mobilization. J Pediatr Orthop 1997;17(5):592–602.

28. Inan M, Gabos PG, Domzalski M, et al. Incomplete transiliac osteotomy in skeletally mature adolescents with cerebral palsy. Clin Orthop Relat Res 2007;462:169–74.

29. Robb JE, Brunner R. A Dega-type osteotomy after closure of the triradiate cartilage in non-walking patients with severe cerebral palsy. J Bone Joint Surg Br 2006;88(7):933–7.

30. Jozwiak M, Koch A. Two-stage surgery in the treatment of spastic hip dislocation–comparison between early and late results of open reduction and derotation-varus femoral osteotomy combined with Dega pelvic osteotomy preceded by soft tissue release. Ortop Traumatol Rehabil 2011;13(2):144–54.

31. Karlen JW, Skaggs DL, Ramachandran M, et al. The Dega osteotomy: a versatile osteotomy in the treatment of developmental and neuromuscular hip pathology. J Pediatr Orthop 2009;29(7):676–82.

32. MacDonald SJ, Hersche O, Ganz R. Periacetabular osteotomy in the treatment of neurogenic acetabular dysplasia. J Bone Joint Surg Br 1999;81(6):975–8.

33. Raphael BS, Dines JS, Akerman M, et al. Long-term followup of total hip arthroplasty in patients with cerebral palsy. Clin Orthop Relat Res 2010;468(7):1845–54.

34. Gabos PG, Miller F, Galban MA, et al. Prosthetic interposition arthroplasty for the palliative treatment of end-stage spastic hip disease in nonambulatory patients with cerebral palsy. J Pediatr Orthop 1999;19(6):796–804.

35. Castle ME, Schneider C. Proximal femoral resection-interposition arthroplasty. J Bone Joint Surg Am 1978;60(8):1051–4.

36. McCarthy RE, Simon S, Douglas B, et al. Proximal femoral resection to allow adults who have severe cerebral palsy to sit. J Bone Joint Surg Am 1988;70(7):1011–6.

37. Egermann M, Doderlein L, Schlager E, et al. Autologous capping during resection arthroplasty of the hip in patients with cerebral palsy. J Bone Joint Surg Br 2009;91(8):1007–12.

38. Hogan KA, Blake M, Gross RH. Subtrochanteric valgus osteotomy for chronically dislocated, painful spastic hips. J Bone Joint Surg Am 2006;88(12):2624–31.

39. McHale KA, Bagg M, Nason SS. Treatment of the chronically dislocated hip in adolescents with cerebral palsy with femoral head resection and subtrochanteric valgus osteotomy. J Pediatr Orthop 1990;10(4):504–9.

40. Leet AI, Chhor K, Launay F, et al. Femoral head resection for painful hip subluxation in cerebral palsy: is valgus osteotomy in conjunction with femoral head resection preferable to proximal femoral head resection and traction? J Pediatr Orthop 2005;25(1):70–3.

41. Senaran H, Holden C, Dabney KW, et al. Anterior knee pain in children with cerebral palsy. J Pediatr Orthop 2007;27(1):12–6.

42. Westberry DE, Davids JR, Jacobs JM, et al. Effectiveness of serial stretch casting for resistant or recurrent knee flexion contractures following hamstring lengthening in children with cerebral palsy. J Pediatr Orthop 2006;26(1):109–14.

43. Macwilliams BA, Harjinder B, Stevens PM. Guided growth for correction of knee flexion deformity: a series of four cases. Strategies Trauma Limb Reconstr 2011;6(2):83–90.

44. Frost HM. Cerebral palsy. The spastic crouch. Clin Orthop Relat Res 1971;80:2–8.

45. Gage JR. Surgical treatment of knee dysfunction in cerebral palsy. Clin Orthop Relat Res 1990;(253): 45–54.

46. Drummond DS, Rogala E, Templeton J, et al. Proximal hamstring release for knee flexion and crouched posture in cerebral palsy. J Bone Joint Surg Am 1974;56(8):1598–602.

47. Bell KJ, Ounpuu S, DeLuca PA, et al. Natural progression of gait in children with cerebral palsy. J Pediatr Orthop 2002;22(5):677–82.

48. Dietz FR, Albright JC, Dolan L. Medium-term follow-up of Achilles tendon lengthening in the treatment of ankle equinus in cerebral palsy. Iowa Orthop J 2006;26:27–32.

49. Borton DC, Walker K, Pirpiris M, et al. Isolated calf lengthening in cerebral palsy. Outcome analysis of risk factors. J Bone Joint Surg Br 2001;83(3): 364–70.

50. Sutherland DH, Cooper L. The pathomechanics of progressive crouch gait in spastic diplegia. Orthop Clin North Am 1978;9(1):143–54.

51. Rethlefsen SA, Yasmeh S, Wren TA, et al. Repeat hamstring lengthening for crouch gait in children with cerebral palsy. J Pediatr Orthop 2013;33(5): 501–4.

52. Stout JL, Gage JR, Schwartz MH, et al. Distal femoral extension osteotomy and patellar tendon advancement to treat persistent crouch gait in cerebral palsy. J Bone Joint Surg Am 2008;90(11): 2470–84.

53. Novacheck TF, Stout JL, Gage JR, et al. Distal femoral extension osteotomy and patellar tendon advancement to treat persistent crouch gait in cerebral palsy. Surgical technique. J Bone Joint Surg Am 2009;91(Suppl 2):271–86.

54. Healy MT, Schwartz MH, Stout JL, et al. Is simultaneous hamstring lengthening necessary when performing distal femoral extension osteotomy and patellar tendon advancement? Gait Posture 2011; 33(1):1–5.

55. Rodda JM, Graham HK, Nattrass GR, et al. Correction of severe crouch gait in patients with spastic diplegia with use of multilevel orthopaedic surgery. J Bone Joint Surg Am 2006;88(12): 2653–64.

56. Waters RL, Garland DE, Perry J, et al. Stiff-legged gait in hemiplegia: surgical correction. J Bone Joint Surg Am 1979;61(6A):927–33.

57. Perry J. Distal rectus femoris transfer. Dev Med Child Neurol 1987;29(2):153–8.

58. Sutherland DH, Davids JR. Common gait abnormalities of the knee in cerebral palsy. Clin Orthop Relat Res 1993;(288):139–47.

59. Muthusamy K, Seidl AJ, Friesen RM, et al. Rectus femoris transfer in children with cerebral palsy: evaluation of transfer site and preoperative indicators. J Pediatr Orthop 2008;28(6):674–8.

60. Ounpuu S, Muik E, Davis RB 3rd, et al. Rectus femoris surgery in children with cerebral palsy. Part I: the effect of rectus femoris transfer location on knee motion. J Pediatr Orthop 1993;13(3):325–30.

61. Dreher T, Wolf SI, Maier M, et al. Long-term results after distal rectus femoris transfer as a part of multilevel surgery for the correction of stiff-knee gait in spastic diplegic cerebral palsy. J Bone Joint Surg Am 2012;94(19). p. e142(1–10).

62. Presedo A, Megrot F, Ilharreborde B, et al. Rectus femoris distal tendon resection improves knee motion in patients with spastic diplegia. Clin Orthop Relat Res 2012;470(5):1312–9.

63. Sutherland DH, Santi M, Abel MF. Treatment of stiff-knee gait in cerebral palsy: a comparison by gait analysis of distal rectus femoris transfer versus proximal rectus release. J Pediatr Orthop 1990; 10(4):433–41.

64. Ounpuu S, Muik E, Davis RB 3rd, et al. Rectus femoris surgery in children with cerebral palsy. Part II: a comparison between the effect of transfer and release of the distal rectus femoris on knee motion. J Pediatr Orthop 1993;13(3):331–5.

65. Miller F, Cardoso Dias R, Lipton GE, et al. The effect of rectus EMG patterns on the outcome of rectus femoris transfers. J Pediatr Orthop 1997; 17(5):603–7.

66. Andreacchio A, Orellana CA, Miller F, et al. Lateral column lengthening as treatment for planovalgus foot deformity in ambulatory children with spastic cerebral palsy. J Pediatr Orthop 2000;20(4):501–5.

67. Dumontier TA, Falicov A, Mosca V, et al. Calcaneal lengthening: investigation of deformity correction in a cadaver flatfoot model. Foot Ankle Int 2005;26(2): 166–70.

68. Mosca VS. Calcaneal lengthening for valgus deformity of the hindfoot. Results in children who had severe, symptomatic flatfoot and skewfoot. J Bone Joint Surg Am 1995;77(4):500–12.

69. Turriago CA, Arbelaez MF, Becerra LC. Talonavicular joint arthrodesis for the treatment of pes planus valgus in older children and adolescents with cerebral palsy. J Child Orthop 2009;3(3): 179–83.

70. Vlachou M, Dimitriadis D. Split tendon transfers for the correction of spastic varus foot deformity: a case series study. J Foot Ankle Res 2010;3:28.

71. O'Byrne JM, Kennedy A, Jenkinson A, et al. Split tibialis posterior tendon transfer in the treatment of spastic equinovarus foot. J Pediatr Orthop 1997; 17(4):481–5.

72. Frost NL, Grassbaugh JA, Baird G, et al. Triple arthrodesis with lateral column lengthening for the treatment of planovalgus deformity. J Pediatr Orthop 2011;31(7):773–82.

73. Koop SE. Scoliosis in cerebral palsy. Dev Med Child Neurol 2009;51(Suppl 4):92–8.

74. Madigan RR, Wallace SL. Scoliosis in the institutionalized cerebral palsy population. Spine 1981; 6(6):583–90.

75. Saito N, Ebara S, Ohotsuka K, et al. Natural history of scoliosis in spastic cerebral palsy. Lancet 1998; 351(9117):1687–92.

76. Thometz JG, Simon SR. Progression of scoliosis after skeletal maturity in institutionalized adults who have cerebral palsy. J Bone Joint Surg Am 1988;70(9):1290–6.

77. Persson-Bunke M, Hagglund G, Lauge-Pedersen H, et al. Scoliosis in a total population of children with cerebral palsy. Spine 2012; 37(12):E708–13.

78. Turi M, Kalen V. The risk of spinal deformity after selective dorsal rhizotomy. J Pediatr Orthop 2000; 20(1):104–7.

79. Johnson MB, Goldstein L, Thomas SS, et al. Spinal deformity after selective dorsal rhizotomy in ambulatory patients with cerebral palsy. J Pediatr Orthop 2004;24(5):529–36.

80. Ginsburg GM, Lauder AJ. Progression of scoliosis in patients with spastic quadriplegia after the insertion of an intrathecal baclofen pump. Spine 2007; 32(24):2745–50.

81. Tsirikos AI, Chang WN, Shah SA, et al. Preserving ambulatory potential in pediatric patients with cerebral palsy who undergo spinal fusion using unit rod instrumentation. Spine 2003;28(5):480–3.

82. Fletcher ND, McClung A, Rathjen KE, et al. Serial casting as a delay tactic in the treatment of moderate-to-severe early-onset scoliosis. J Pediatr Orthop 2012;32(7):664–71.

83. White KK, Song KM, Frost N, et al. VEPTR growing rods for early-onset neuromuscular scoliosis: feasible and effective. Clin Orthop Relat Res 2011;469(5):1335–41.

84. McElroy MJ, Sponseller PD, Dattilo JR, et al. Growing rods for the treatment of scoliosis in children with cerebral palsy: a critical assessment. Spine 2012;37(24):E1504–10.

85. Gau YL, Lonstein JE, Winter RB, et al. Luque-Galveston procedure for correction and stabilization of neuromuscular scoliosis and pelvic obliquity: a review of 68 patients. J Spinal Disord 1991;4(4): 399–410.

86. Miller F. Cerebral palsy. 2005; x, 1055 p. ill. (some col.) 1029 cm. + 1051 CD-ROM (1054 1053/1054 in.). Available at: Publisher description http://www. loc.gov/catdir/enhancements/fy0662/2003065734-d.html. Table of contents only http://www.loc.gov/catdir/enhancements/fy0818/2003065734-t.html. Accessed January 4, 2005.

87. Polly DW Jr, Sturm PF. Traction versus supine side bending. Which technique best determines curve flexibility? Spine 1998;23(7):804–8.

88. Vaughan JJ, Winter RB, Lonstein JE. Comparison of the use of supine bending and traction radiographs in the selection of the fusion area in adolescent idiopathic scoliosis. Spine 1996; 21(21):2469–73.

89. Auerbach JD, Spiegel DA, Zgonis MH, et al. The correction of pelvic obliquity in patients with cerebral palsy and neuromuscular scoliosis: is there a benefit of anterior release prior to posterior spinal arthrodesis? Spine 2009;34(21):E766–74.

90. Tsirikos AI, Chang WN, Dabney KW, et al. Comparison of one-stage versus two-stage anteroposterior spinal fusion in pediatric patients with cerebral palsy and neuromuscular scoliosis. Spine 2003; 28(12):1300–5.

91. Piazzolla A, Solarino G, De Giorgi S, et al. Cotrel-Dubousset instrumentation in neuromuscular scoliosis. Eur Spine J 2011;20(Suppl 1):S75–84.

92. Tsirikos AI, Lipton G, Chang WN, et al. Surgical correction of scoliosis in pediatric patients with cerebral palsy using the unit rod instrumentation. Spine 2008;33(10):1133–40.

93. Boachie-Adjei O, Lonstein JE, Winter RB, et al. Management of neuromuscular spinal deformities with Luque segmental instrumentation. J Bone Joint Surg Am 1989;71(4):548–62.

94. Lonstein JE, Koop SE, Novachek TF, et al. Results and complications after spinal fusion for neuromuscular scoliosis in cerebral palsy and static encephalopathy using luque galveston instrumentation: experience in 93 patients. Spine 2012; 37(7):583–91.

95. Mattila M, Jalanko T, Puisto V, et al. Hybrid versus total pedicle screw instrumentation in patients undergoing surgery for neuromuscular scoliosis: a comparative study with matched cohorts. J Bone Joint Surg Br 2012;94(10):1393–8.

96. Yazici M, Asher MA, Hardacker JW. The safety and efficacy of Isola-Galveston instrumentation and arthrodesis in the treatment of neuromuscular spinal deformities. J Bone Joint Surg Am 2000;82(4): 524–43.

Elbow Fractures and Dislocations

Kevin J. Little, MD[a,b,*]

KEYWORDS

- Supracondylar • Lateral condyle • Medal epicondyle • Elbow dislocations • Radial neck
- Olecranon • Monteggia

KEY POINTS

- Elbow fractures are common in pediatric patients.
- Most injuries to the pediatric elbow are stable and require simple immobilization; however, more severe fractures can occur, often requiring operative stabilization and/or close monitoring.
- Careful clinical and radiographic evaluation can lead to an accurate diagnosis and prompt, appropriate treatment.
- Although many injuries about the elbow present pitfalls during diagnosis and treatment, most children recover excellent function and are able to return to premorbid activities with no limitations.

INTRODUCTION

Young children are at a significant risk for traumatic injuries that can lead to morbidity and mortality. Approximately 70% of fractures involve the upper extremity, with 8% to 10% involving the distal humerus or proximal radius and ulna.[1,2] In 2005 alone, trauma to the upper extremity in children less than 19 years of age resulted in approximately $8 billion in direct health care costs and loss of estimated future income.[3] The shoulder and elbow are the 2 joints responsible for positioning the hand in space for functional use. These actions allow infants and children to explore and interact with the world around them but place the upper extremity at risk for injury. The incidence of various fractures about the elbow peaks at different ages for children and depends highly on the specific activities performed as well as the maturity of the elbow.

The distal humerus physis develops as 4 distinct ossification centers, whereas the proximal radius and ulna each contribute 1 ossification center. The sequence of ossification is fairly predictable: the capitellum appears first between 1 and 2 years of age, followed by the radial head at 2 to 4 years of age, then the medial epicondyle at 4 to 6 years of age, the trochlea at 9 to 10 years of age, the olecranon at 9 to 11 years of age, and lateral epicondyle at 9.5 to 11.5 years of age. The appearance of the radial head is occasionally preceded by the medial epicondyle in girls, whose ossification centers typically appear 1 to 2 years earlier than boys. The trochlea, lateral epicondyle, and capitellum ossification centers fuse into the distal humeral epiphysis at around 11 years of age in girls and 13 to 14 years of age in boys. The radial head and olecranon ossification centers close at 12 to 13 years of age in girls and 14 to 15 years of age in boys. The medial epicondyle is the last to fuse to the distal humerus at 13 to 14 years of age in girls and 15 years of age in boys.[4]

SUPRACONDYLAR HUMERUS FRACTURES

Supracondylar humerus fractures are the most common pediatric elbow fracture, accounting for 3.3% of all pediatric fractures[5] and 60% of

The author has nothing to disclose.
[a] Division of Pediatric Orthopaedics, Hand and Upper Extremity Surgery, Cincinnati Children's Hospital Medical Center, 3333 Burnet Avenue, ML 2017, Cincinnati, OH 45229, USA; [b] Department of Orthopaedic Surgery, University of Cincinnati College of Medicine, 231 Albert Sabin Way, Cincinnati, OH 45229, USA
* Division of Pediatric Orthopaedics, Hand and Upper Extremity Surgery, Cincinnati Children's Hospital Medical Center, 3333 Burnet Avenue, ML 2017, Cincinnati, OH 45229.
E-mail address: Kevin.little@cchmc.org

Orthop Clin N Am 45 (2014) 327–340
http://dx.doi.org/10.1016/j.ocl.2014.03.004
0030-5898/14/$ – see front matter © 2014 Elsevier Inc. All rights reserved.

pediatric elbow fractures.[6] Biomechanically, the supracondylar region of the humerus is prone to injury because of the thin sheet of bone that sits between the medial and lateral columns. During a fall, children will attempt to brace themselves with their hand and wrist, which can transmit the force of the fall through an extended elbow joint to the supracondylar area. Tension on the anterior joint capsule, via elbow hyperextension, acts to further displace the fracture.[7] Extension-type injuries resulting from a fall onto an outstretched hand (FOOSH) make up 97% of supracondylar fractures, whereas flexion-type injuries from a direct blow to the posterior olecranon compose the rest.[8] Transphyseal injures have been described in infants and should be considered in patients with elbow swelling and pain before the development of ossification centers, especially in the setting of suspected or confirmed nonaccidental trauma.[9] This injury is difficult to diagnose on plain radiographs, although it can be apparent as a misalignment of the humerus and ulna; ultrasound is a useful adjunct modality to confirm a suspected diagnosis. Because of this misalignment, transphyseal injuries can be misinterpreted as an elbow dislocation. However, the latter is exceedingly rare in infants and toddlers. The treatment of transphyseal injuries is the same as that in displaced supracondylar fractures. Closed reduction and percutaneous pinning are the mainstay of treatment, and an elbow arthrogram can assist with identifying appropriate landmarks during pinning to ensure that anatomic alignment is obtained.[9]

The peak age for supracondylar fractures is between 5 and 7 years.[3] The child presents with elbow pain, edema, and variable ecchymosis, often with significant deformity in severe injuries. Open fractures are noted in up to 3% of patients; concomitant injuries, typically involving the forearm or wrist, are seen in 11% of patients. Occult fractures are common in the developing elbow, typically presenting as painful, swollen elbows without definitive radiographic evidence of fracture. An anterior and/or posterior fat pad sign (Fig. 1A) is often the only indication of occult injury. A careful physical examination including palpation of the radial neck, olecranon, medial and lateral epicondyles, and supracondylar region will often reveal the location of an occult fracture, which is often only manifested radiographically as a healing fracture on routine follow-up radiographs. A careful neurologic and vascular examination must be performed in the emergency department and documented, such that it can be compared with a postreduction or postoperative examination in displaced fractures. Any evidence of vascular

compromise or insufficiency to the hand, especially in patients with a cool, white, pulseless extremity, is considered an indication for emergent reduction and surgical fixation. Nerve injuries are present in 11.3% of supracondylar fractures, most commonly in the anterior interosseous nerve, median nerve, and radial nerve for extension-type injuries and the ulnar nerve in flexion-type injuries.[10]

Standard anteroposterior (AP) and lateral radiographs are obtained to evaluate the injured elbow. Once a supracondylar humerus fracture is identified, AP and lateral forearm and posteroanterior and lateral wrist radiographs are mandatory for the evaluation of concomitant injuries to the forearm or wrist. The diagnosis of an additional forearm or wrist fracture, a pediatric floating elbow, imparts a substantially increased risk of compartment syndrome and indicates surgical fixation of unstable radius and ulna fractures, which could otherwise be managed nonoperatively with closed reduction and casting.[11] Preoperative grading of supracondylar humerus fractures is based on the lateral view (Table 1). A line drawn along the anterior cortex of the humerus shaft (anterior humeral line) should intersect or touch the capitellum.[12] On the AP view, a postreduction determination of the angle between the long axis of the humerus shaft and the proximal capitellum ossification center, known as the Baumann angle, is typically performed. This angle, also known as the shaft-capitellum angle, normally lies between 64° and 81°; an increasing angle correlates with increasing clinical cubitus varus. It should be noted that there is confusion in the literature as to which angle Baumann was referring[13]; the Baumann angle has been frequently described, incorrectly, as the angle between a line perpendicular to the humeral shaft line and the superior border of the capitellum (the complement of the true Baumann angle).

Treatment in children is based on the Gartland classification, with type I fractures requiring only above-elbow cast treatment for 3 to 4 weeks until radiographic healing is noted. The treatment of type II injuries (see Fig. 1B) remains controversial as some researchers advocate closed reduction and casting, whereas others advocate closed reduction and percutaneous pinning. Type II fractures, whereby the anterior humeral line touches the capitellum, can be treated in an above-elbow cast with weekly radiographs to ensure maintenance of alignment. Parikh[14] noted that in type II injuries, closed reduction and casting in 90° to 100° of flexion resulted in adequate maintenance of alignment in 72% of patients; those that lost alignment during subsequent weekly follow-up were successfully converted to operative fixation

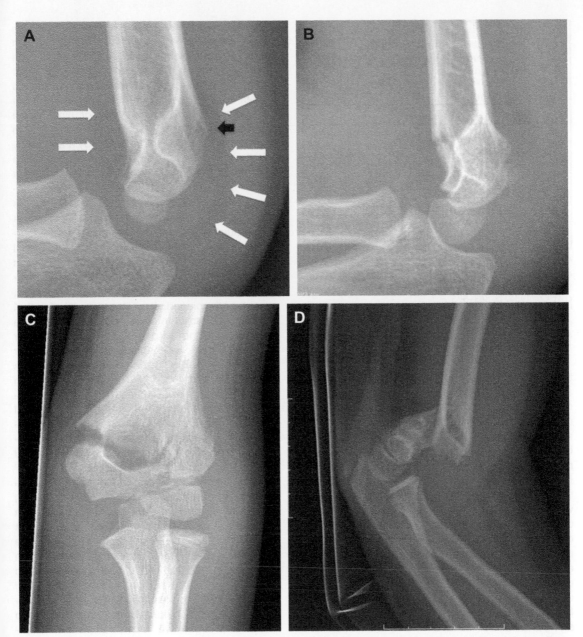

Fig. 1. Supracondylar humerus fractures: (*A*) Lateral view of Gartland type I with associated fat pad sign (*large white arrows*) and subtle posterior cortical buckling (*small black arrow*) indicating the fracture line. (*B*) Lateral view of Gartland type IIA fracture with posterior angulation and intact posterior hinge. (*C*) Anteroposterior view of Gartland type IIB fracture with medial instability without complete displacement. (*D*) Lateral view of Gartland type III fracture with complete dissociation of fracture fragments.

when necessary. O'hara[15] showed that closed reduction and plaster immobilization in type IIB (see **Fig. 1**C) and III (see **Fig. 1**D) fractures resulted in a 26% loss of reduction and surgical fixation. Type III injuries require expedient closed reduction and percutaneous pinning. In patients without neurovascular compromise, fixation can be delayed beyond 8 hours without an increased risk

of patient morbidity and complications, allowing for patients presenting overnight to be treated the following morning, provided a qualified physician or assistant is available for close neurovascular monitoring.[16]

Patients with type II and III injuries with neurovascular compromise or with concomitant unstable injury to the ipsilateral extremity should be

Table 1
Wilkins modification of the Gartland classification for extension-type supracondylar humerus fractures

Type[a]	Description
I	Nondisplaced fracture
IIA	Displaced fracture with intact posterior cortical hinge
IIB	Displaced fracture with malrotation or lateral displacement without loss of cortical contact
III	Completely displaced fracture
IV[b]	Completely displaced fracture with multidirectional instability

[a] *Data from* Wilkins KE. Fractures and dislocations of the elbow region. In: Rockwood CA, Wilkins KE, King RE, editors. Fractures in children, vol. 3. Philadelphia: JB Lippincott Co; 1984. p. 363–575.
[b] *Data from* Leitch KK, Kay RM, Femino JD, et al. Treatment of multidirectionally unstable supracondylar humeral fractures in children: a modified Gartland type-IV fracture. J Bone Joint Surg Am 2006;88:980–5.

taken to the operating room urgently for reduction and pinning. Indications for open reduction include open fractures and when interposed periosteum or neurovascular structures prevent anatomical alignment. This soft tissue interposition can often be detected during reduction maneuvers as a rubbery feeling instead of normal crepitus between fracture fragments. Any worsening of the vascular status of patients after reduction and pinning warrants an immediate surgical exploration by a qualified hand or vascular surgeon. Invasive vascular studies will delay diagnosis and add cost and possible morbidity while providing limited additional information that can be used in clinical decision making.[17] In most cases of vascular compromise, the artery is simply tethered to the fracture by a supratrochlear branch of the brachial artery; however, arterial thrombus and intimal tear injuries can be seen and require exploration and repair or interpositional vein grafting.[18]

During closed reduction, the fracture can be reduced via a milking procedure to remove interposed periosteum or brachialis muscle. The fracture is then distracted and flexed with anterior pressure on the olecranon. AP alignment can be verified via the Baumann angle, and lateral alignment is verified using the anterior humeral line. Typically, 2 divergent percutaneous 0.062-in Kirschner (K) wires are then placed through the lateral condyle into the medial metadiaphyseal distal humerus. One pin is fixated into the medial column, just above the fracture line, while the other is passed superior to the olecranon fossa to hold fixation into the lateral column. In patients with significant medial comminution or unstable reduction during fluoroscopic evaluation, a third pin can be placed either from a lateral or medial entry point. If a medial pin is used, 2 steps are performed to protect the ulnar nerve. First the elbow is brought into extension to decrease anterior ulnar nerve subluxation; secondly, a small incision is made to dissect down to the medial epicondyle and verify that the pin does not transect or impinge on the ulnar nerve during motion.[19] The placement of a medial and lateral pin (cross pinning) is biomechanically equivalent in torsional stability to the placement of 2 divergent lateral pins in anatomically reduced fractures but provides superior fixation in malreduced fractures and those with medial comminution.[20,21] In patients whereby reduction is blocked by soft tissue or edema, and the previously described milking procedure does not help, a posteriorly placed, percutaneous intrafocal K wire can be placed to assist with reduction. Care must be taken not to penetrate past the anterior cortex and risk damaging the neurovascular bundle. Open reduction is reserved for patients with arterial injury or when anatomic reduction cannot be obtained via closed methods. Compartment syndrome has been noted in 0.5% of all supracondylar fractures[22] and in up to 6% of patients with questionable vascular status.[18] In children, compartment syndrome is best diagnosed using the 3 As (anxiety, agitation, and analgesia).[23] The first sign of impending compartment syndrome is an increasing need for narcotic analgesia, and sedating medications are contraindicated in the postoperative period as they can mask this need. This diagnosis is made clinically, and the measurement of compartment pressure often confuses the picture in that the natural diastolic pressure in children is often around 30 mm Hg. However, the measurement of compartment pressure can be useful in the operating room in order to compare preoperative and postoperative measurements, whereby a significant decrease in pressures can indicate that adequate release has been performed.

Nerve injuries associated with supracondylar humerus fractures typically resolve spontaneously over time. However, if no clinical or electromyographic recovery is noted after 5 months, exploration is warranted.[24] Excellent recovery is typically noted with neurolysis, and sural nerve grafting is only required if a complete transection is identified. Cubitus varus or valgus can be seen in patients with inadequate initial reduction or inadequate fixation resulting in a loss of reduction. Symptomatic cubitus varus initially presents as a loss of carrying angle and painless, cosmetic deformity but can lead to tardy posterolateral elbow instability.[25] The preferred treatment of cubitus varus is a closing wedge osteotomy, whereas more severe cubitus varus requires a step-cut osteotomy[26] or dome osteotomy[27] to prevent lateral prominence. Superficial pin tract infections are seen in approximately 1% of patients; deep infections, including osteomyelitis and septic arthritis, are noted in 0.2%.[22]

Postoperative management includes the placement of a plaster splint or loose above-elbow cast in 50° to 60° of flexion. Patients with a neurovascular abnormality or at risk for compartment syndrome are admitted for frequent neurovascular checks. The cast is removed at 4 weeks, and pins are pulled if fracture healing is noted on postoperative radiographs. Gentle elbow range of motion is begun and continued until full motion is obtained.

INTRAARTICULAR HUMERUS FRACTURES

Fractures involving the articular surface of the distal humerus are the second most common elbow fractures, accounting for approximately 20% of all elbow fractures.[6] Lateral condyle fractures are the most common at 16.9% of elbow fractures, followed by medial condyle fractures.[6] Lateral condyle fractures occur when a varus force is directed across an extended elbow, leading to an avulsion force across the distal humerus physis via the lateral collateral ligament complex. The fracture line travels through the epiphysis and will sometimes dissipate before reaching the articular cartilage surface because of the inherent pliability of this structure. Medial condyle fractures occur via a valgus-directed force through a similar mechanism, although the trochlea does not ossify until 9 to 10 years of age, making this fracture difficult to identify on radiographs in young children.

Occasionally, the only sign of injury is a small avulsion fracture noted on plain radiographs, which frequently represents a large osteochondral avulsion fracture (**Fig. 2**). Waters and colleagues[28] termed these as *TRASH* lesions (The Radiographic Appearance Seemed Harmless) and recommended a low threshold for further imaging studies, including ultrasound, arthrography, or magnetic resonance imaging (MRI). In young children who require sedation for MRI, the author recommends an elbow arthrogram under anesthesia in the operating theater, with the plan for subsequent surgical fixation in the same setting as indicated by the radiographic findings.

The incidence of lateral condyle fractures peaks at 6 years of age, whereas the peak for medial condyle fractures is between 8 and 10 years of age.[29] Patients complain of swelling and tenderness about the elbow following a fall from substantial height. AP and lateral radiographic images are often misleading with these injuries because of the oblique posterior fracture plane. The internal oblique view is usually the best view to detect a lateral condyle fracture and to evaluate displacement[30]; therefore, 4 views of the elbow, including AP, lateral, internal, and external oblique, are advised for suspected or confirmed condylar fractures.

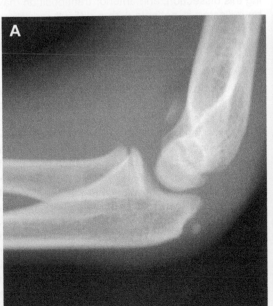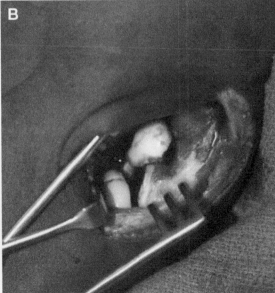

Fig. 2. (*A*) Small avulsion fracture in the anterior elbow, which (*B*) corresponds to a large osteochondral capitellar shear fracture on exploration of the joint.

Computed tomography (CT) scans have been advocated by some as it allows for 3-dimensional (3D) visualization of the displacement seen in this complex fracture pattern; however, it does not allow for visualization of the articular surface and is not routinely recommended.[31]

Lateral condylar fractures of the humerus were originally classified by Milch[32] as entering the joint surface through the trochlea-capitellar groove (type I) or through the lateral wall of the trochlea (type II). Although this scheme postulated that type I fractures were more stable than type II, this was not borne out in later studies, which additionally showed a 52% rate of disagreement between radiographs and surgical findings.[33] More recent classification schemes are based on the amount of displacement seen on the internal oblique radiograph[34] and can be used to indicate surgical treatment (**Table 2**). Fractures displaced less than 2 mm can be treated with close observation in an above-elbow cast until radiographic healing is noted (**Fig. 3**A). Weekly radiographs can be obtained in the cast to assess for changes in alignment; but the practitioner should have a low threshold for obtaining out-of-cast images, in cases when such assessment is difficult. Late fracture displacement, even 2 to 3 weeks after injury, can be seen (see **Fig. 3**B), often in patients with initial examination findings of significant soft tissue swelling or pain out of proportion to the radiographic findings.

Type II and type III injuries require surgical fixation because of the high rates of nonunion and malunion seen following closed treatment of these injuries. Intraoperative arthrogram is useful for assessing joint surface congruity following closed reduction in type II injuries. Although type II injuries can be treated with closed reduction if adequate reduction is identified, most researchers would advocate open reduction through a direct lateral approach in type III injuries.[35] Dissection posteriorly along the capitellum should be avoided because of the increased risks of damaging the blood supply to the developing capitellum ossific nucleus. Song and colleagues[36] recently published good results with closed reduction under arthrogram and pinning of significantly displaced type III injuries; however, they warned that the technique was difficult to master and should not be undertaken by those unfamiliar with the treatment of pediatric lateral condyle injuries.

Medial condyle fractures were originally described and classified by Milch,[32] but the classification was expanded by Kilfoyle[37] to include indications for surgical treatment. Type I injuries are incomplete and dissipate at the physis, whereas type II injuries progress through to the articular surface without displacement. Type III injuries are complete and unstable, typically with the fragment being pulled anteriorly and medially because of the pull of the flexor-pronator mass. Nondisplaced injuries, such as those seen in type I and type II fractures, can be treated in an above-elbow cast, with close follow-up to ensure the fracture remains aligned. Unstable injuries, including type II fractures that subsequently displace and type III fractures, should be treated with open reduction and internal fixation through a medial approach.[38] Care must be taken to protect the ulnar nerve during this dissection, and anterior transposition may be indicated in patients with a difficult reduction. Extensive posterior and medial dissection should be avoided as it can lead to the development of trochlear osteonecrosis and subsequent fishtail deformity (see **Fig. 3**C).

The surgical technique for condylar fractures is similar to supracondylar fractures. The c-arm can be used as a hand table or, alternatively, the patient's arm can be placed on a hand table. The author's preferred method for the arthrogram is via a posterior approach into the olecranon fossa just superior to the tip of the flexed olecranon. In comparison with the standard approach into the soft spot between the radial head, lateral epicondyle, and olecranon, this approach minimizes the risk of extravasated dye hindering the assessment of articular congruity because of the more superior entry portal. Patients are managed in a cast for 4 to 6 weeks postoperatively, until fracture healing is noted on radiographs and percutaneous pins can be pulled. Range-of-motion exercises are then recommended with the addition of occupational or physical therapy as needed. Stiffness is

Table 2
Jakob-Skaggs classification for lateral condyle fractures

Type	Displacement	Treatment
I	<2 mm	Cast with weekly follow-up
II	>2 mm with intact cartilage hinge seen on arthrogram	Closed reduction and percutaneous pinning
III	>2 mm with complete disruption of articular surface	Open reduction and pinning or internal fixation

Adapted from Weiss JM, Graves S, Yang S, et al. A new classification system predictive of complications in surgically treated pediatric humeral lateral condyle fractures. J Pediatr Orthop 2009;29(6):602–5; with permission.

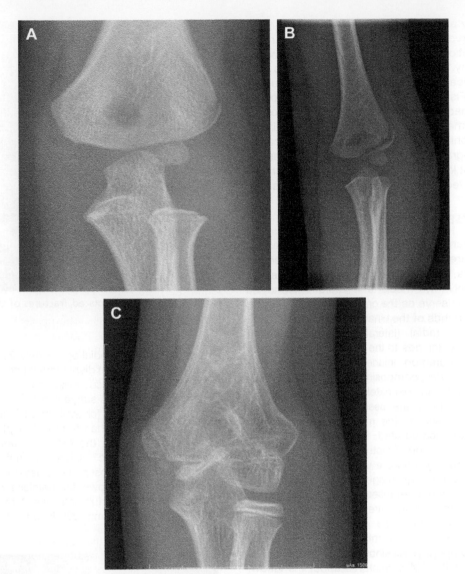

Fig. 3. Lateral condyle fractures: (*A*) Minimally displaced fracture of the lateral condyle. (*B*) Displaced lateral condyle fracture consistent with an unstable fracture pattern. (*C*) Fishtail deformity 2 years after open reduction and internal fixation of the fracture noted in Fig. 3B.

a frequent complication following articular injury in the elbow and occupational or physical therapy is often required, even after nonoperative treatment. Other complications in condylar fractures included malunion and nonunion, especially following lateral condyle injury whereby the fragment migrates in a superolateral direction. This complication results in significant cubitus valgus, which is initially a painless deformity but can develop into tardy ulnar nerve palsy or symptomatic arthritis. Surgical treatment of established nonunions and malunions is difficult because of the high rates of complications, such as stiffness, osteonecrosis of the capitellum, and persistent nonunion. A recent report by

Bauer and colleagues[39] evaluating intraarticular osteotomy to treat established malunions of lateral condyle fractures demonstrated an improvement in the end range of motion of the elbow but noted that the procedure was technically demanding and not without risk. The indications for open reduction and internal fixation of the lateral condyle nonunions are narrow and include patients with a large metaphyseal fragment; less than 1 cm of joint line displacement; and an open, viable lateral condylar physis.[40] Patients that do not meet these criteria could be considered candidates for in situ fusion of the displaced articular surface and subsequent varus osteotomy to correct the valgus deformity at the elbow. Those patients with tardy ulnar nerve palsy undergo anterior ulnar nerve transposition in addition to a supracondylar varus osteotomy.[40] Medial condyle nonunion is rare and typically presents as a painless cubitus varus.[38] Fishtail deformities can develop following lateral, medial, or supracondylar fractures of the distal humerus and often present as a painless radiographic finding (see **Fig. 3**C). In most cases, the radiographic deformity does not progress to functional losses or cosmetic findings and should be observed radiographically on a yearly basis.

APOPHYSEAL ELBOW INJURIES

The olecranon, medial epicondyle, and lateral epicondyle are apophyseal centers of attachment for the triceps, flexor/pronator, and extensor muscles, respectively. The medial and lateral epicondyles additionally serve as the origin of the anterior and posterior bands of the ulnar (medial) collateral ligament and radial (lateral) collateral ligament, respectively. Injuries to the medial epicondyle are the most common injuries to the apophyseal elbow structures, composing 14% of distal humerus fractures. Approximately 50% of medial epicondyle fractures are associated with pediatric elbow dislocations, the most serious of which involve an incarcerated fragment in the joint following reduction. Fractures of the lateral epicondyle are rare and are usually only diagnosed during a narrow age range when the epicondyle is ossified but not yet fused to the trochlea. Olecranon apophyseal fractures are associated with osteogenesis imperfecta (OI) in approximately 50% of cases.[41] In patients with a suspected or confirmed apophyseal elbow injury, there is an association with MORE fractures about the elbow: *m*edial epicondyle, *o*lecranon, *r*adial head, lateral *e*picondyle (**Fig. 4**).

Medial epicondyle fractures are seen with a fall or sports injury inducing a valgus stress across the elbow, often resulting in an elbow dislocation, which can spontaneously reduce. The most common presenting symptom is swelling and ecchymosis about the medial elbow, whereas injury to the ulnar nerve is rare despite significant trauma in the region. Anatomically, the medial epicondyle sits posteriorly along the distal ulna. Most commonly, the avulsed fragment translates anteriorly and inferiorly, making a true radiographic determination of displacement difficult.[42] AP and lateral radiographs of the elbow are the first step in diagnosis, although internal oblique radiographs serve as a better approximation of true displacement. The 3D CT scan has been shown to be the most precise method for the measurement of displacement.[43]

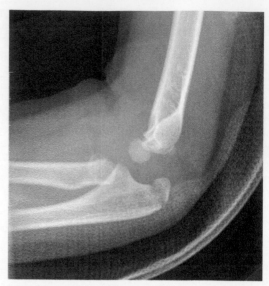

Fig. 4. Concomitant displaced fractures of the radial neck and olecranon.

The treatment of medial epicondyle fractures is based on the amount of displacement noted; however, a lack of consensus exists as to how much displacement warrants surgical intervention. Cast treatment is indicated for avulsions of the medial epicondyle with less than 5 mm of displacement as measured on both the AP and lateral radiographs. Radiographic union is not always apparent; however, most patients develop a stable fibrous union that allows for painless range of motion and return to full activities.[44] In patients with greater than 15-mm displacement (**Fig. 5**),

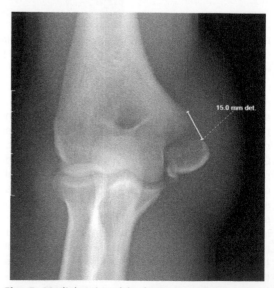

Fig. 5. Medial epicondyle fracture with 15 mm of displacement.

nonoperative treatment yields a high rate of persistent valgus elbow instability.[45] The controversy lies with the treatment of fractures with 5 to 15 mm of displacement whereby some researchers have shown good functional results with closed treatment,[46] whereas others have shown a higher incidence of instability, especially in gymnasts or athletes who compete in throwing sports.[45] In patients with incarcerated epicondyle fractures, prompt diagnosis and treatment is essential to prevent articular necrosis. Closed reduction under sedation or anesthesia via the Robert maneuver (placing a valgus stress across the elbow with wrist and finger flexion to extract the fragment) is occasionally successful, and open reduction is often performed concomitantly with internal fixation. In young patients with small fragments, internal fixation is typically performed with divergent K wires, whereas partially threaded, cannulated screws plus a washer are advised in older children.

Lateral epicondyle fractures are rare and are typically associated with a varus force directed across the elbow leading to avulsion via the lateral collateral ligament. Occasionally, these fractures are associated with medial elbow dislocations and present with tenderness and swelling about the lateral elbow. It is important to differentiate between fractures of the radial neck, lateral epicondyle, and supracondylar humerus based on the exact location of tenderness, especially in cases when radiographs are inconclusive. Additionally, the lateral epicondyle ossifies peripherally first, then proceeds centrally, such that the normal ossification pattern can be mistaken for a displaced fracture on AP elbow radiographs. Advanced imaging, such as MRI or ultrasound, can be used to confirm the diagnosis. Most lateral epicondyle fractures are minimally displaced and can be treated with a cast or brace until symptoms subside, although incarcerated lateral epicondyle fragments requiring open reduction have been reported with medial elbow dislocations.[47]

Olecranon apophyseal avulsion fractures are rare in children, except in patients with OI. Nondisplaced fractures can be treated in an above-elbow cast, although in patients with OI, there is a high rate of refracture even after radiographic healing, such that operative fixation should be considered in these patients. Fractures with more than 3 to 5 mm of displacement are indicated for surgical stabilization. The fracture is exposed from a posterior approach and coapted using a tension band construct. In patients with OI, consideration should be taken to leave the hardware in place in order to reduce the refracture risk.[41,48]

ELBOW DISLOCATIONS

Dislocations of the elbow joint are rare in the first decade of life and become more common in older children involved in sporting activities, with a peak age noted at around 12 years old.[49] These injuries are more common in boys and typically involve the nondominant extremity.[24] In patients less than 2 years of age without a capitellum ossific nucleus, displaced transphyseal fractures are often confused with elbow dislocations. This differentiation is important, as the former requires a child abuse work-up and closed reduction and pinning of the fracture. Elbow dislocations are classified based on the direction of dislocation, which includes straight posterior, posterolateral, posteromedial, lateral, medial, and anterior.

Concomitant fractures (medial and lateral epicondyles, coronoid, radial head, radial neck, and osteochondral avulsion fractures) to the elbow are common and should be assessed before and after reduction. Conscious sedation or general anesthesia is typically required for reductions and the stability of the elbow should be assessed after joint relocation. Advanced imaging, such as CT or MRI, is indicated in patients with incongruent reductions or significant instability to assess for occult injuries or incarcerated articular shear injuries.

Simple, stable dislocations can be treated conservatively with a splint or cast for 2 to 3 weeks, followed by active range-of-motion exercises, or formal occupational or physical therapy. Medial, lateral, or straight posterior dislocations can be treated using a hinged elbow brace that blocks terminal extension at the angle noted to maintain stability, which allows for immediate range of motion to mitigate stiffness. Surgical fixation is usually limited to patients in whom concomitant displaced elbow fractures are noted or in patients with incongruent reductions.[49]

Complex dislocations involving separation of the proximal radioulnar joint, so-called divergent elbow dislocations,[50] or those involving translocation of the radius and ulna[51] have been described in pediatric patients. Although these injuries seem to involve significant destabilizing forces about the elbow, simple closed reduction and brief immobilization is often sufficient for treatment provided that they are promptly and accurately diagnosed. Open reduction is indicated in patients with incongruent reductions or unstable concomitant fractures. The most common complication following elbow dislocation is a loss of terminal motion in extension or flexion, which can be ameliorated by encouraging early, protected range of motion within the limits of stability.[49]

Ligamentous injuries to the elbow are common in children, especially in early childhood. The most common injury results from a pulled arm, whereby the radial head subluxes out of the annular ligament leading to pain and decreased motion.[52] This injury has been termed a *nursemaid's elbow*, and patients typically present with their arm held in a flexed and pronated posture at the elbow. Radiographs of the elbow are taken to rule out true fracture or dislocation but are not suggestive of radiocapitellar subluxation as has been previously suggested.[53] The reduction technique involves elbow flexion and hyperpronation, which has been shown to be less painful and more successful than elbow flexion and supination.[54] Following successful reduction, patients are typically able to use the elbow without pain; any subsequent refusal to use the arm should warrant splinting and close follow-up to rule out associated cartilaginous or ligamentous injury to the elbow.

PROXIMAL RADIUS AND ULNA FRACTURES

Fractures of the proximal radius and ulna account for approximately 7% and 6% of elbow fractures, respectively.[55] The radial neck can be injured during impaction against the capitellum with longitudinal compression or a valgus force. Transphyseal fractures of the radial neck can occur during reduction of elbow dislocations if the head gets caught on the posterior capitellum during anterior translation. Age differences in injury pattern are present with physeal or metaphyseal compression injuries occurring in younger children, whereas articular surface fractures typically occur in older children. Most fractures occur following a FOOSH injury and present with elbow pain, swelling, and tenderness over the radial neck. AP and lateral radiographs are typically sufficient for diagnosis, although minor fractures may have subtle findings. A radial neck view can be obtained to confirm the diagnosis when radiographs are inconclusive or to verify displacement.

Radial neck fractures were classified by Judet[56] and are based on displacement and angulation noted on AP radiographs (**Table 3**). Judet type I and II injuries are nondisplaced or angulated less than 30°, respectively, and can be treated in an above-elbow cast. In children with greater than 30° of angulation (Judet III and IV), closed reduction under conscious sedation or general anesthesia should be performed. Various reduction techniques have been described,[57] and reduction is frequently successful. Following failed closed reduction, a percutaneous pin can be inserted into the fracture site and used for leverage and/or fixation of the fragment.[58] Additionally, a distally

Table 3
Judet classification of radial neck fractures

Type	Description
I	Nondisplaced or horizontal shift of epiphysis
II	<30° angulation
III	30°–60° angulation
IV a	60°–80° angulation
IV b	>80° angulation or complete dislocation of epiphysis

Adapted from Judet H, Judet J. Fractures et orthopédie de l'enfant. Paris, France: Libraire Maloine; 1974. p. 31–9; with permission.

inserted flexible intramedullary nail can be used to assist with fracture reduction and for definitive fixation until healing is noted.[59,60] Open reduction is only indicated following failed closed reduction and leads to an increased risk of complications, including stiffness, nonunion, or avascular necrosis. Following open reduction, internal fixation with either a flexible nail or K wires should be performed to lessen the risk of postoperative radial head avascular necrosis.[61]

Radial head fractures are rare in children and are predominantly found following closure of the radial neck physis. In skeletally immature children, radial neck fractures are associated with progressive subluxation of the radiocapitellar joint and arthrosis,[62] such that even nondisplaced injuries should be followed closely. Thus, a low threshold for surgical fixation is advised in these injuries. Operative indications are similar to those seen in adults and include greater than 50% involvement of the articular surface or greater than 2-mm articular step-off. Fractures are fixed from either a posterolateral (Kocher) approach between the anconeus and extensor carpi ulnaris (ECU) muscles or a lateral approach between the extensor digitorum communis and ECU muscles. Radial head excision is not advised in children because of bony overgrowth of the radial shaft, and every attempt should be made to fix even comminuted articular fractures in these patients.

Olecranon fractures often occur following a direct blow to the proximal ulna and present with posterior elbow pain, swelling, and olecranon tenderness. AP and lateral radiographs of the elbow are typically sufficient. In rare cases, osteochondral sleeve injuries involving a substantial portion of the articular surface are possible and are best diagnosed using MRI.[63] Minimally displaced fractures can be treated in an above-elbow cast. Olecranon fractures with 1 to 3 mm of displacement are often stable because of the thick periosteum found in children and can be casted in slight extension to alleviate undue tension on the fracture from the triceps muscle. Fractures with displacement of more than 3 mm along the articular surface should be reduced and fixed with a tension band construct. The use of a nonabsorbable suture for the figure-of-8 band has been advocated in children in order to limit the dissection necessary during hardware removal.[64]

MONTEGGIA FRACTURES

Giovanni Monteggia first described a fracture of the proximal ulna with dislocation of the radial head in 1814, before the advent of radiography. Bado[65] subsequently classified these injuries based on the direction of the radial head dislocation (Table 4). Additionally, because of the presence of incomplete fractures and open physes in children, Bado also described Monteggia-equivalent fractures in skeletally immature patients. Type I equivalents involve greenstick or plastic deformation fractures of the ulna and are the most common.[65] Less common equivalent types include both-bone proximal-third forearm fractures with the radial fracture more proximal than the ulnar fracture, elbow dislocations with an ulnar diaphyseal fracture with or without a proximal radius fracture, and isolated radial neck fractures with radiocapitellar dislocation. Patients often present with forearm pain following a FOOSH injury, which often masks the elbow pain caused by the radiocapitellar dislocation, making it easy to miss the Monteggia component both clinically and radiographically. Standard AP and lateral radiographs of the forearm are obtained along with AP and lateral views of the elbow. Both sets of radiographic films are recommended during the initial and subsequent evaluations, as it is important to follow both fracture healing and radiocapitellar alignment throughout the treatment regimen. The radiocapitellar line has been used to verify appropriate radiographic alignment but has been shown to be unreliable, especially in younger patients.[66] Additionally, a line should be drawn along the posterior cortex of the ulna on the lateral view (Fig. 6A). The ulnar bow sign is found if any portion of the ulna lies anterior to this line, which indicates that there is a pathologic lesion, such as plastic deformation or malunion of the ulna.[67] Furthermore, congenital radial head dislocations have been described in patients with proximal ulna fractures. A careful radiographic assessment of the radial head will reveal a concave radial head in acute dislocations and a convex radial head in chronic injuries.

Monteggia fractures are treated based on the ulnar fracture with careful consideration as to the direction of dislocation as identified with the Bado classification.[68] Closed reduction under conscious sedation or general anesthesia should be attempted for all angulated incomplete fractures. Plastic deformation injuries often require significant force over a bolster to achieve reduction. In complete injuries, the ulnar fracture should be brought out to length followed by correction of the angular deformity, which often will lead to relocation of the radiocapitellar joint. If spontaneous reduction is not achieved, the elbow can be flexed to 90° and the forearm can be fully supinating in Bado I injuries and pronating in Bado II and III injuries to assist with reduction. Following reduction, the fracture should be immobilized in a splint or cast in 100° to 110° of flexion in full supination or pronation (based on the reduction maneuver) to increase stability. If closed treatment is chosen, the fracture should be monitored with weekly biplanar forearm and elbow radiographs to ensure that late fracture displacement or radiocapitellar subluxation does not occur. Operative fixation is often required in patients with short oblique or transverse injuries to the proximal ulna metadiaphysis because of the inherent instability seen with these fractures. Internal fixation is typically performed with K wires or a plate-and-screw construct to maintain alignment, whereas in type IV injuries intramedullary fixation of the radius and ulna are often required.

Monteggia fracture/dislocations often present as missed Monteggia lesions in cases when the initial treating physician missed the dislocation or when progressive subluxation of the radiocapitellar joint occurs over time because of a malunited ulna fracture. Most often these are Bado I injuries because an anterior radial head dislocation is often clinically silent. An ulnar bow sign is often present in these patients, and early operative intervention is indicated in order to prevent the development of radial head dysplasia. The operative technique involves a tricortical osteotomy of the ulna at the apex of deformity and open reduction of the radiocapitellar joint (see Fig. 6B). The osteotomy should

Table 4
Bado classification of Monteggia fractures

Type	Description
I	Anterior dislocation of radial head
II	Posterior dislocation of radial head
III	Lateral dislocation of radial head
IV	Anterior dislocation of radial head with concomitant radial shaft fracture

Adapted from Bado JL. The Monteggia lesion. Clin Orthop Relat Res 1967;50:71–8; with permission.

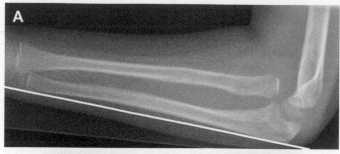

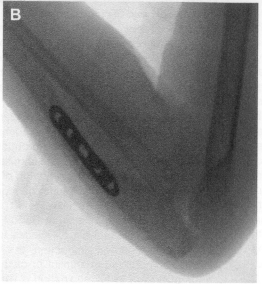

Fig. 6. (*A*) Missed Monteggia fracture equivalent with greenstick fracture of the ulna and anterior dislocation of the radial head. Note the positive ulnar bow sign (*white line*). (*B*) Following tricortical osteotomy, the anterior dislocation of the radial head has been reduced and maintained after open reduction. Note the air arthrogram confirming true cartilaginous alignment.

be progressively angulated until the radiocapitellar articulation is stable throughout the entire range of elbow motion, both in pronosupination and flexion/extension.[69] Reconstruction of the annular ligament is seldom required unless persistent instability remains.

SUMMARY

Injuries to the elbow are common in children and occur throughout all age groups. Careful clinical and radiographic evaluation can lead to an accurate diagnosis and prompt, appropriate treatment. Although many injuries about the elbow present pitfalls during diagnosis and treatment, most children recover excellent function and are able to return to premorbid activities with no limitations.

REFERENCES

1. Hedstrom EM, Svennson O, Bergstrom U, et al. Epidemiology of fractures in children and adolescents. Acta Orthop 2010;81(1):148–53.

2. Randsborg PH, Gulbrandsen P, Saltytė Benth J, et al. Fractures in children: epidemiology and activity-specific fracture rates. J Bone Joint Surg Am 2013;95(7):e42.

3. National Center for Injury Prevention and Control. (n.d.). (C. F. Control, Producer). Available at: http://www.cdc.gov/ncipc/wisqars. Accessed June 13, 2013.

4. Patel B, Reed M, Patel S. Gender-specific pattern differences of the ossification centers in the pediatric elbow. Pediatr Radiol 2009;39(3):226–31.

5. Landin LA. Fracture patterns in children: analysis of 8,682 fractures with special reference to incidence, etiology and secular changes in a Swedish urban population, 1950-1979. Acta Orthop Scand Suppl 1983;202:1–109.

6. Landin L, Danielsson L. Elbow fractures in children: an epidemiological analysis of 589 cases. Acta Orthop Scand 1986;57:309–12.

7. Omid R, Choi PD, Skaggs DL. Supracondylar humeral fractures in children. J Bone Joint Surg Am 2008;90:1121–32.

8. Farnsworth CL, Silva PD, Mubarak SJ. Etiology of supracondylar humerus fractures. J Pediatr Orthop 1998;18:38–42.

9. Sherr-Lurie N, Bialik GM, Ganel A, et al. Fractures of the humerus in the neonatal period. Isr Med Assoc J 2011;13(6):363–5.

10. Babal JC, Mehlman CT, Klein G. Nerve injuries associated with pediatric supracondylar humeral fractures: a meta-analysis. J Pediatr Orthop 2010; 30:253–63.

11. Ring D, Waters PM, Hotchkiss RN, et al. Pediatric floating elbow. J Pediatr Orthop 2001;21(4):456–9.

12. Herman MJ, Boardman MJ, Hoover JR, et al. Relationship of the anterior humeral line to the capitellar ossific nucleus: variability with age. J Bone Joint Surg Am 2009;91:2188–93.

13. Acton JD, McNally MA. Baumann's confusing legacy. Injury 2001;32(1):41–3.

14. Parikh SN, Wall EJ, Foad S, et al. Displaced type II extension supracondylar humerus fractures: do they all need pinning? J Pediatr Orthop 2004;24: 380–4.

15. O'Hara LJ, Barlow JW, Clarke NM. Displaced supracondylar fractures of the humerus in children. J Bone Joint Surg Br 2000;82:204–10.

16. Mehlman CT, Strub WM, Roy DR, et al. The effect of surgical timing on the perioperative complications of treatment of supracondylar humeral fractures in children. J Bone Joint Surg Am 2001;83: 323–7.

17. Griffin KJ, Walsh SR, Markar S, et al. The pink pulseless hand: a review of the literature regarding management of vascular complications of supracondylar humeral fractures in children. Eur J Vasc Endovasc Surg 2008;36(6):697–702.

18. Choi PD, Melikian R, Skaggs DL. Risk factors for vascular repair and compartment syndrome in the pulseless supracondylar humerus fracture in children. J Pediatr Orthop 2010;30(1):50–6.

19. Yen YM, Kocher MS. Lateral entry compared with medial and lateral entry pin fixation for completely displaced supracondylar humeral fractures in children. Surgical technique. J Bone Joint Surg Am 2008;90(Suppl 2 Pt 1):20–30.

20. Bloom T, Robertson C, Mahar AT, et al. Biomechanical analysis of supracondylar humerus fracture pinning for slightly malreduced fractures. J Pediatr Orthop 2008;28(7):766–72.

21. Larson L, Firoozbakhsh K, Passarelli R, et al. Biomechanical analysis of pinning techniques for pediatric supracondylar humerus fractures. J Pediatr Orthop 2006;26(5):573–8.

22. Bashyal RK, Chu JY, Schoenecker PL, et al. Complications after pinning of supracondylar distal humerus fractures. J Pediatr Orthop 2009;29:704–8.

23. Bae DS, Kadiyala RK, Waters PM. Acute compartment syndrome in children: contemporary diagnosis, treatment, and outcome. J Pediatr Orthop 2001;5:680–8.

24. Henrikson B. Supracondylar fractures of the humerus in children. Acta Chir Scand Suppl 1966; 369:1–72.

25. O'Driscoll SW, Spinner RJ, McKee MD, et al. Tardy posterolateral rotatory instability of the elbow due to cubitus varus. J Bone Joint Surg Am 2001;83: 1358–69.

26. Davids JR, Lamoreaux DC, Brooker RC, et al. Translation step-cut osteotomy for the treatment of posttraumatic cubitus varus. J Pediatr Orthop 2011;31(4):353–65.

27. Pankaj A, Dua A, Malhotra R, et al. Dome osteotomy for posttraumatic cubitus varus: a surgical technique to avoid lateral condylar prominence. J Pediatr Orthop 2006;26(1):61–6.

28. Waters PM, Beaty J, Kasser J. Elbow "TRASH" (the radiographic appearance seemed harmless) lesions. J Pediatr Orthop 2010;30(Suppl 2):S77–81.

29. Peterson CA, Peterson HA. Analysis of the incidence of injuries to the epiphyseal growth plate. J Trauma 1972;12(4):275–81.

30. Song KS, Kang CH, Min BW, et al. Internal oblique radiographs for diagnosis of nondisplaced or minimally displaced lateral condylar fractures of the humerus in children. J Bone Joint Surg Am 2007; 89(1):58–63.

31. Chapman VM, Grottkau BE, Albright M, et al. Multidetector computed tomography of pediatric lateral condylar fractures. J Comput Assist Tomogr 2005; 29(6):842–6.

32. Milch H. Fractures and fracture dislocations of the humeral condyles. J Trauma 1964;4:592–607.

33. Mirsky EC, Karas EH, Weiner LS. Lateral condyle fractures in children: evaluation of classification and treatment. J Orthop Trauma 1997;11(2):117–20.

34. Weiss JM, Graves S, Yang S, et al. A new classification system predictive of complications in surgically treated pediatric humeral lateral condyle fractures. J Pediatr Orthop 2009;29(6):602–5.

35. Mintzer CM, Waters PM, Brown DJ, et al. Percutaneous pinning in the treatment of displaced lateral condyle fractures. J Pediatr Orthop 1994;14(4): 462–5.

36. Song KS, Shin YW, Oh CW, et al. Closed reduction and internal fixation of completely displaced and rotated lateral condyle fractures of the humerus in children. J Orthop Trauma 2010;24(7):434–8.

37. Kilfoyle RM. Fractures of the medial condyle and epicondyle of the elbow in children. Clin Orthop Relat Res 1965;41:43–50.

38. Leet AI, Young C, Hoffer MM. Medial condyle fractures of the humerus in children. J Pediatr Orthop 2002;22(1):2–7.

39. Bauer AS, Bae DS, Brustowicz KA, et al. Intra-articular corrective osteotomy of humeral lateral condyle

malunions in children: early clinical and radiographic results. J Pediatr Orthop 2013;33(1):20–5.

40. Shimada K, Masada K, Tada K, et al. Osteosynthesis for the treatment of non-union of the lateral humeral condyle in children. J Bone Joint Surg Am 1997;79(2):234–40.

41. Gwynne-Jones DP. Displaced olecranon apophyseal fractures in children with osteogenesis imperfecta. J Pediatr Orthop 2005;25(2):154–7.

42. Pappas N, Lawrence JT, Donegan D, et al. Intraobserver and interobserver agreement in the measurement of displaced humeral medial epicondyle fractures in children. J Bone Joint Surg Am 2010; 92(2):322–7.

43. Edmonds EW. How displaced are "nondisplaced" fractures of the medial humeral epicondyle in children? Results of a three-dimensional computed tomography analysis. J Bone Joint Surg Am 2010; 92(17):2785–91.

44. Josefsson PO, Danielsson LG. Epicondylar elbow fracture in children. 35-year follow-up of 56 unreduced cases. Acta Orthop Scand 1986;57(4): 313–5.

45. Lee HH, Shen HC, Chang JH, et al. Operative treatment of displaced medial epicondyle fractures in children and adolescents. J Shoulder Elbow Surg 2005;14(2):178–85.

46. Farsetti P, Potenza V, Caterini R, et al. Long-term results of treatment of fractures of the medial humeral epicondyle in children. J Bone Joint Surg Am 2001; 83(9):1299–305.

47. Pouliart N, De Boeck H. Posteromedial dislocation of the elbow with associated intraarticular entrapment of the lateral epicondyle. J Orthop Trauma 2002;16(1):53–6.

48. Zionts LE, Moon CN. Olecranon apophysis fractures in children with osteogenesis imperfecta revisited. J Pediatr Orthop 2002;22(6):745–50.

49. Carlioz H, Abols Y. Posterior dislocation of the elbow in children. J Pediatr Orthop 1984;4(1):8–12.

50. Eylon S, Lamdan R, Simanovsky N. Divergent elbow dislocation in the very young child: easily treated if correctly diagnosed. J Orthop Trauma 2011;25(1):e1–4.

51. Combourieu B, Thevenin-Lemoine C, Abelin-Genevois K, et al. Pediatric elbow dislocation associated with proximal radioulnar translocation: a report of three cases and a review of the literature. J Bone Joint Surg Am 2010;92(8):1780–5.

52. Browner EA. Nursemaid's elbow (annular ligament displacement). Pediatr Rev 2013;34(8):366–7.

53. Eismann EA, Cosco ED, Wall EJ. Absence of radiographic abnormalities in nursemaid's elbows. J Pediatr Orthop 2013. [Epub ahead of print].

54. Krul M, van der Wouden JC, van Suijlekom-Smit LW, et al. Manipulative interventions for reducing pulled elbow in young children. Cochrane Database Syst Rev 2012;(1):CD007759.

55. Maylahn DJ, Fahey JJ. Fractures of the elbow in children. JAMA 1958;166:220–8.

56. Judet H, Judet J. Fractures et orthopédie de l'enfant. Paris: Maloine; 1974. p. 31–9.

57. Neher CG, Torch MA. New reduction technique for severely displaced pediatric radial neck fractures. J Pediatr Orthop 2003;23(5):626–8.

58. Schmittenbecher PP, Haevernick B, Herold A, et al. Treatment decision, method of osteosynthesis, and outcome in radial neck fractures in children: a multicenter study. J Pediatr Orthop 2005;25(1): 45–50.

59. Metaizeau JP, Prevot J, Schmitt M. Reduction and fixation of fractures of the neck of the radius be centro-medullary pinning. Original technique. Rev Chir Orthop Reparatrice Appar Mot 1980; 66:47–9.

60. Eberl R, Singer G, Fruhmann J, et al. Intramedullary nailing for the treatment of dislocated pediatric radial neck fractures. Eur J Pediatr Surg 2010; 20(4):250–2.

61. Waters PM, Stewart SL. Radial neck fracture nonunion in children. J Pediatr Orthop 2001;21(5): 570–6.

62. Van Zeeland NL, Bae DS, Goldfarb CA. Intra-articular radial head fracture in the skeletally immature patient: progressive radial head subluxation and rapid radiocapitellar degeneration. J Pediatr Orthop 2011;31(2):124–9.

63. Ohta T, Itoh S, Okawa A, et al. Osteochondral flap fracture of the olecranon with subluxation of the elbow in a child. J Orthop Sci 2010;15(5):686–9.

64. Gortzak Y, Mercado E, Atar D, et al. Pediatric olecranon fractures: open reduction and internal fixation with removable Kirschner wires and absorbable sutures. J Pediatr Orthop 2006;26(1): 39–42.

65. Bado JL. The Monteggia lesion. Clin Orthop Relat Res 1967;50:71–86.

66. Kunkel S, Cornwall R, Little K, et al. Limitations of the radiocapitellar line for assessment of pediatric elbow radiographs. J Pediatr Orthop 2011;31(6): 628–32.

67. Lincoln TL, Mubarak SJ. "Isolated" traumatic radial-head dislocation. J Pediatr Orthop 1994; 14(4):454–7.

68. Ring D, Waters PM. Operative fixation of Monteggia fractures in children. J Bone Joint Surg Br 1996;78(5):734–9.

69. Nakamura K, Hirachi K, Uchiyama S, et al. Long-term clinical and radiographic outcomes after open reduction for missed Monteggia fracture-dislocations in children. J Bone Joint Surg Am 2009;91(6):1394–404.

Evidence-based Management of Developmental Dysplasia of the Hip

Anthony Philip Cooper, MBChB, FRCS (Tr&Orth)[a],
Siddesh Nandi Doddabasappa, MBBS, MS(Ortho), FRCS(Glasg)[a],
Kishore Mulpuri, MBBS, MS(Ortho), MHSc(Epi)[b],*

KEYWORDS

- Developmental dysplasia hip (DDH) • Management • Treatment • Evidence

KEY POINTS

- Developmental dysplasia of the hip (DDH) is a common condition of childhood.
- The overall quality of evidence for the management of DDH is low, with most studies being retrospective.
- There remains considerable controversy regarding the optimal treatment of DDH in the current body of evidence. It is not possible to recommend or reject most treatment options.

INTRODUCTION

Developmental dysplasia of the hip (DDH) is a spectrum of hip disorders that range from a mildly dysplastic but concentrically reduced and stable hip, to a hip that is frankly dislocated and severely dysplastic (**Fig. 1**).[1–3] The goal in the management of DDH is to achieve a stable, concentric reduction of the hip to ensure that any dysplasia is adequately corrected and to avoid the complications of treatment, the most significant of which is avascular necrosis (AVN) of the femoral head.

The treatment options for DDH vary depending on the age at presentation and where along the spectrum of disease the patient's condition lies. This article reviews the evidence for the treatment of DDH. The major outcome measures assessed are the failure of reduction or redislocation, additional surgery, and AVN.

PAVLIK HARNESS

Arnold Pavlik first reported the use of the Pavlik[4] harness in 1946 and revolutionized the treatment of hip dysplasia. His theory was that hip abduction and knee flexion would maintain hip motion and result in the gentle reduction of the hip.[4] Successful treatment, defined as reduction of a dislocated hip or maintenance of a reduced but dysplastic hip, has been reported at rates of 80.2% to 100% (**Table 1**). It is stated that treatment should be started as soon as the diagnosis of hip dysplasia is made.[12] The earlier the diagnosis, the higher the success rate, with statistically significant improvements seen if treatment is started before 7 weeks of age.[13,14] The natural history of hip instability is one of potential spontaneous resolution in the early weeks of life and, as such, the effect size of the Pavlik harness may be overestimated. Several studies, including

No external funding was received for the completion of this work.
a Department of Orthopaedics, BC Children's Hospital, 1D-05, 4480 Oak Street, Vancouver, British Columbia V6H 3N1, Canada; b Department of Orthopaedics, BC Children's Hospital, 1D-66, 4480 Oak Street, Vancouver, British Columbia V6H 3N1, Canada
* Corresponding author.
E-mail address: kmulpuri@cw.bc.ca

Orthop Clin N Am 45 (2014) 341–354
http://dx.doi.org/10.1016/j.ocl.2014.03.005
0030-5898/14/$ – see front matter © 2014 Elsevier Inc. All rights reserved.

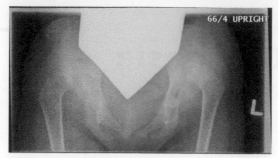

Fig. 1. AP radiograph of 4-year-old pelvis showing bilateral dislocated hips.

1 level of evidence at level 2 and 1 at level 3,[15] have compared immediate bracing with ultrasonographic examination and observation only, which have shown no difference in outcome if bracing is delayed for 2 weeks from birth.

The reported duration of treatment in the Pavlik harness varied from 11 to 28 weeks,[16] with no consensus on the duration of treatment. Some investigators recommend weaning of the brace following 6 weeks of location of the hip.[8] Reported time to reduction varied from 2 weeks [17] to 32 weeks.[16] Ultrasonography is an important tool for the surveillance of treatment and to determine when treatment should be discontinued either because of successful or unsuccessful treatment.[18–20]

The AVN rate following treatment with the Pavlik harness has been reported at rates varying from 0% to 28%.[21–23] Two studies have suggested a correlation between increasing severity of dislocation and AVN rate.[9,24] Femoral nerve palsy is a known complication of Pavlik harness treatment. Murnaghan and colleagues[25] reported an AVN rate of 2.5% of 1218 patients and a 70% chance of failure of Pavlik treatment in the presence of a femoral nerve palsy.

Residual acetabular dysplasia has been reported following Pavlik harness treatment. Harris and colleagues[26] reported a 5% rate of acetabular dysplasia in 550 patients at 2 years. Fujioka and colleagues[27] examined 158 hips at a minimum of 20 years' follow-up and found that 26.6% of patients were dysplastic as defined by a Severin classification of grade III or higher, with 2.5% classified as grade V (in which the femoral head articulates with a pseudoacetabulum).[28] Yoshitaka and colleagues[29] found similar results with 26.3% of 262 hips rated as Severin class III or IV at a mean follow-up of 19 years. Tucci and colleagues[30] found that 17% of 74 hips initially treated by Pavlik harness for acetabular dysplasia had what were described as mild abnormalities of the acetabular roof at an average of 10 years' follow-up. According to the Severin classification, 1 hip was class II and 1 hip was class III. All patients had normal radiographs at ages 1 and 5 years.

The Pavlik harness has been compared with other methods of treatment. Atar and colleagues[31] compared the Pavlik harness with the Frejka pillow in a nonrandomized case series, evaluating reduction and AVN rate. The case series found a failure rate of 12% for the Pavlik and 10% for the Frejka with corresponding AVN rates of 6% and 7%. Czubak and colleagues[32] compared patients older than 6 months; 143 patients using the Frejka pillow and 95 using the Pavlik harness. Results showed that 89% of the hips treated with the Frejka pillow and 95% treated with the Pavlik harness were successfully reduced, with AVN rates of 7% in the Frejka group and 12% in the Pavlik group, and it was concluded that there were better results for the Frejka pillow. However, Brurås and colleagues[33] found no difference in rates of dysplasia in a randomized control trial of Frejka pillow followed by rigid abduction bracing compared with surveillance only at 6 years.

Table 1
Summary of evidence using the Pavlik harness for treatment of DDH

Study	No. of Hips (No. of Dislocated Hips)	Success Rate (%)	AVN Rate (%)	Level of Evidence
Pavlik & Peltier[5]	1912 (632)	84	0	4
Wada et al[6]	2481 (1523)	80.2 81.9	14.3 11.5	4
Walton et al[7]	123 (43)	90	2.4	4
Cashman et al[8]	546 (118)	96.7	1	4
Grill et al[9]	3611 (2519)	92	2.38	4
Johnson et al[10]	91 (20)	90	0	4
Filipe & Carlioz[11]	74	—	5.4	4

Wilkinson and colleagues[34] retrospectively compared the efficacy of the Pavlik harness, the Craig splint, and the von Rosen splint with no splint in the treatment of neonatal hip dysplasia. In this nonrandomized study treatment was decided on by the treating orthopedic surgeon. They concluded that the von Rosen splint resulted in better radiological appearance and fewer secondary interventions than the other forms of treatment; however, the numbers were small (the largest study arm had only 43 hips) with multiple potential confounding factors.

The von Rosen splint has been reported to have a success rate (defined as no requirement for further intervention) between 92% and 100%, with an AVN rate of 0.6% to 0.8% (**Table 2**).[34–39] These outcome measures have limitations: the study groups were heterogenous, timing of treatment varied, and the presence of AVN was not routinely recorded.

Summary

The evidence for the use of Pavlik harness in the treatment of dislocated hips is low because of potential risk of selection and performance bias, inconsistency in study designs, imprecision of statistical reporting, and the absence of randomized control trials. Given that the natural history of hip instability often resolves spontaneously in the early weeks of life, the effectiveness of the Pavlik harness may have been overestimated.

The evidence for the use of the Pavlik harness in the treatment of acetabular dysplasia rather than dislocation is low, with long-term studies reporting persistent dysplasia rates of up to 26%.

There is no consensus from the data regarding the timing of Pavlik harness treatment. It is likely that Pavlik harness treatment in the first 6 weeks of life results in overtreatment of some patients. Initiation of treatment beyond 4 months of life is associated with increased risk of failure.

Ultrasonography may be useful in the surveillance of treatment in the Pavlik harness. However, there is no consensus from the available evidence regarding the optimal timing for cessation of Pavlik treatment.[8]

The evidence for the use of alternatives to the Pavlik harness, such as the von Rosen splint and Craig splint, is scant, because of the small number of poorly designed observational studies with low patient numbers. As a result, this area warrants further study.

CLOSED REDUCTION

The closed reduction of the dislocated hip was first described in 1838 by Pravez and often involves examination under anesthesia, an arthrogram either with or without an adductor tenotomy, followed by immobilization of the hip, usually using a spica cast. Preoperative traction can be used as an aid to reduction.

Failed reduction following closed reduction has been reported at rates varying from 0% to 25%, with redislocation rates reported between 2.8% and 13.6%.[40–44] Rates of AVN have been reported as 2.6% and 60%, with the variation largely caused by differences in the definitions of AVN and the timing of follow-up evaluation.[40–46] The rate of further surgical procedures is again highly variable and is based on the different treatment rationales and thresholds for surgical intervention. These rates have been reported between 10% and 101%.[40–42,44] For example, Terjesen and Halvorsen[41] reported 79 procedures in 78 patients, largely because of their practice of performing derotation osteotomies of the proximal femur as a staged procedure following closed reduction.

Traction has been described either as a definitive method of reducing a dislocated hip[47,48] or as a preoperative adjunct to closed reduction. The evidence for preoperative traction is conflicting. Gregosiewicz and Wosko[49] reported a rate

Table 2
Summary of evidence for use of von Rosen splint for treatment of DDH

Study	No. of Hips	Success Rate (%)	AVN Rate (%)	Level of Evidence
Finlay et al[35]	81 dislocated or able to be dislocated	95	Not reported	4
Fredensborg[36]	111 unstable hips	100	0.9	4
Mitchell[37]	100	92	Not reported	4
Heikkilä[38]	180	99.4	0.6	4
Wilkinson et al[34]	26	100	0	3
Lauge-Pedersen et al[39]	275	97.8	Not reported	3

of AVN of 6.5% with traction compared with 16% without traction. DeRosa and Feller[50] were proponents of preoperative traction as an aid to reducing the hips of 60 of 66 patients with no AVN. Daoud and Saighi-Bououina[51] also reported a successful closed reduction rate in older children (mean age of 33 months) of 76% of 50 hips with an AVN rate of 7.9% and a redislocation rate of 7.9%. Neither of these studies had a control group for comparison.

Langenskiöld and Paavilainen[52] compared 176 hips treated with preoperative traction with a historical group of 86 hips treated before the introduction of traction in their hospital. The AVN rate in the patients with traction was 21.6% and without traction it was higher at 83.7%.[52] Sibiński and colleagues[53] compared 107 hips treated with preliminary traction and closed reduction with a historical cohort of 48 hips treated without traction. They reported a 42% rate of AVN in the group treated without traction compared with a 29% rate in those treated with traction. However, because of the large difference in group size between the two groups, caution should be exercised in interpreting these data. Kutlu and colleagues[54] reported their results of 2 cohorts consisting of 89 hips treated with preliminary traction and 65 hips treated without preliminary traction and found no statistically significant differences in the rates of AVN between the two groups. Brougham and colleagues[45] also found no significant difference in the rate of AVN between 42 hips treated without traction, 86 hips treated with traction at 60°, and 82 hips treated with traction at 90°.

There remains controversy regarding the timing of closed reduction and the relationship to the presence or absence of the ossific nucleus. Clarke and colleagues[55] stated that before ossification the vasculature of the capital femoral epiphysis is vulnerable to compression and ischemia and, as such, reduction should be delayed until the ossific nucleus is visible because it provides mechanical strength and indicates the establishment of a collateral circulation. Segal and colleagues[56] supported these findings with a porcine and finite element model. Segal and colleagues[57] reported a 4% rate of AVN following reduction in the presence of an ossific nucleus compared with 53% if reduction was performed before the development of the ossific nucleus as identified on radiographs in their retrospective review of 57 hips. Clarke and colleagues[55] proposed a treatment algorithm for delaying surgical intervention until the ossific nucleus is present radiographically. The noncontrolled series delayed treatment until the ossific nucleus was present or the patient reached 13 months of age and showed no increase in AVN compared with other series. However, Luhmann and colleagues[58,59] found no difference in the rates of AVN with respect to the presence or absence of the ossific nucleus. These results were supported by the same findings from a series by Cooke and colleagues. Both series were retrospective (**Table 3**).

Summary

A consensus is required in the reporting and classification of AVN in DDH in order to effectively compare outcomes of treatment of DDH.

There is insufficient evidence to recommend or reject the use of preoperative traction as an adjunct to closed reduction.

There is insufficient evidence to recommend or reject waiting for the presence of the ossific nucleus to be evident before closed reduction.

OPEN REDUCTION

Open reduction of the dislocated hip can be performed through various approaches. The medial approach, first described by Ludloff[60] in 1908 and its subsequent modifications[61,62] remain

Table 3
Summary of evidence for closed reduction in DDH

Study	No. of Hips	Failed Reduction/ Redislocation	AVN Rate	Further Procedures	Level of Evidence
Murray et al[40]	35	2 (5.7%)	4 (12%)	10 (30.3%)	4
Terjesen & Halvorsen[41]	78	4 (5%)/2 (2.8%)	11 (14%)	79	4
Race & Herring[42]	59	8 (13.6%)	20 (33.9%)	6	4
Brougham et al[45]	210	Not reported	99 (47%)	Not reported	4
Ishii & Ponseti[43]	40	0	12 (30%)	Not reported	4
Zionts & MacEwen[44]	51	13 (25%)/2 (3.9%)	1 (2.6%)	29 (76.3%)	4
Malvitz & Weinstein[46]	152	Not reported	91 (60%)	Not reported	4

controversial. Advocates recommend it for the cosmetic scar, the ability to avoid damage to the abductors and the iliac apophysis, less joint stiffness, direct access to the obstacles to reduction, low blood loss, and the ability to perform bilateral surgery in 1 sitting.[63–66] However, it is also criticized because there is a potential risk of AVN caused by damage to the medial circumflex vessels, the acetabulum is not easily visualized, and a capsulorrhaphy or simultaneous secondary procedures cannot be performed.[64,67,68]

The redislocation rate for this technique varies between 0% and 6.1% (**Table 4**), with rates of AVN varying from 8.9% to 45.4%. There is variation from 11.1% to 85.4% in the reported rates of reoperation. There is no clear association between ligation of the medial femoral circumflex vessels and the rate of AVN.[64,74]

Compared with the evidence for the medial approach to reduction, less has been published on the anterior or Smith-Peterson approach, likely because it is easier to combine the anterior approach with concomitant osteotomies compared with the medial approach. Doudoulakis and Cavadias[76] reported a series of 69 hips reduced using the Smith-Peterson approach and found 1 redislocated hip, an AVN rate of 13%, and a reoperation rate of 18 cases (26%). Dhar and colleagues[77] reported a series of 99 hips treated by open reduction via a Smith-Peterson approach. The rate of AVN was 23.2%, with a redislocation rate of 1.8% and 24 further operative procedures. In their series of 113 hips, Szepesi and colleagues[78] found a redislocation rate of 2.7% (3 hips), a 21.2% rate of further procedures, and a rate of AVN of approximately 11%. At a mean follow-up of 18 years, Varner and colleagues[79] reported 82% excellent, 3% good, 10%

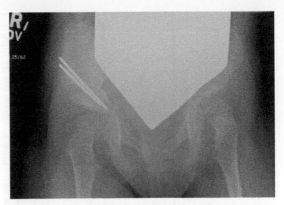

Fig. 2. AP radiograph of a pelvis after SIO.

fair, and 5% poor Iowa hip scores following anterior open reduction and, if required, femoral or acetabular osteotomy. Cordier and colleagues[80] reported on the Tonnis anterior approach in 118 hips with a redislocation rate of 11% and AVN rate of 6%.[80,81]

There is conflicting evidence regarding the timing of medial open reduction in relation to the age of the patient. Okano and colleagues[69] found unacceptable radiological results and AVN rates in patients more than 17 months of age. In contrast, Altay and colleagues[82] found no correlation between age at time of surgery and rate of AVN.

Summary

The quality of evidence for open reduction is low. Most cases are observational retrospective case series. Because open reduction is often performed after failure of closed reduction it is difficult to accurately attribute rates of AVN to the open reduction in certain studies. There are no randomized control trials of the different approaches for

Table 4
Evidence for the use of the medial approach for open reduction

Study	No. of Hips	Redislocation	AVN Rate	Further Procedures	Level of Evidence
Okano et al[69]	45	1 (2.2%)	13 (29%)	5 (11.1%)	4
Ucar et al[70]	44	0	9 (20%)	11 (25%)	4
Konigsberg et al[71]	40	1 (2.5%)	11 (27.5%)	8 (20%)	4
Morcuende et al[64]	97	2 (2.1%)	44 (45.4%)	16 (16.5%)	4
Koizumi et al[68]	35	0	15 (42.9%)	16 (45.7%)	4
Mankey et al[63]	66	1 (1.5%)	7 (10.6%)	22 (33%)	4
Sosna & Rejholec[72]	62	0	22 (35.5%)	53 (85.4%)	4
Bache et al[62]	109	3 (2.8%)	45 (41.3%)	44 (40%)	4
Kiely et al[73]	49	3 (6.1%)	7 (14.3%)	8 (16.3%)	4
Tumer et al[74]	56	0	5 (8.9%)	13 (23.2%)	4
Mergen et al[75]	31	0	3 (9.7%)	5 (16.1%)	4

Table 5
Summary of evidence for pelvic osteotomies

Study	Technique	No. of Hips	Mean Follow-up (mo)	Additional Surgery	AVN	Severin Class[27]
Böhm et al[85]	Salter	73	30.9	7 (9.6%)	44 (60%)	Class I, 79% (of 63 hips) Class 2, 9.5% Class 3, 3.2% Class 4, 4.8% Class 5, 1.6% Class 6, 1.6%
Thomas et al[86]	Salter	80	45	24 THR	Not reported	Class I, 17.6% (of 51 hips) Class 2, 64.7% Class 3, 15.7% Class 4, 2.0% Class 5, 0 Class 6, 0
Roth et al[101]	Salter	123	63	Not reported	3.8%	Class I, 67.5% (of 123 hips) Class 2, 17.9% Class 3, 11.4% Class 4, 3.3% Class 5, 0 Class 6, 0
Barrett et al[87]	Salter	68	100	11 (16.2%)	4 (7.4%)	Not reported
Haidar et al[88]	Salter & open reduction	37	7.6	2 (5.4%) subluxation	3 (8.1%)	Class I, 32.4% (of 37 hips) Class 2, 51.4% Class 3, 10.8% Class 4, 5.4% Class 5, 0 Class 6, 0
Eyre-Brook et al[102]	Pemberton +/− OR	37	6	Not reported	1 (2.7%)	Not reported
Aydin et al[89]	Pemberton	91	60	Not reported	17 (18.6%)	Not reported

Wu et al[90]	OR & Pemberton	49	134.6	Excluded	25 (51%)	Class 1a, 55.1% (of 49 hips) Class 1b, 4.1% Class 2, 26.5% Class 3, 10.2% Class 4, 0 Class 5, 4.1% Class 6, 0
Szepesi et al[91]	Pemberton +/− femoral osteotomy	80	64	1 (wedge displacement)	—	Class 1, 8.8% (of 80 hips) Class 2, 70.0% Class 3, 16.3% Class 4, 5.0% Class 5, 0 Class 6, 0
Faciszewski et al[92]	Pemberton osteotomy	52	120	Not reported	0	Class 1a, 80.8% Class 1b, 3.8% Class 2a, 9.6% Class 2b, 3.8% Class 3, 1.9% Class 4, 0 Class 5, 0 Class 6, 0
Reichel & Hein[96]	Modified Dega & intertrochanteric osteotomy	70	182	6 repeat varus osteotomy 2 bone wedge resorption 2 fixation femoral fracture	18 patients	Unable to determine from data provided
Karlen et al[97]	Dega & multiple procedures	50 (26 DDH, 24 neuromuscular)	51	1 closed reduction (posttraumatic)	2 (8%)	Not reported
Aksoy et al[98]	Dega +/− OR & femoral shortening	43	58	1 containment	6 (14.0%)	Not reported

Abbreviations: OR, open reduction; THR, Total hip replacement.

open reduction and, as such, it is not possible to recommend one approach rather than another.

PELVIC OSTEOTOMIES

Multiple pelvic and periacetabular osteotomies have been described for the treatment of DDH. They can be classified into reorienting osteotomies, volume-reducing osteotomies, and salvage procedures.

Salter[83] first described the innominate osteotomy to redirect and stabilize the dislocated hip in children aged 18 months to 6 years or to treat residual dysplasia or recurrent dislocation in 1961. Pemberton reported his pericapsular osteotomy in 1965. This procedure is an incomplete transiliac osteotomy hinged about the triradiate cartilage that has the ability to improve both anterior and lateral coverage of the femoral head.[84] Böhm and colleagues[85] reported the long-term outcome of the Salter innominate osteotomy (SIO), noting that increasing severity of dislocation was associated with worse outcome, with a possible increase in the risk of AVN if the SIO and open reduction were performed concomitantly. Thomas and colleagues[86] reported on the 45-year follow-up of Salter's[83] series of patients undergoing surgery between 18 months and 4.7 years and found that bilateral hip dislocation and postoperative complications were negative predictive factors and that there was an overall failure rate, defined as total joint arthroplasty, of 46%. Age at the time of index surgery did not affect outcome, although the investigators conceded that this may be because of type II error. Barrett and colleagues[87] found no difference in outcome for patients treated with a concomitant open reduction with those treated with a prior open reduction and an SIO at a later stage. However, there was a worse outcome for those patients more than 4 years of age. Haidar and colleagues[88] had similar results in their series (Fig. 2).

The Pemberton pericapsular osteotomy (PPO) is claimed to provide superior correction compared with other procedures because this osteotomy is performed closer to the origin of the deformity in DDH.[84] Aydin and colleagues[89] found a statistically significant increase in the rate of AVN with increasing level of dislocation. Wu and colleagues[90] found that there was a correlation between AVN and worsening lateral hip subluxation and concluded that the percentage of inferior displacement correlates and predicts the probability of osteonecrosis in the femoral head.

Szepesi and colleagues[91] reported the results of 80 Pemberton osteotomies with 1 to 15 years of follow-up and found that, at ages greater than 7 years, the results reduced from 84% good or excellent to 58%. In addition, placement of patients in the frog-leg position in plaster casts was detrimental to outcome. Faciszewski and colleagues[92] found that preexisting AVN was detrimental to outcome with only 2 out of 10 hips with preexisting AVN achieving a Severin rating of Ia at latest follow-up.

The SIO is a complete redirectional osteotomy of the acetabulum that results in reorientation of the triradiate cartilage from its origin just medial to the femoral head to a superior position. In contrast, the PPO is an incomplete reshaping osteotomy of the acetabular roof hinged at the triradiate cartilage beginning between the anterior iliac spines and results in relative retroversion of the acetabulum.[93] The PPO has a theoretic risk of increasing pressure on the femoral head resulting in an increased risk of osteonecrosis.[90] Only 1 study was identified that compared the SIO and PPO and this study compared radiological outcomes alone.[93] The investigators found a significant difference in the acetabular depth ratio between the two surgical procedures, indicating that the PPO resulted in an increase in the depth of the acetabulum but a decrease in its width. In contrast, no significant difference in center-edge angle of Wiberg or Reimer index was identified between the two groups. No clinical outcome differences were investigated in this study.

The Dega osteotomy was first described in 1969.[94] It is an incomplete transiliac osteotomy that hinges on the posteromedial iliac cortex and sciatic notch.[95] Reichel and Hein[96] reported the largest series of 70 patients treated with a modified Dega and combined intertrochanteric osteotomy. Eighty percent had good or very good results at 15 years, with no redislocations and satisfactory correction in patients aged between 0.7 and 7 years, and the investigators postulated that there is insufficient remodeling potential beyond the age of 7 years.[96]

Karlen and colleagues[97] reported on a series of 50 hips with 53 months of follow-up: 26 hips diagnosed with DDH had an AVN rate of 8%; it was concluded that this was a safe and effective single-stage treatment of DDH. Aksoy and colleagues[98] retrospectively reviewed 43 hips with 58 months' follow-up to evaluate the improvement in acetabular index (AI). The mean preoperative AI was 35° and postoperative AI was 20°. Following initial correction, they found a mean improvement of 7°, with no worsening of AI in any patient.

El-Sayed and colleagues[99] reported a series of 109 hips, 61 of which underwent an SIO and 48 of which underwent a Dega acetabuloplasty based on the treating surgeon's preference. The worst

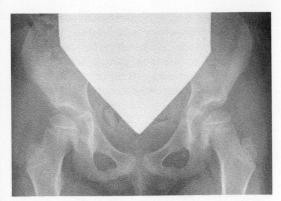

Fig. 3. AP radiograph of pelvis with bilateral hip dysplasia in a 5-year-old female patient.

outcome was seen in the group less than 4 years of age treated by Dega osteotomy, and this was attributed to the more technically demanding procedure of the smaller ilium. The overall results showed a favorable outcome in 90.16% treated by SIO and 79.16% treated by Dega. Despite this there was a significant difference in the AI improvement, favoring the Dega. The investigators attributed the difference in outcome to the learning curve of the, at that time, newly introduced Dega acetabuloplasty, and this, in conjunction with the lack of randomization, limits the significance of these results.

In contrast, Lopez-Carreno and colleagues[100] found a statistically significant difference in favor of the Dega compared with the SIO in a non-randomized retrospective review of 99 hips (43 Dega, 56 SIO) in terms of joint mobility, gait, and improvement in AI. A greater percentage of hips treated with Dega were classified as Severin type I compared with the SIO; however, no statistical test of significance was applied to this difference.

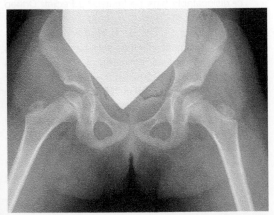

Fig. 4. Abduction internal rotation radiograph of the pelvis with bilateral hip dysplasia in a 5-year-old female patient.

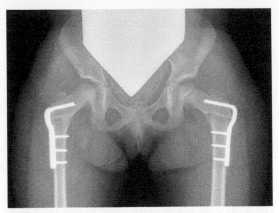

Fig. 5. AP radiograph of the pelvis after bilateral varus derotation osteotomies of 5-year-old girl with bilateral hip dysplasia.

Summary

The quality of evidence for type of pelvic osteotomy performed for residual dysplasia or management of primary hip dislocation is low. Most cases are observational retrospective case series and, as such, it is not possible to recommend one procedure rather than another. Two retrospective nonrandomized trials comparing SIO with Dega may favor the Dega, but a randomized prospective trial is required to establish this.

Treatment of DDH with either SIO, PPO, or Dega has better results when performed before the age of 8 years. A summary of evidence for pelvic osteotomies is given in **Table 5**.

FEMORAL OSTEOTOMIES

Multiple studies have reported the use of the femoral osteotomy, either as a shortening, derotation, or valgus osteotomy (**Figs. 3–7**).[64,69,91,96,97] These procedures can be intertrochanteric or subtrochanteric. However, these studies are reported

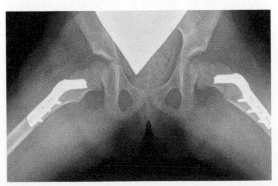

Fig. 6. Frog-leg lateral radiograph after bilateral varus derotation osteotomies of 5-year-old girl with bilateral hip dysplasia.

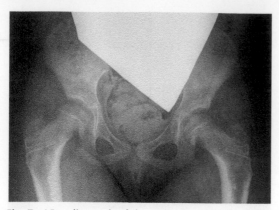

Fig. 7. AP radiograph of the pelvis 3 years after bilateral varus derotation osteotomies.

in conjunction with multiple additional procedures, often as an adjunct to previous index procedures and, as such, no studies were identified that compared the effectiveness of these procedures.

SUMMARY

The overall body of evidence for the management of DDH consists largely of retrospective case series reporting the results of single surgeons. There is a lack of prospective randomized comparative trials. The future direction of research into the management of DDH should include prospective randomized multicentre trials.

REFERENCES

1. Aronsson DD, Goldberg MJ, Kling TF, et al. Developmental dysplasia of the hip. Pediatrics 1994; 94(2 pt 1):201–8.

2. Wright JG, Swiontkowski MF, Heckman JD. Introducing levels of evidence to the journal. J Bone Joint Surg Am 2003;85(1):1–3.

3. Balshem H, Helfand M, Schünemann HJ, et al. GRADE guidelines: 3. Rating the quality of evidence. J Clin Epidemiol 2011;64(4):401–6. http://dx.doi.org/10.1016/j.jclinepi.2010.07.015.

4. Mubarak SJ, Bialik V. Pavlik: the man and his method. J Pediatr Orthop 2003;23(3):342–6.

5. Pavlik A, Peltier LF. The functional method of treatment using a harness with stirrups as the primary method of conservative therapy for infants with congenital dislocation of the hip. Clin Orthop Relat Res 1992;(281):4–10.

6. Wada I, Sakuma E, Otsuka T, et al. The Pavlik harness in the treatment of developmentally dislocated hips: results of Japanese multicenter studies in 1994 and 2008. J Orthop Sci 2013;18(5):749–53. http://dx.doi.org/10.1007/s00776-013-0432-z.

7. Walton MJ, Isaacson Z, McMillan D, et al. The success of management with the Pavlik harness for developmental dysplasia of the hip using a United Kingdom screening programme and ultrasound-guided supervision. J Bone Joint Surg Br 2010; 92(7):1013–6. http://dx.doi.org/10.1302/0301-620X. 92B7.23513.

8. Cashman JP, Round J, Taylor G, et al. The natural history of developmental dysplasia of the hip after early supervised treatment in the Pavlik harness. A prospective, longitudinal follow-up. J Bone Joint Surg Br 2002;84(3):418–25. http://dx.doi.org/10. 1302/0301-620X.84B3.12230.

9. Grill F, Bensahel H, Canadell J, et al. The Pavlik harness in the treatment of congenital dislocating hip: report on a multicenter study of the European Paediatric Orthopaedic Society. J Pediatr Orthop 1988;8(1):1–8.

10. Johnson AH, Aadalen RJ, Eilers VE, et al. Treatment of congenital hip dislocation and dysplasia with the Pavlik harness. Clin Orthop Relat Res 1981;(155):25–9.

11. Filipe G, Carlioz H. Use of the Pavlik harness in treating congenital dislocation of the hip. J Pediatr Orthop 1982;2(4):357–62.

12. Weinstein SL, Mubarak SJ, Wenger DR. Developmental hip dysplasia and dislocation part II. Instr Course Lect 2004;53:531–42.

13. Atalar H, Sayli U, Yavuz OY, et al. Indicators of successful use of the Pavlik harness in infants with developmental dysplasia of the hip. Int Orthop 2007;31(2):145–50.

14. Gardiner HM, Dunn PM. Controlled trial of immediate splinting versus ultrasonographic surveillance in congenitally dislocatable hips. Lancet 1990; 336(8730):1553–6.

15. Lorente Moltó FJ, Gregori AM, Casas LM, et al. Three-year prospective study of developmental dysplasia of the hip at birth: should all dislocated or dislocatable hips be treated? J Pediatr Orthop 2002;22(5):613–21.

16. van der Sluijs JA, De Gier L, Verbeke JI, et al. Prolonged treatment with the Pavlik harness in infants with developmental dysplasia of the hip. J Bone Joint Surg Br 2009;91(8):1090–3. http://dx.doi.org/10.1302/0301-620X.91B8.21692.

17. Malkawi H. Sonographic monitoring of the treatment of developmental disturbances of the hip by the Pavlik harness. J Pediatr Orthop B 1998;7(2): 144–9.

18. Taylor GR, Clarke NM. Monitoring the treatment of developmental dysplasia of the hip with the Pavlik harness. J Bone Joint Surg Br 1997;79(5):719–23.

19. Sochart DH, Paton RW. Role of ultrasound assessment and harness treatment in the management of developmental dysplasia of the hip. Ann R Coll Surg Engl 1996;78(6):505–8.

20. Elbourne D, Dezateux C, Arthur R, et al. Ultrasonography in the diagnosis and management of developmental hip dysplasia (UK Hip Trial): clinical and economic results of a multicentre randomised controlled trial. Lancet 2002;360(9350):2009–17.

21. Suzuki S, Kashiwagi N, Kasahara Y, et al. The incidence of avascular necrosis in three types of congenital dislocation of the hip as classified by ultrasound. J Bone Joint Surg Br 1996;78(4):631–5.

22. Suzuki S, Yamamuro T. Avascular necrosis in patients treated with the Pavlik harness for congenital dislocation of the hip. J Bone Joint Surg Am 1990;72(7):1048–55.

23. Iwasaki K. Treatment of congenital dislocation of the hip by the Pavlik harness. Mechanism of reduction and usage. J Bone Joint Surg Am 1983;65(6):760–7.

24. Suzuki S, Seto Y, Futami T, et al. Preliminary traction and the use of under-thigh pillows to prevent avascular necrosis of the femoral head in Pavlik harness treatment of developmental dysplasia of the hip. J Orthop Sci 2000;5(6):540–5.

25. Murnaghan ML, Browne RH, Sucato DJ, et al. Femoral nerve palsy in Pavlik harness treatment for developmental dysplasia of the hip. J Bone Joint Surg Am 2011;93(5):493–9. http://dx.doi.org/10.2106/JBJS.J.01210.

26. Harris IE, Dickens R, Menelaus MB. Use of the Pavlik harness for hip displacements. When to abandon treatment. Clin Orthop Relat Res 1992;(281):29–33.

27. Fujioka F, Terayama K, Sugimoto N, et al. Long-term results of congenital dislocation of the hip treated with the Pavlik harness. J Pediatr Orthop 1995;15(6):747–52.

28. Severin EA. Contribution to the knowledge of congenital dislocation of the hip joint. Late results of closed reduction and arthrographic studies of recent cases. Acta Chir Scand 1941;84(63):1–142.

29. Yoshitaka T, Mitani S, Aoki K, et al. Long-term follow-up of congenital subluxation of the hip. J Pediatr Orthop 2001;21(4):474–80.

30. Tucci JJ, Kumar SJ, Guille JT, et al. Late acetabular dysplasia following early successful Pavlik harness treatment of congenital dislocation of the hip. J Pediatr Orthop 1991;11(4):502–5.

31. Atar D, Lehman WB, Tenenbaum Y, et al. Pavlik harness versus Frejka splint in treatment of developmental dysplasia of the hip: bicenter study. J Pediatr Orthop 1993;13(3):311–3.

32. Czubak J, Piontek T, Niciejewski K, et al. Retrospective analysis of the non-surgical treatment of developmental dysplasia of the hip using Pavlik harness and Frejka pillow: comparison of both methods. Ortop Traumatol Rehabil 2004;6(1):9–13.

33. Brurås KR, Aukland SM, Markestad T, et al. Newborns with sonographically dysplastic and potentially unstable hips: 6-year follow-up of an RCT. Pediatrics 2011;127(3):e661–6. http://dx.doi.org/10.1542/peds.2010-572.

34. Wilkinson AG, Sherlock DA, Murray GD. The efficacy of the Pavlik harness, the Craig splint and the von Rosen splint in the management of neonatal dysplasia of the hip. A comparative study. J Bone Joint Surg Br 2002;84(5):716–9.

35. Finlay HV, Maudsley RH, Busfield PI. Dislocatable hip and dislocated hip in the newborn infant. Br Med J 1967;4(5576):377–81.

36. Fredensborg N. The results of early treatment of typical congenital dislocation of the hip in Malmö. J Bone Joint Surg Br 1976;58(3):272–8.

37. Mitchell GP. Problems in the early diagnosis and management of congenital dislocation of the hip. J Bone Joint Surg Br 1972;54(1):4–12.

38. Heikkilä E. Comparison of the Frejka pillow and the von Rosen splint in treatment of congenital dislocation of the hip. J Pediatr Orthop 1988;8(1):20–1.

39. Lauge-Pedersen H, Gustafsson J, Hägglund G. 6 weeks with the von Rosen splint is sufficient for treatment of neonatal hip instability. Acta Orthop 2006;77(2):257–61. http://dx.doi.org/10.1080/17453670610045993.

40. Murray T, Cooperman DR, Thompson GH, et al. Closed reduction for treatment of development dysplasia of the hip in children. Am J Orthop 2007;36(2):82–4.

41. Terjesen T, Halvorsen V. Long-term results after closed reduction of late detected hip dislocation: 60 patients followed up to skeletal maturity. Acta Orthop 2007;78(2):236–46. http://dx.doi.org/10.1080/17453670710013744.

42. Race C, Herring JA. Congenital dislocation of the hip: an evaluation of closed reduction. J Pediatr Orthop 1983;3(2):166–72.

43. Ishii Y, Ponseti IV. Long-term results of closed reduction of complete congenital dislocation of the hip in children under one year of age. Clin Orthop Relat Res 1978;(137):167–74.

44. Zionts LE, MacEwen GD. Treatment of congenital dislocation of the hip in children between the ages of one and three years. J Bone Joint Surg Am 1986;68(6):829–46.

45. Brougham DI, Broughton NS, Cole WG, et al. Avascular necrosis following closed reduction of congenital dislocation of the hip. Review of influencing factors and long-term follow-up. J Bone Joint Surg Br 1990;72(4):557–62.

46. Malvitz TA, Weinstein SL. Closed reduction for congenital dysplasia of the hip. Functional and radiographic results after an average of thirty years. J Bone Joint Surg Am 1994;76(12):1777–92.

47. Yamada N, Maeda S, Fujii G, et al. Closed reduction of developmental dislocation of the hip by

prolonged traction. J Bone Joint Surg Br 2003; 85(8):1173–7.

48. Rampal V, Sabourin M, Erdeneshoo E, et al. Closed reduction with traction for developmental dysplasia of the hip in children aged between one and five years. J Bone Joint Surg Br 2008;90(7):858–63. http://dx.doi.org/10.1302/0301-620X.90B7.20041.

49. Gregosiewicz A, Wosko I. Risk factors of avascular necrosis in the treatment of congenital dislocation of the hip. J Pediatr Orthop 1988;8:17–9.

50. DeRosa GP, Feller N. Treatment of congenital dislocation of the hip. Clin Orthop Relat Res 1987;(225): 77–85. http://dx.doi.org/10.1097/00003086-1987 12000-00008.

51. Daoud A, Saighi-Bououina A. Congenital dislocation of the hip in the older child. The effectiveness of overhead traction. J Bone Joint Surg Am 1996; 78(1):30–40.

52. Langenskiöld A, Paavilainen T. The effect of prereduction traction on the results of closed reduction of developmental dislocation of the hip. J Pediatr Orthop 2000;20(4):471–4.

53. Sibiński M, Murnaghan C, Synder M. The value of preliminary overhead traction in the closed management of DDH. Int Orthop 2006;30(4): 268–71.

54. Kutlu A, Ayata C, Ogün TC, et al. Preliminary traction as a single determinant of avascular necrosis in developmental dislocation of the hip. J Pediatr Orthop 2000;20(5):579–84.

55. Clarke NM, Jowett AJ, Parker L. The surgical treatment of established congenital dislocation of the hip. J Pediatr Orthop 2005;25(4):434–9. http://dx. doi.org/10.1097/01.bpo.0000158003.68918.28.

56. Segal LS, Schneider DJ, Berlin JM, et al. The contribution of the ossific nucleus to the structural stiffness of the capital femoral epiphysis: a porcine model for DDH. J Pediatr Orthop 1999;19(4): 433–7.

57. Segal LS, Boal DK, Borthwick L, et al. Avascular necrosis after treatment of DDH: the protective influence of the ossific nucleus. J Pediatr Orthop 1999;19(2):177–84.

58. Luhmann SJ, Schoenecker PL, Anderson AM, et al. The prognostic importance of the ossific nucleus in the treatment of congenital dysplasia of the hip. J Bone Joint Surg Am 1998;80(12): 1719–27.

59. Cooke SJ, Rees R, Edwards DL, et al. Ossification of the femoral head at closed reduction for developmental dysplasia of the hip and its influence on the long-term outcome. J Pediatr Orthop B 2010; 19(1):22–6. http://dx.doi.org/10.1097/BPB.0b013e 32832fc8ca.

60. Ludloff K. The open reduction of the congenital hip dislocation by an anterior incision. J Bone Joint Surg Am 1913;10(3):438–54.

61. Ferguson AB. Primary open reduction of congenital dislocation of the hip using a median adductor approach. J Bone Joint Surg Am 1973;55(4): 671–89.

62. Bache CE, Graham HK, Dickens DR, et al. Ligamentum teres tenodesis in medial approach open reduction for developmental dislocation of the hip. J Pediatr Orthop 2008;28(6):607–13. http:// dx.doi.org/10.1097/BPO.0b013e318184202c.

63. Mankey MG, Arntz GT, Staheli LT. Open reduction through a medial approach for congenital dislocation of the hip. A critical review of the Ludloff approach in sixty-six hips. J Bone Joint Surg Am 1993;75(9):1334–45.

64. Morcuende JA, Meyer MD, Dolan LA, et al. Long-term outcome after open reduction through an anteromedial approach for congenital dislocation of the hip. J Bone Joint Surg Am 1997;79(6): 810–7.

65. Weinstein SL, Ponseti IV. Congenital dislocation of the hip. J Bone Joint Surg Am 1979;61(1):119–24.

66. Zamzam MM, Khoshhal KI, Abak AA, et al. One-stage bilateral open reduction through a medial approach in developmental dysplasia of the hip. J Bone Joint Surg Br 2009;91(1):113–8. http://dx. doi.org/10.1302/0301-620X.91B1.21429.

67. Kalamchi A, Schmidt TL, MacEwen GD. Congenital dislocation of the hip. Open reduction by the medial approach. Clin Orthop Relat Res 1982;(169): 127–32.

68. Koizumi W, Moriya H, Tsuchiya K, et al. Ludloff's medial approach for open reduction of congenital dislocation of the hip. A 20-year follow-up. J Bone Joint Surg Br 1996;78(6):924–9.

69. Okano K, Yamada K, Takahashi K, et al. Long-term outcome of Ludloff's medial approach for open reduction of developmental dislocation of the hip in relation to the age at operation. Int Orthop 2009; 33(5):1391–6. http://dx.doi.org/10.1007/s00264-009-0800-7.

70. Ucar DH, Işiklar ZU, Stanitski CL, et al. Open reduction through a medial approach in developmental dislocation of the hip: a follow-up study to skeletal maturity. J Pediatr Orthop 2004;24(5): 493–500.

71. Konigsberg DE, Karol LA, Colby S, et al. Results of medial open reduction of the hip in infants with developmental dislocation of the hip. J Pediatr Orthop 2003;23(1):1–9.

72. Sosna A, Rejholec M. Ludloff's open reduction of the hip: long-term results. J Pediatr Orthop 1992; 12(5):603–6.

73. Kiely N, Younis U, Day JB, et al. The Ferguson medial approach for open reduction of developmental dysplasia of the hip. A clinical and radiological review of 49 hips. J Bone Joint Surg Br 2004; 86(3):430–3.

74. Tumer Y, Ward WT, Grudziak J. Medial open reduction in the treatment of developmental dislocation of the hip. J Pediatr Orthop 1997;17(2):176–80.

75. Mergen E, Adyaman S, Omeroglu H, et al. Medial approach open reduction for congenital dislocation of the hip using the Ferguson procedure. Arch Orthop Trauma Surg 1991;110(3):169–72. http://dx.doi.org/10.1007/BF00395803.

76. Doudoulakis JK, Cavadias A. Open reduction of CDH before one year of age. 69 hips followed for 13 (10-19) years. Acta Orthop Scand 1993;64(2):188–92.

77. Dhar S, Taylor JF, Jones WA, et al. Early open reduction for congenital dislocation of the hip. J Bone Joint Surg Br 1990;72(2):175–80.

78. Szepesi K, Biró B, Fazekas K, et al. Preliminary results of early open reduction by an anterior approach for congenital dislocation of the hip. J Pediatr Orthop B 1995;4(2):171–8.

79. Varner KE, Incavo SJ, Haynes RJ, et al. Surgical treatment of developmental hip dislocation in children aged 1 to 3 years: a mean 18-year, 9-month follow-up study. Orthopedics 2010;33(3). http://dx.doi.org/10.3928/01477447-20100129-05.

80. Cordier W, Tönnis D, Kalchschmidt K, et al. Long-term results after open reduction of developmental hip dislocation by an anterior approach lateral and medial of the iliopsoas muscle. J Pediatr Orthop B 2005;14(2):79–87.

81. Tönnis D. Surgical treatment of congenital dislocation of the hip. Clin Orthop Relat Res 1990;(258):33–40.

82. Altay M, Demirkale I, Senturk F, et al. Results of medial open reduction of developmental dysplasia of the hip with regard to walking age. J Pediatr Orthop B 2013;22(1):36–41. http://dx.doi.org/10.1097/BPB.0b013e3283587631.

83. Salter RB. Innominate osteotomy in the treatment of congenital dislocation and subluxation of the hip. J Bone Joint Surg Br 1961;43(3):518–39.

84. Pemberton PA. Pericapsular osteotomy of the ilium for the treatment of congenital subluxation and dislocation of the hip. J Bone Joint Surg Am 1965;47:65–86.

85. Böhm P, Brzuske A. Salter innominate osteotomy for the treatment of developmental dysplasia of the hip in children: results of seventy-three consecutive osteotomies after twenty-six to thirty-five years of follow-up. J Bone Joint Surg Am 2002;84-A(2):178–86.

86. Thomas SR, Wedge JH, Salter RB. Outcome at forty-five years after open reduction and innominate osteotomy for late-presenting developmental dislocation of the hip. J Bone Joint Surg Am 2007;89(11):2341–50.

87. Barrett WP, Staheli LT, Chew DE. The effectiveness of the Salter innominate osteotomy in the treatment of congenital dislocation of the hip. J Bone Joint Surg Am 1986;68(1):79–87.

88. Haidar RK, Jones RS, Vergroesen DA, et al. Simultaneous open reduction and Salter innominate osteotomy for developmental dysplasia of the hip. J Bone Joint Surg Br 1996;78(3):471–6.

89. Aydin A, Kalali F, Yildiz V, et al. The results of Pemberton's pericapsular osteotomy in patients with developmental hip dysplasia. Acta Orthop Traumatol Turc 2012;46(1):35–41.

90. Wu KW, Wang TM, Huang SC, et al. Analysis of osteonecrosis following Pemberton acetabuloplasty in developmental dysplasia of the hip: long-term results. J Bone Joint Surg Am 2010;92(11):2083–94. http://dx.doi.org/10.2106/JBJS.I.01320.

91. Szepesi K, Rigó J, Biró B, et al. Pemberton's pericapsular osteotomy for the treatment of acetabular dysplasia. J Pediatr Orthop B 1996;5(4):252–8.

92. Faciszewski T, Kiefer GN, Coleman SS. Pemberton osteotomy for residual acetabular dysplasia in children who have congenital dislocation of the hip. J Bone Joint Surg Am 1993;75(5):643–9.

93. Ertürk C, Altay MA, Işikan UE. A radiological comparison of Salter and Pemberton osteotomies to improve acetabular deformations in developmental dysplasia of the hip. J Pediatr Orthop B 2013;22(6):527–32. http://dx.doi.org/10.1097/BPB.0b013e32836337cd.

94. Dega W. Selection of surgical methods in the treatment of congenital dislocation of the hip in children. Chir Narzadow Ruchu Ortop Pol 1969;34(3):357–66.

95. Grudziak JS, Ward WT. Dega osteotomy for the treatment of congenital dysplasia of the hip. J Bone Joint Surg Am 2001;83-A(6):845–54.

96. Reichel H, Hein W. Dega acetabuloplasty combined with intertrochanteric osteotomies. Clin Orthop Relat Res 1996;(323):234–42.

97. Karlen JW, Skaggs DL, Ramachandran M, et al. The Dega osteotomy: a versatile osteotomy in the treatment of developmental and neuromuscular hip pathology. J Pediatr Orthop 2009;29(7):676–82. http://dx.doi.org/10.1097/BPO.0b013e3181b7691a.

98. Aksoy C, Yilgor C, Demirkiran G, et al. Evaluation of acetabular development after Dega acetabuloplasty in developmental dysplasia of the hip. J Pediatr Orthop B 2013;22(2):91–5. http://dx.doi.org/10.1097/BPB.0b013e32835c2a7d.

99. El-Sayed M, Ahmed T, Fathy S, et al. The effect of Dega acetabuloplasty and Salter innominate osteotomy on acetabular remodeling monitored by the acetabular index in walking DDH patients between 2 and 6 years of age: short- to middle-term follow-up. J Child Orthop 2012;6(6):471–7. http://dx.doi.org/10.1007/s11832-012-0451-x.

100. Lopez-Carreno E, Carillo H, Gutierrez M. Dega versus Salter osteotomy for the treatment of developmental dysplasia of the hip. J Ped Ortho B 2008; 17(5):213–21.

101. Roth A, Gibson DA, Hall JE. The experience of five orthopedic surgeons with innominate osteotomy in the treatment of congenital dislocation and subluxation of the hip. Clin Orthop Relat Res 1974;(98):178–82.

102. Eyre-Brook AL, Jones DA, Harris FC. Pemberton's acetabuloplasty for congenital dislocation or subluxation of the hip. J Bone Joint Surg Br 1978;60(1):18–24.

Upper Extremity

Preface
Upper Extremity

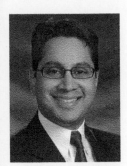

Asif M. Ilyas, MD
Editor

In this issue of the *Orthopedic Clinics of North America*, we present several interesting articles in the Upper Extremity section, reviewing a number of sports-oriented topics.

Paxton and colleagues present a discussion on shoulder instability in the elderly. Although uncommon, a shoulder dislocation in advancing age can result in significant dysfunction and demonstrates a higher association with fractures and rotator cuff tears than in the younger patient. The authors present its incidence, mechanism of injury, diagnosis, associated injuries, and treatment options.

Kinsella and colleagues and Patel and colleagues present a detailed review of throwing injuries of the shoulder and elbow, respectively. Overhead throwers, in particular, baseball players, expose the shoulder and elbow to significant forces, lending them susceptible to a number of injuries that can compromise play and function. The authors present detailed reviews of the mechanism of injury, risk factors, anatomy, diagnosis, classification, and both surgical and nonsurgical treatment options.

Asif M. Ilyas, MD
Rothman Institute
Thomas Jefferson University
925 Chestnut Street
Philadelphia, PA 19107, USA

E-mail address:
asif.ilyas@rothmaninstitute.com

The Thrower's Elbow

Ronak M. Patel, MD[a], T. Sean Lynch, MD[a], Nirav H. Amin, MD[a],
Gary Calabrese, PT[a], Stephen M. Gryzlo, MD[b], Mark S. Schickendantz, MD[a],*

KEYWORDS

- Overhead throwing athlete • Ulnar collateral ligament • Tommy John • Ulnar subluxation
- Olecranon impingement • Capitellar OCD

KEY POINTS

- Most elbow injuries occur as a result of the stresses incurred during the acceleration phase.
- During overhead throwing, a large valgus force on the elbow created by humeral torque is countered by rapid elbow extension, creating significant tensile stress along the medial compartment, shear stress in the posterior compartment, and compressive stress in the lateral compartment.
- The docking technique in ulnar collateral ligament (UCL) reconstruction demonstrated a lower complication rate and a greater rate of return to play compared with the Jobe technique.
- During surgical management of valgus extension overload syndrome, it is recommended that only the osteophyte and no native olecranon be removed to prevent iatrogenic instability.

INTRODUCTION

The elbow undergoes significant stress during the throwing motion of an overhead athlete. The forces generated in the various phases of the throwing arc are distributed through the soft tissue and bone of the elbow joint. In athletes, such as baseball players, repetition leads to attritional damage to the elbow. The specific constellation of injuries suffered in baseball and other overhead sports, such as softball, football, tennis, and javelin, are well documented. These injuries include (1) medial UCL tears, (2) ulnar neuritis, (3) flexor-pronator injury, (4) medial epicondyle apophysitis or avulsion, (5) valgus extension overload syndrome with olecranon osteophytes, (6) olecranon stress fractures, (7) osteochondritis dissecans (OCD) of the capitellum, and (8) loose bodies.[1]

Approximately 55% of high school students participate in sports, and in 2013, softball and baseball ranked as the forth and third most popular high school sports for girls and boys, respectively.[2] More than 2 million high school athletes are seen for sports-related injuries on an annual basis. Although the rate of elbow injuries is relatively low, the total number of such injuries is significant due to the high number of participants. With increasing rates of adolescent and young adults participating in athletics, knowledge regarding the diagnosis and treatment of thrower's elbow remains prudent. The elbow joint is complex, however, and understanding the management of thrower's elbow injuries begins with understanding the anatomy and pathophysiology.

The purpose of this review article is to describe the biomechanics of the throwing motion, the examination of the elbow, the diagnostic evaluation, and the diagnosis and treatment of the spectrum of elbow injuries common to a thrower (**Box 1**).

FUNCTIONAL ANATOMY

The elbow is a ginglymus joint that allows flexion-extension through the ulnohumeral articulation and pronation-supination through the radiocapitellar articulation. It is one of the most congruent joints in the body, with the trochlea covered by articular cartilage over a 300° arc. The bony anatomy of the proximal ulna and olecranon fossa provides primary stability at opposite ends of terminal

[a] Sports Health, Department of Orthopaedic Surgery, The Cleveland Clinic Foundation, 5555 Transportation Boulevard, Garfield Heights, OH 44125, USA; [b] Department of Orthopaedic Surgery, Feinberg School of Medicine, Northwestern University, 676 North St. Clair, #1350, Chicago, IL, USA
* Corresponding author.
E-mail address: SCHICKM@ccf.org

Orthop Clin N Am 45 (2014) 355–376
http://dx.doi.org/10.1016/j.ocl.2014.03.007
0030-5898/14/$ – see front matter © 2014 Elsevier Inc. All rights reserved.

orthopedic.theclinics.com

Box 1
Thrower's elbow pain differential diagnosis

UCL injury

Ulnar neuropathy

Flexor-pronator injury

Medial apophysitis or epicondyle avulsion

Valgus extension overload syndrome

Olecranon stress fracture

OCD of the capitellum

motion: less than 20° and greater than 120° of flexion. The radial head provides secondary restraint to valgus stress at 30°. The primary stability during the functional arc of an overhead athlete (20°–120°) emanates from the soft tissue restraints.[3–5] Furthermore, much of the stability derived from the osseous structure resists against varus stress with the elbow in extension.[5–7]

The soft tissue structures that provide static valgus elbow stability vital to overhead throwing include the anterior joint capsule, the UCL complex, and the radial collateral ligament complex. The UCL is composed of 3 bundles: an anterior, a transverse oblique and a posterior. The anterior bundle provides valgus stability throughout the entire range of motion (ROM) and consists of anterior and posterior bands that originate from the inferior aspect of the medial epicondyle and insert at the sublime tubercle on the medial aspect of the coronoid process (**Fig. 1**A–D).[5–8] The anterior band provides primary stability against valgus stress from full extension to 90° of flexion and secondary restraint at flexion greater than 90°. The posterior band, which is nearly isometric, provides functionally important restraint between 60° and full flexion, an arc of motion pivotal in the motion of an overhead throwing athlete.[9,10]

The oblique bundle (transverse ligament) lies at the distal-medial aspect of the joint capsule and does not actually cross the elbow joint. The posterior bundle is thinner and weaker than the anterior bundle and provides secondary elbow stability at greater than 90° of flexion.[5,6,9]

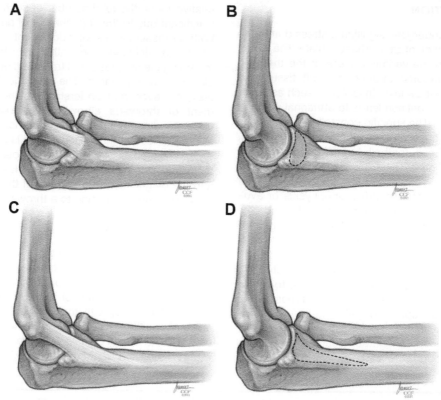

Fig. 1. Anatomy of the anterior bundle of the medial UCL of the elbow. Illustrations demonstrating traditional anatomy of the medial ulnar collateral ligament anterior band (*A*), traditional ulnar footprint (dashed line) (*B*). Illustrations of recently identified anatomy of the medial ulnar collateral ligament anterior band (*C*) and footprint at an osseous ridge that extends from the sublime tubercle to just medial to the ulnar insertion of the brachialis muscle tendon[160] (outlined with dashed line) (*D*). (*Courtesy of* Clinic Center for Medical Art & Photography © 2014, Cleveland. All Rights Reserved; with permission.)

The dynamic elbow stabilizers consist of the muscles in the flexor-pronator mass that originate off the medial epicondyle. This mass consists of the pronator teres, flexor carpi radialis, palmaris longus, flexor digitorium superficialis, and flexor carpi ulnaris (FCU), which functionally stabilize against valgus stress during active motion.[11]

Lastly, the ulnar nerve courses the medial elbow joint emanating from the arcade of Struthers and passing into the posterior compartment of the arm through the medial intermuscular septum. The nerve, along with a rich plexiform of vessels, enters the cubital tunnel just posterior to the medial epicondyle. The UCL complex forms the floor of the cubital tunnel whereas the roof is composed of the arcuate (Osborne) ligament. Distally, the ulnar nerve passes between the 2 heads of the FCU and rests on the flexor digitorum profundus.

BIOMECHANICS OF THROWING

Overhead throwing sports are typically grouped together because the general motion is similar. Thus, a baseball pitcher's throwing motion, which is the most heavily investigated model, serves as the basis for understanding biomechanics. The baseball pitch is divided into 6 stages of coordinated upper extremity, trunk, and lower extremity movements (**Fig. 2**).[7,12–18] The stages specific to elbow motion include

I.   Wind-up: the elbow is flexed and the forearm is pronated as the arm is initially overhead and returns to an adducted position.
II. Early cocking: the elbow maintains flexion and forearm pronation as the glenohumeral joint is abducted and externally rotated and the leading lower extremity is advanced.
III. Late cocking: involves increasing elbow flexion between 90° and 120° and forearm pronation to 90° while maximizing shoulder abduction and external rotation.
IV. Acceleration: the elbow is rapidly extended as the humerus adducts and internally rotates during a coordinated forward movement of the upper extremity and trunk. This stage terminates with ball release over 40 to 50 milliseconds, during which the elbow accelerates as much as 600,000°/s.[5,19]
V.   Deceleration: rapid deceleration occurs at a rate of 500,000°/s^2 over a time span of 50 milliseconds as excess kinetic energy is dissipated.[7,12–16,19]
VI. Follow-through: the elbow reaches full extension and throwing motion terminates.

Most elbow injuries occur as a result of the stresses incurred during stage IV or the acceleration phase where valgus forces reach as high as 64 Nm.[20] The valgus torque concentrate to the medial elbow, primarily the anterior bundle of the UCL.[11,14] Approximately 300 N of shear force is experienced by the medial elbow.[20] Concomitantly, compressive forces at the lateral radiocapitellar joint reach 500 N.[20] Nevertheless, modification to throwing biomechanics may not necessarily lead to improved clinical outcomes because the stresses from repetitive throwing may be the driving force to injury.

DEVELOPMENTAL CHANGES OF THE ELBOW

The repetitive stresses at the elbow and shoulder from throwing can lead to developmental changes, and, eventually, injury in young athletes. Small adaptive changes proximally may affect more distal segments of the kinetic chain.[21] For instance, Garrison and colleagues[22] found deficits

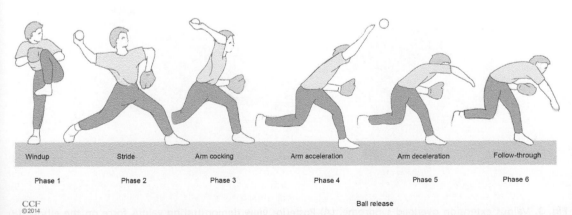

| Windup | Stride | Arm cocking | Arm acceleration | Arm deceleration | Follow-through |

| Phase 1 | Phase 2 | Phase 3 | Phase 4 | Phase 5 | Phase 6 |

Ball release

Fig. 2. Overhead throwing phases. (*Courtesy of* Clinic Center for Medical Art & Photography © 2014, Cleveland. All Rights Reserved; with permission.)

in total ROM of the shoulder were associated with UCL tears in a cross-sectional study of high school and collegiate baseball players. Changes in the shoulder include increase in external rotation from humeral retroversion and capsular laxity as well as decrease in internal rotation from osseous adaptations.[23–26] Polster and colleagues[27] demonstrated that the mean dominant arm humeral torsion in professional pitchers was 38.5° ± 8.9° (range, 23.0°–53.9°) compared with 27.6° ± 8.0° (range, 11.8°–45.0°) in the nondominant arm. This adaptation may be protective because the investigators found a higher incidence of severe injuries in players with lower degrees of dominant torsion. Burkhart and colleagues[28] proposed that increased humeral torsion leads to greater external rotation of the shoulder during late cocking, thus providing a longer throwing arc and potentially a greater peak velocity that increases the stresses experienced by the elbow. Distally at the elbow, Hang and colleagues[29] found that 94% of competitive young baseball players had radiographic signs of medial epicondylar apophyseal hypertrophy.

In overhead throwing athletes, understanding the difference between commonly seen asymptomatic adaptive changes and clinically significant pathology is critical in providing proper care to these athletes.[30] In a study of asymptomatic professional baseball players, Kooima and colleagues[31] found an 87% prevalence of chronic UCL injury and an 81% prevalence of posteromedial osteochondral injury. In asymptomatic major league baseball pitchers, increased medial laxity on valgus stress is not uncommon.[32,33] In a skeletally immature or adolescent thrower, the physis or apophysis absorbs the stresses of throwing and undergoes changes.[29,34] With time, asymptomatic changes may progress to symptomatic pathology with increased stress or frequency beyond reparative potential.

PATHOPHYSIOLOGY OF ELBOW INJURIES

King and colleagues[35] described a spectrum of elbow injuries in baseball pitchers from medial tension overload to extension overload to lateral compression overload. These injury patterns can be explained by one mechanism: valgus extension overload syndrome.[36] During overhead throwing, a large valgus force on the elbow created by humeral torque is countered by rapid elbow extension creating significant tensile stress along the medial compartment, shear stress in the posterior compartment, and compressive stress in the lateral compartment.[20,30] Repetitive, near-failure tensile stresses create microtrauma and attenuation anterior bundle of the UCL, leading to progressive valgus instability. Continued shear stress and impingement in the posterior compartment lead to olecranon tip osteophytes, loose bodies, and articular damage to the posteromedial trochlea in the continuum of valgus extension overload syndrome (**Fig. 3**A, B). As the UCL becomes incompetent, the osseous constraints of the posteromedial elbow become important stabilizers during throwing. Subtle laxity in the UCL also leads to stretch of the other medial structures, including the flexor-pronator mass and ulnar nerve. Extrinsic valgus stresses and intrinsic muscular contractions of the flexor-pronator mass lead to tendonitis. Completing the spectrum of thrower's elbow,

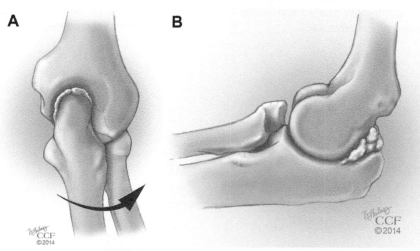

Fig. 3. Valgus extension overload syndrome. (*A*) Posterior view demonstrating valgus force on the elbow. (*B*) Lateral view demonstrating posterior olecranon osteophytes. (*Courtesy of* Clinic Center for Medical Art & Photography © 2014, Cleveland. All Rights Reserved; with permission.)

ulnar neuropathy is common given the superficial position of the nerve. The nerve is susceptible to injury from traction, compression, and irritation at the medial aspect of the elbow. In any overhead throwing athlete, UCL attenuation or failure must be ruled out but should not be the only pathology considered.

HISTORY AND PHYSICAL EXAMINATION

A thorough history starts with knowing the patients, their sport, and their level of competition. Asking an athlete specifically about the chief complaint may help delineate between primary (ie, decreased velocity on pitch from UCL attenuation) and secondary processes (ie, pain from posteromedial impingement). Complaints may include pain, decreased motion, mechanical symptoms (clicking, locking, popping, and so forth), instability, and paresthesias as well as throwing-specific symptoms. Changes in accuracy, velocity, stamina, and strength aid in diagnosis and serve as markers to measure improvement. Timing of symptoms may not always be clear; however, if a specific injury or event occurred, it is important to know when, how, and whether there were any antecedent or prodromal symptoms. Any changes in a training or throwing regimen should be noted, including pitch counts, innings pitched, games pitched, and rest between pitching for baseball players.

The timing, onset, and frequency of pain are important to determine.[20,37] In athletes with valgus instability, approximately 85% experience pain during the late cocking and early acceleration phases of throwing.[38]

Physical examination starts with inspection of an athlete's posture, arm position, muscle mass, and skin. Any asymmetries compared with contralateral extremity should be detected. Elbow flexion to approximately 70° allows the greatest intracapsular volume and may be an indication of effusion.[6] Flexion, at a lesser degree, may be secondary to an extension block from posteromedial olecronan osteophytes. With the elbow in extension and forearm in full supination, the carrying angle can be determined. The normal carrying angle is 11° in men and 13° in women.[39] Lastly, inspect the skin for any ecchymoses or prior incisions.

Palpate the olecranon, medial and lateral epicondyles, radial head, and soft spot to establish the important landmarks of the elbow. Tenderness on palpation of these landmarks may indicate acute fracture, stress fracture, or tendonitis. In skeletally immature athletes, tenderness may indicate injury to the apophysis or physis. Lateral olecranon tenderness to palpation may indicate a stress fracture whereas proximal medial tenderness may be related to impingement. Lastly, palpation of the radial head during an arc of passive supination and pronation can help identify osteochondral defects, joint incongruency, and injury to the annular ligament.

Tenderness over the insertions of the various tendons around the elbow can indicate microtrauma or inflammation. The flexor-pronator mass lies just distal to the medial epicondyle with the arm at 90°. Having patients actively flex the wrist helps identify the tendinous mass, accentuate any pain, and differentiate from UCL pathology. Ranging the elbow from 90° of flexion to approximately 50° to 70° of flexion helps to displace the flexor-pronator mass anterior and exposing the UCL just posterior. Focal swelling and tenderness along the UCL should be concerning. As discussed previously, the UCL has 3 distinct bundles, with the anterior bundle running from the inferior aspect of the medial epicondyle to the medial aspect of the coronoid process.

Directly posterior and distal to the medial epicondyle lies the cubital tunnel, which encloses the ulnar nerve. Palpation of the ulnar nerve from proximal at the arcade of Struthers to distal at the FCU should not elicit any pain. Furthermore, percussion of the nerve should be benign (Tinel sign), but radiating symptoms into the ulnar hand and 2 digits indicate ulnar nerve pathology. The ulnar nerve may be symptomatic, however, even if tenderness is not appreciated. The elbow should be fully extended and then flexed with and without pressure on the nerve proximal to the medial epicondyle. Anterior subluxation of the ulnar nerve can cause local or radiating discomfort.[40,41]

Stability of the elbow can be assessed with patients in either the supine or seated position. In the supine position, the humerus is stabilized in maximal external rotation and 30° of flexion.[4,42,43] With the forearm fully pronated and the elbow flexed 20° to 30° to unlock the olecranon from the olecranon fossa, valgus stress is gradually applied to the elbow and opening is assessed.[44] Less than 1 mm of opening and a firm endpoint should normally be appreciated during the manual valgus stress test. Physiologic laxity may be present, however, and it is more appropriate to compare the stability with the contralateral extremity. Increased opening of the joint space or reproduction of a patient's pain should raise suspicion of injury to the anterior band of the anterior bundle of the UCL.[7,38,44]

The milking maneuver tests the posterior band of the anterior bundle of the UCL. In this maneuver, the forearm is supinated fully and the elbow is flexed beyond 90° (approximately 120°) and the humerus is at the athlete's side (Fig. 4).[7] The

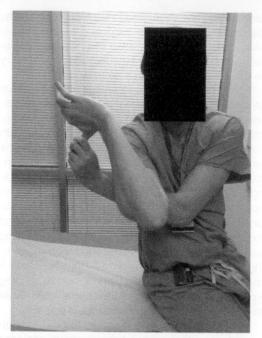

Fig. 4. Milking maneuver for evaluation of the UCL. The forearm is supinated fully and the elbow is flexed beyond 90°. The thumb is then pulled laterally by the athlete's contralateral extremity, creating a valgus force on the elbow. Pain, instability, or apprehension is indicative of injury to the UCL.

thumb is then pulled laterally by the examiner or the athlete's contralateral extremity, creating a valgus force on the elbow. Pain, instability, or apprehension is indicative of injury to the UCL.

Lastly, with the patient in the seated position and the forearm supinated, the elbow is slightly flexed. With one hand on the posterior aspect of the distal humerus and the other hand on the volar forearm, the elbow is rapidly extended while applying a valgus stress.[36] Pain with this valgus extension overload test indicates impingement of the posteromedial tip of the olecranon on the medial wall of the olecranon fossa.

IMAGING MODALITIES

Standard anteroposterior, lateral, and oblique radiographs are obtained of the elbow. Radiographs may demonstrate calcification of the UCL, osteophytes adjacent to the UCL, olecranon fossa osteophytes, sclerotic OCD lesions, and/or loose bodies. Fluoroscopy is useful in assessing for medial instability by stressing the elbow and comparing with the contralateral extremity. Asymmetry alone, however, may not be enough to diagnose acute injury to the UCL because asymptomatic pitchers have been found to have some laxity in pitching elbow compared with the

contralateral extremity.[33,45] Nevertheless, greater than 3 mm of opening is concerning for UCL injury and valgus instability.[5,7]

Conventional radiographs are not sensitive for detecting stress injuries in bone. The sensitivity of initial radiographs is as low as 15% and becomes positive over time in only 50% of patients.[46,47]

Radionuclide bone scanning is sensitive but less specific for detecting osseous stress injuries, even in their early stages.[48–52] Radionuclide technetium Tc 99m diphosphonate triple-phase scanning can provide the diagnosis as early as 2 to 8 days after the onset of symptoms.[53]

CT can help differentiate between stress fractures and other conditions that may show increased uptake on bone scan (**Fig. 5**). A CT scan is not sensitive, however, in detecting stress injuries in their early stages.[54]

MRI can detect early stress changes as well as muscle and tendon changes, loose bodies, osteochondral injuries, olecranon osteophytes, and neurologic changes to thrower's elbow. MRI is useful in evaluating UCL avulsions, partial ligamentous injuries, midsubstance tears, and the status of the surrounding soft tissues (**Fig. 6**). MRI has been found 57% sensitive and 100% specific in detecting UCL injuries.[55–58] MRI arthrography seems to improve the sensitivity of detection of UCL tears, with saline injection improving the

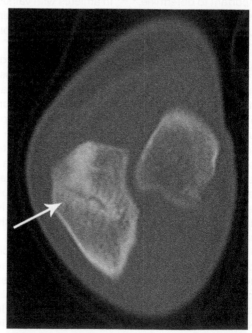

Fig. 5. Axial slice of a CT scan of a professional pitcher demonstrating a stress fracture of the olecranon (*arrow*).

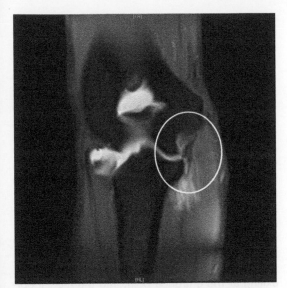

Fig. 6. Coronal slice of an MRI demonstrating a medial UCL tear (*circle*).

sensitivity of UCL detection to 92%.[56] Potter[58] and Gaary and colleagues[57] have reported similar sensitivity and specificity with nonarthrogram MRI using special sequences at the Hospital for Special Surgery. Timmerman and colleagues[59] compared CT arthrogram with both contrast-enhanced MRI and nonenhanced MRI and found a sensitivity of 86% and specificity of 91%.

ULNAR COLLATERAL LIGAMENT INJURIES

Depending on the extent of damage to the UCL, specific treatment programs can be implemented. Complete disruption of the anterior bundle of the UCL can destabilize the elbow against valgus stress encountered during the throwing motion. Partial tears of the UCL can be managed nonoperatively in low-demand patients[3,60]; however, results in overhead throwing athletes have not been promising.[61] Overall, treatment options for UCL injury include nonoperative rehabilitation, direct ligament repair, or free-tendon graft reconstruction.

Nonoperative Treatment

After a complete evaluation and diagnosis of a UCL injury through physical examination and radiologic studies, physician and athlete must agree on the appropriate course of care. Nonsurgical treatment measures are indicated for the initial treatment of sprains of the medial UCL in the vast majority of cases. Patients who present with findings consistent with a partial tear of the UCL, grade I and some grade II, should be initially

placed on a period of active rest for 6 to 12 weeks. It is important to protect the elbow from valgus stress, including throwing, for a minimum of 6 weeks. Using a criteria-based rehabilitation program assures that a patient's progress is appropriate for individual rehabilitation potential at each criteria stage.

Initially, athletes are treated with cryotherapy, pain-modulating electrotherapy modalities, antiinflammatory medication, and a hinged elbow brace restricting full extension because relief of pain and reduced inflammation dictate the subsequent rehabilitation strategies. The early focus of rehabilitation is in regaining or maintaining elbow and shoulder ROM in conjunction with shoulder-strengthening exercises. Scapular-based exercises are initiated immediately for both nonoperative and operative UCL rehabilitation programs. Patients can continue core- and lower quarter–strengthening exercises performed without gripping heavy weight or resistance. Once a patient has regained full pain-free elbow ROM, there is a progression from isometric to isotonic upper arm–based to a forearm-based resistance program focusing on strengthening the medial dynamic stabilizers with emphasis on the pronator teres, FCU, and flexor digitorum superficialis. Hamilton and colleagues[13] found that when UCL stabilizing capabilities are compromised, activity of these medially based muscles is decreased. A criteria-based return-to-throw program is initiated when functional patterns, with resistance, consistent for pitching are pain-free and valgus stress testing is negative. Retting and colleagues[62] evaluated 31 throwing athletes treated nonoperatively for a UCL injury with a minimum of 3 months of rest with rehabilitation. They reported a 42% return to competitive throwing at the same level or higher at an average of 24.5 weeks.

Recent interest in platelet-rich plasma (PRP) has led to a broad array of applications. Podesta and colleagues[63] evaluated their outcomes in 34 athletes with partial UCL tears who received 1 PRP injection to the elbow after failing 2 months of typical nonoperative management; 30 of the 34 returned to play at preinjury level at an average of 12 weeks.

Operative Treatment

Overhead throwing athletes with complete disruption of the anterior bundle of the UCL are candidates for surgical intervention if they wish to return to preinjury level of play. Athletes with partial tears unable to return to competitive throwing (or other overhead sport) due to continued medial elbow pain despite completion of an adequate course of nonoperative treatment are considered candidates for surgical treatment as well. The goal of surgical reconstruction of the medial UCL is restoration of valgus stability to the elbow.

Direct primary repair of the UCL is reserved for acute avulsion injuries from either the humeral origin or coronoid insertion.[38,64,65] UCL injuries in throwing athletes are typically present, however, as attenuated ligaments or midsubstance tears. Chronic repetitive microtrauma leads to significant scarring and subsequent inability for effective primary repair of the UCL.[61,66] Limited studies of results after primary repair of medial UCL injuries exist.[38,67,68] Level IV retrospective series have shown inconsistency in documentation of athletic level and return to play.[65,66] A case series of 47 adolescent athletes (mean age 17.2 years) by Savoie and colleagues[68] reported 93% good to excellent results after primary repair of proximal and distal ligament avulsion injuries using suture anchors or bone tunnels.

Meanwhile, studies comparing repair with reconstructive techniques have shown better results with the latter. Conway and colleagues[38] treated 14 overhead throwing athletes with UCL deficiency with primary repair and 56 with graft reconstruction. In the repaired group, 50% of the athletes returned to preinjury level of sport, and, overall, 71% had good or excellent results. In the reconstruction group, 68% returned to preinjury level of sport, whereas 80% had good or excellent results. Andrews and Timmerman[69] evaluated 72 professional baseball players who underwent elbow surgery and found that neither of the 2 athletes who underwent primary repair of the UCL returned to sport, whereas 12 of the 14 who underwent reconstruction were able to return to play. Lastly, Azar and colleagues[45] reported results of 67 patients treated with UCL primary repair or reconstruction with 12- to 72-month follow-up; 5 of the 8 patients (63%) treated with repair returned to preinjury level of play compared with 48 of 59 (81%) in the reconstruction group.

Frank Jobe first performed reconstruction of the elbow medial UCL on September 25, 1974, on Los Angeles Dodgers left-handed pitcher Tommy John. John returned to pitching in 1976 and over the next 13 seasons went on to pitch 2500 innings, compiling a record of 164 wins and 125 loses, and never having another significant problem with his elbow. John's successful return to pitching after surgery revolutionized the treatment of athletes with injuries to the medial UCL and popularized the procedure, known as *Tommy John surgery*.

In the Jobe 3-ply technique, the ipsilateral palmaris longus tendon is harvested as a graft.[38,64] Other suitable options for graft material include the contralateral palmaris longus tendon and gracilis tendon. Allograft gracilis tendon may also be used. Savoie and colleagues[70] performed hamstring allograft medial UCL reconstruction in 116 overhead athletes. Of these 116 athletes, 110 returned to play with 88% playing at or above preinjury level.

Two converging drill holes are created in the sublime tubercle of the proximal ulna, creating a bone tunnel, and 2 divergent drill holes are created in the medial epicondyle (**Fig. 7**). With the assistance of a suture passer, the graft is passed first through the bone tunnel in the ulna. It is then crossed over itself as the posterior limb of the graft is passed up the anterior tunnel into the medial epicondyle with the anterior limb going into the posterior tunnel. The limb within the posterior tunnel is then brought up around the back of the epicondyle and passed distally back into the anterior tunnel, exiting at the entrance point into the medial epicondyle. With the elbow positioned in approximately 30° of flexion and the forearm in neutral rotation, with a slight varus moment applied to the elbow, the graft is tensioned and sutured to itself, resulting in a 3-ply graft reconstruction. Any remaining native ligament is then incorporated into the graft, reinforcing the construct.

The classic Jobe surgical technique involves exposing the UCL by reflecting the flexor-pronator origin off the medial epicondyle and anteriorly transposing the ulnar nerve in a submuscular position. Early published results of medial UCL reconstructions performed using this technique reported a high incidence of postoperative ulnar nerve complications.[38,64] Thompson and colleagues reported a 31% incidence of postoperative ulnar nerve dysfunction whereas Smith and colleagues found an incidence of 21%. In an effort to minimize these complications, contemporary techniques use a muscle-splitting approach through the FCU.[71,72] Additionally, most surgeons currently reserve ulnar nerve transposition for those athletes with clinically significant ulnar nerve instability.[72]

Several modifications of the Jobe original 3-ply technique have been developed over the past decade.[73] In addition, a variety of graft fixation methods have been investigated in both the clinical and laboratory settings. These include interference screws, suture anchors, flip-buttons, and combinations of these fixation methods, along with variations in tunnel placement both proximally and distally.[73–87] An arthroscopically assisted technique has been studied in the laboratory and has shown biomechanically promising results.[85]

The most widely applied and studied of these newer techniques is the docking procedure.[74,76,77,83,84,86,88,89] In the docking technique,

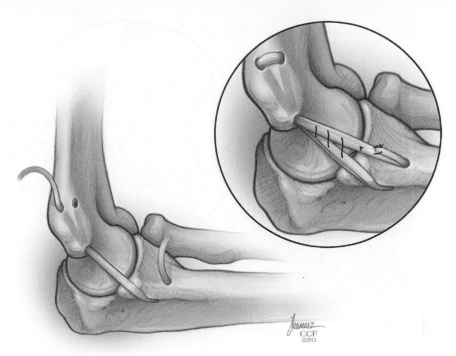

Fig. 7. Illustration of classic 3-ply medial UCL reconstruction technique as described by Jobe. Inset: Completed reconstruction. (*Courtesy of* Clinic Center for Medical Art & Photography © 2014, Cleveland. All Rights Reserved; with permission.)

converging drill holes are used to create a tunnel at the level of the sublime tubercle of the proximal ulna as in the Jobe 3-ply method. Instead of divergent tunnels in the medial epicondyle of the humerus, however, a single blind-ended tunnel (socket) is created (**Fig. 8**). At the end of this socket, 2 small exit holes are created to allow for passage of sutures that have been sutured to end of the graft. These sutures are used to pull the graft into the humeral socket where it is seated at the base. The passing sutures are then tied to each other over the back of the epicondyle. This method of fixation eliminates the suture/graft interface that is present in the 3-ply reconstruction and has been shown in biomechanical studies to have higher peak load to failure values compared with Jobe and interference screw techniques.[74,83] A recent systematic review by Watson and colleagues[90] found that the docking technique and a suspensory button technique most commonly failed secondary to suture failure, whereas the most common modes of failure for the Jobe technique and interference screw technique were ulnar tunnel fractures and graft ruptures, respectively.

A modification of the docking technique has recently been introduced. The DANE TJ UCL reconstruction uses traditional docking fixation proximally into a socket within the medial epicondyle of the humerus.[82,91] Distally, however, instead of a tunnel in the ulna, another socket is created

(**Fig. 9**). Fixation of the ulnar end of the graft is achieved with an interference screw, whereas fixation proximally is performed with 2 sutures exiting the end of the humeral socket and tied to each other, as in the traditional docking technique. To augment proximal fixation of the graft, some surgeons place an interference screw within the medial epicondyle socket. The addition of an interference screw for fixation proximally has been shown to result in less gap formation under valgus loading in the laboratory setting, perhaps allowing for better healing of the graft within the humeral bone socket.[78–80] Aperture fixation, as is achieved with interference screws, may also result in increased graft isometry and increased stiffness of the overall construct.[75] Concerns with this type of fixation include low initial fixation strength and the potential for graft slippage in the early postoperative period.[78]

Surgical reconstruction of the UCL dictates a reduced pace of rehabilitation and is a lengthy process. Therefore, the postoperative management varies depending on the surgical procedure performed. The initial goals of the program center on protection of the UCL graft, decreasing pain and effusion, and maintaining muscular strength in the forearm-based musculature.

Patients are fit postoperatively with a posteriorly based elbow splint fixed at 90° of flexion for immobilization and a compression dressing during the

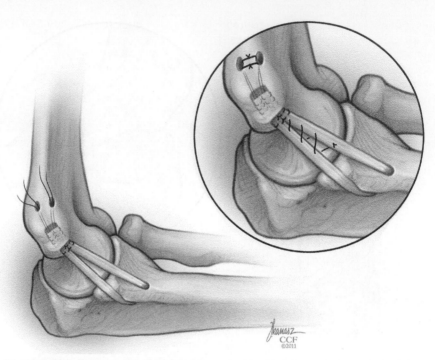

Fig. 8. Schematic of original docking technique for UCL reconstruction. Inset: Completed reconstruction. (*Courtesy of* Clinic Center for Medical Art & Photography © 2014, Cleveland. All Rights Reserved; with permission.)

acute phase of healing. During the immediate postoperative, acute phase of healing, the athlete is started on a program emphasizing wrist flexion and extension active ROM gripping exercises, while maintaining a neutral wrist position, and submaximal isometric exercises for the hand, wrist, and elbow in all directions. The initiation of the subacute phase of rehabilitation, usually 2 to

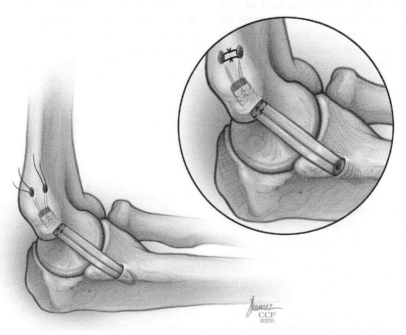

Fig. 9. Drawing of the DANE TJ modification of the docking technique. Inset: Completed reconstruction. (*Courtesy of* Clinic Center for Medical Art & Photography © 2014, Cleveland. All Rights Reserved; with permission.)

4 weeks, occurs as patients are transferred from the posterior splint to a hinged elbow brace that allows between 40° and 100° of elbow motion. The ROM is gradually increased so that full elbow ROM is achieved by postoperative week 5 to 6, at which time the hinged elbow brace usage is discontinued. Isometric exercise progression is advanced to include moderately applied force and light resistance isotonic exercises. Initiating the isotonic exercises while maintaining decreased valgus load allows for maximum support of the elbow as a new exercise procedure is introduced into the rehabilitation program. The athlete is advanced in the scapular stabilization and shoulder exercise program to include light to moderate resistance below 90° of shoulder elevation. Manual resistance is used for scapular stabilization exercises and short arc proprioceptive neuromuscular facilitation upper extremity patterns are initiated with resistance placed proximal to the elbow.

During the intermediate phase of rehabilitation, 6 to 10 weeks, the exercise program is advanced to include shoulder positioning into external rotation coupled with scapular retraction, shoulder elevation greater than 90°, biceps and triceps isotonic resistance, wrist pronation and supination, and core stabilization. Eccentric loading is initiated manually between 9 and 10 weeks postoperatively. Emphasis is placed on exercises that activate the FCU and flexor digitorum superficialis because they are believed to assist the UCL in medial elbow stabilization. Plyometric exercises are initiated after successful performance of manual and active resisted eccentric loading exercises. The athlete couples the exercise progression with nonthrowing baseball pitching–specific drills for balance point position, arm path to shoulder/elbow 90/90 positioning, and stride direction and length. The shoulder rotator cuff and scapulothoracic exercises incorporate functional chain positioning of the lower extremity and trunk to maximize complex movement patterns necessary for a successful return to throwing. A return-to-throw progression and interval throwing program is initiated at week 16.

Outcomes after UCL reconstruction have shown generally favorable results, with reported return-to-play rates as high as 95%.[38,45,64,67,72,77,84,88,89,91,92] A systematic review of the literature by Vitale and Ahmad[93] concluded that overall 83% of patients (493) had excellent results (return to the same level of play for at least 1 year). An overall complication rate of 10% is reported, with ulnar nerve complications the most common. Better results were seen with a muscle-splitting surgical approach, no ulnar nerve

transposition, and utilization of the docking technique. Also, adolescent athletes do not fare as well as college and professional athletes after surgical reconstruction of the UCL. In a retrospective study of 27 high school athletes who had undergone UCL reconstruction, Petty and colleagues[94] reported that only 74% were able to return to the same level of play after surgery. They identified grossly positive stress radiographs, sublime tubercle avulsion fractures, and ossicles within the proximal end of the ligament as poor prognostic indicators.

In a more recent systematic review of more than 1300 patients, Watson and colleagues[90] found the docking technique demonstrated a lower complication rate (6.0%) compared with the Jobe technique (51.4%) ($P = 4.48 \times 10^{-6}$). Additionally, there was a trend toward a greater rate of return to play with the docking technique compared with the Jobe technique at 90.4% and 66.7%, respectively ($P = 1.29 \times 10^{-5}$).

Revision surgery for the treatment of failed reconstructed ligaments is technically challenging and is associated with a high incidence of complications and generally poor outcomes.[95,96] In a recent case series, Dines and colleagues[96] reported that only 33% of athletes were able to return to play after revision medial UCL reconstruction, with 40% of patients experiencing complications.

ULNAR NEUROPATHY

Ulnar neuropathy at the elbow is the second most prominent neuropathy of the upper extremity, and its superficial location makes it particularly susceptible to injury in throwing athletes. The ulnar nerve is susceptible to several mechanical factors, including compression, traction, and irritation of the nerve.[44] During the acceleration phase of the throwing motion, the ulnar nerve is subject to longitudinal traction.[97] Potential sites of compression proximal to the cubital tunnel include the arcade of Struthers and the medial intermuscular septum. Distal sites of potential compression include the area between the FCU and the medial forearm musculature. Recently, Li and colleagues[98] even reported compression through the anconeus epitrochlearis, which may be hypertrophied in overhead throwing athletes. Aoki and colleagues[99] found a hypertrophic medial head of the triceps impinging on the ulnar nerve as the elbow was flexed greater than 90° in a series of adolescent baseball players with ulnar neuropathy. Osborne ligaments represent the predominant compression site in the cubital tunnel, which is bordered laterally by the elbow, anteriorly by the medial epicondyle, and medially by the origin of the FCU,[100,101] although compression may also occur from osteophytes, loose bodies, or synovitis.

Repetitive throwing motions can cause both physiologic and pathologic responses that may be the primary cause of ulnar neuropathy.[102,103] Many secondary causes exist. More than 40% of athletes with valgus instability experience ulnar neuritis secondary to irritation from the inflammation of the UCL as well as increased stretch from valgus stress. Approximately 60% of athletes with medial epicondylitis develop ulnar nerve symptoms.[38,44,104] Osteophytes from valgus extension overload and friction from ulnar nerve subluxation can serve as underlying etiologies as well.[105]

Intraneural pressure within the ulnar nerve varies with wrist, elbow, and shoulder position. Pechan and Julis[106] found the pressure within the nerve to be 3 times the resting level when the elbow was flexed and the wrist extended. Continuation of the throwing motion with further elbow flexion and shoulder abduction causes the intraneural pressure to rise 6 times the resting level. This increased pressure is attributed to nerve stretch, tightening of the cubital tunnel, and compression.[107] Repetitive motions can induce chronic changes to the ulnar nerve and surrounding soft tissues, potentially leading to nerve fibrosis and ischemia.

In addition to the history and examination discussed previously, the elbow flexion test with the elbow maintained in maximum flexion and wrist in extension for 1 minute should be conducted. Symptoms of ulnar neuritis consist of an aching pain along the ulnar side of the forearm radiating into the ulnar 2 digits of the hand. Reports of clumsiness or numbness should be evaluated further. Monofilament testing can detect early sensory changes, and hand intrinsic atrophy or weakness represents the earliest motor changes.

Electrodiagnostic testing may be useful in diagnosing ulnar neuropathy; however, changes may not be seen until disease has advanced. Wei and colleagues[108] performed nerve conduction velocity testing in baseball pitchers and did not find a significant difference between the dominant and nondominant arms among injured pitchers. A negative electrodiagnostic test, however, does not rule out ulnar neuritis.[41,102]

Nonoperative Treatment

Nonoperative management typically begins with activity restriction, antiinflammatories, cryotherapy, and physical therapy. Ulnar subluxation or dislocation may require a brief period of immobilization. After resolution of symptoms, a gradual return-to-throw program can be initiated. Symptoms from superficial irritation of the nerve can be treated with elbow pads. Ulnar neuropathy in overhead throwing athletes typically stems, however, from an underlying cause, and as throwing is resumed, symptoms likely resurface.

Operative Treatment

Indications for operative management include failed nonoperative treatment, persistent ulnar-nerve subluxation, symptomatic tension neuropraxia, and concomitant medial elbow problems that require surgery.[107] The surgical options for treatment include decompression (in situ) of the ulnar nerve, medial epicondilectomy, and anterior transposition of the nerve (submuscular, intramuscular, or subcutaneous). Simple decompression and medial epicondilectomy are prone to failure in overhead throwing athletes. Decompression may address some of the compressive forces within and around the cubital tunnel but does not address irritation from traction and repetitive motion. Furthermore, in cases of ulnar nerve subluxation, decompression fails to stabilize the nerve. Medial epicondilectomy aims to prevent traction irritation to the nerve as it passes posterior to the medial epicondyle. Well-recognized complications include, however, nerve instability, valgus instability from iatrogenic injury to the UCL, and weakness from disruption of the flexor-pronator mass.

Anterior transposition of the ulnar nerve is the mainstay of surgical management of ulnar neuritis. Subcutaneous transposition has the advantage of less surgical morbidity to the flexor-pronator mass and may be recommended in patients undergoing concomitant UCL reconstruction.[45,109,110] The main disadvantage of the subcutaneous technique is its susceptibility to direct trauma.[44,102,103] Other concerns include potential for developing instability and recurrence of symptoms from new compression under the subcutaneous fasciodermal sling. Anterior submuscular transposition involves greater surgical dissection in the medial soft tissues and a lengthier postoperative rehabilitation course but provides thorough decompression of the nerve while protecting it from direct and indirect trauma. In submuscular transfer, the nerve sits deep to the medial flexor mass and arises superficial to the pronator muscle mass. The outcomes of ulnar nerve transposition in overhead athletes support both approaches in throwing athletes. Studies comparing the results of these techniques, including 2 meta-analyses, have not found a significant difference between the procedures in terms of postoperative clinical outcomes or motor nerve conduction velocities; however, these were not specific to throwing athletes.[111,112]

Del Pizzo and colleagues[41] reported their findings on 19 baseball players who underwent anterior subcutaneous ulnar nerve transposition for recalcitrant ulnar neuritis; 9 of 15 athletes (60%) evaluated at 3 to 58 months postoperatively were able to return to play. Rettig and Ebben[110] performed 21 anterior subcutaneous transposition procedures in 20 athletes for failed conservative management of cubital tunnel syndrome. All athletes returned to play at an average of 12.6 weeks. The investigators recommended subcutaneous transposition in light of faster postoperative recovery and rehabilitation.

The senior authors' (SMG and MSS) preference is subcutaneous anterior transposition of the ulnar nerve supported by facial slings, paying particular care to preserve the motor branches to the FCU. A 4- to 6-cm curvilinear incision is made just posterior to the medial epicondyle along the path of the ulnar nerve. Dissection is carried out, taking care to protect any branches of the medial antebrachial cutaneous nerve. The ulnar nerve is identified in the cubital tunnel by opening the cubital tunnel at its midsection just posterior to the medial epicondyle. The distal one-half of the cubital tunnel is then released, including the Osborne ligament and any compressive fibers in the proximal FCU. The proximal cubital tunnel is then released, extending proximally to the arcade of Struthers. Two fascial slings are developed from the superficial flexor-pronator muscle fascia, and the fascia is closed. The ulnar nerve is transposed anterior to the medial epicondyle and held loosely in place by suturing the fascial slings to the flexor fascia. The posterior triceps fascia is then sutured to the medial epicondyle to close the cubital tunnel, and the FCU fascial split is reapproximated loosely. The elbow is splinted in 90° of elbow flexion for the 7 to 10 days postoperatively to allow soft tissue healing, followed by progressive motion and rehabilitation to return to play.

FLEXOR-PRONATOR INJURY

The flexor-pronator muscle mass at the medial side of the elbow provides dynamic stability against valgus forces.[13–16] Repetitive contraction of the flexor-pronator muscles occurs during the acceleration phase of throwing as well as with wrist flexion during ball release.[16] An acute complete rupture of the common flexor-pronator origin from the medial epicondyle is an uncommon injury in overhead athletes; rather, athletes may develop a spectrum of injuries from mild muscular overuse

to chronic tendinitis or acute partial muscle tears (**Fig. 10**).[65] The typical presentation includes an athlete with medial elbow pain during the late cocking or acceleration phase of throwing with continuation during ball release as the forearm is pronated and the wrist flexed. With complete ruptures of the flexor-pronator muscle mass, players may recall general prodromal symptoms followed by a single event leading to a pop sensation or sound.

The main differential diagnosis in these cases should include injury to the UCL. In flexor-pronator injuries, athletes have tenderness to palpation just distal to the medial epicondyle along the common origin. Meanwhile, in UCL injuries, the tenderness is typically posterior and distal to that of flexor-pronator pain along the sublime tubercle. Lastly, pain with flexor-pronator injury should be exacerbated with wrist flexion and elbow extension. Nevertheless, clinical differentiation between these 2 entities can be difficult and an MRI aids in diagnosis. Combined UCL and flexor-pronator injuries are not uncommon.

Overuse tendonitis and partial tears of the flexor-pronator muscle mass can be treated with active rest, ice, antiinflammatory medications, physical therapy, and gradual return to throwing. Corticosteroids are generally avoided given the proximity of the UCL. No data are currently available on the efficacy of PRP injections for flexor-pronator injury in overhead throwing athletes. Complete ruptures of the flexor-pronator origin require prolonged rest and rehabilitation. Splinting the wrist in neutral position may alleviate acute

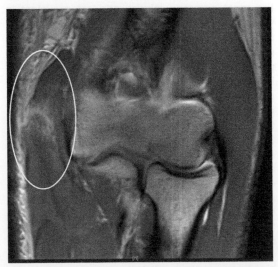

Fig. 10. Coronal slice of an MRI of a minor league reliever demonstrating a tear of the flexor-pronator mass near the proximal origin (*circle*).

pain during the first 7 to 10 days after injury. Rehabilitation with emphasis on ROM first followed by resistance training is necessary before interval throwing is initiated. If pain or weakness reoccurs with throwing, then surgical repair may be necessary. Because surgical treatment is rarely required, failure of nonoperative treatment should heighten awareness of other underlying pathology.

Overhead throwers are also vulnerable to pronator syndrome, which is compression of the median nerve caused by hypertrophy of pronator teres secondary to repetitive activity. Athletes complain of vague, fatigue-like pain over the proximal volar aspect of forearm exacerbated by resisted forearm pronation and wrist flexion. If nonoperative management with activity modification and antiinflammatory medications fails, then surgical exploration with division of superficial head of the pronator teres and decompression of the median nerve may be required. Similarly, hypertrophy of the flexor-pronator mass can cause a localized compartment syndrome induced by repetitive throwing. Medial elbow and forearm pain is associated specifically with throwing and resolves with rest. This condition may be difficult to diagnose but typically responds well to adequate stretching, interval rests, and adherence to proper pitching mechanics.[3]

MEDIAL EPICONDYLE AVULSION OR APOPHYSITIS

Little League elbow is a general term referring to medial-sided stress injuries that can occur in skeletally immature throwing athletes.[113,114] Medial epicondyle avulsion injury and apophysitis are the most common injuries and are prevalent in youth baseball. Hang and colleagues[29] found that 52% of Little League players in Taiwan reported medial elbow pain or soreness at some point during the course of a season. Grana and Rashkin[115] reported that 58% of older adolescent pitchers experience elbow pain or injury at some point during the season. In skeletally immature throwers, both the static (UCL) and dynamic (flexor-pronator muscle group) medial stabilizers attach to the medial epicondyle, thus conferring all of the static and dynamic stress to the medial epicondylar physis. Valgus and contractile forces across the elbow that result in ligament and tendon injury in the adult thrower lead to injury to the weaker medial epicondyle apophyseal plate in the skeletally immature thrower. Symptomatic injury is associated with the combination of repetitive forces on the medial elbow and inadequate intervals of rest.[116–118] The use of breaking pitches in this age group and improper throwing

mechanics have also been suggested as possible causes but not proved.[117–119] Bennett coined the term, Little Leaguer's elbow, to describe the clinical and radiographic changes associated with these medial-sided traction injuries in skeletally immature athletes.[120] Repetitive valgus loading can lead to apophyseal fragmentation or avulsion of the medial epicondyle apophysis as well as changes in the radiocapitellar joint laterally.

Medial epicondylar apophysitis should be suspected in young athletes with point tenderness over the medial epicondyle and pain with valgus stress of the elbow. Patients with avulsion fractures typically have significant swelling and decreased ROM. Radiographs may show a subtle widening of the physeal plate and comparison views of the uninvolved limb are vital. MRI typically shows more findings than radiographs; however, these do not necessarily have clinical correlation and do not change management.[121]

Initial treatment consists of an extended period of rest and cryotherapy until symptoms resolve and a gradual return to throwing. Harada and colleagues[122] found that athletes noncompliant with pitching restrictions and who returned to rigorous activity prior to bone union on radiographs had significant delays in bone union at both 6 months and 1 year compared with athletes who waited until complete bone union prior to resuming rigorous throwing. Although activity modification is successful in apophysitis, treatments of epicondylar avulsions remain controversial.[123]

In cases of complete avulsion of the medial epicondyle, most investigators recommend open reduction and internal fixation if the fragment is displaced 5 mm or greater. Nonoperative management is successful in the management of minimally displaced fractures without instability. These injuries can be treated with splint immobilization for 5 to 7 days, followed by early motion.[124–126] Lawrence and colleagues[127] recommend nonoperative management in young athletes with low-energy medial epicondyle avulsions, a stable elbow, and minimal fracture displacement (5.3 ± 2.0 mm). Open reduction and internal fixation can be successful in athletes who sustain more significant trauma, who have elbow laxity or instability, or who have significant fracture fragment displacement (7.1 ± 2.9 mm) after a fracture of the medial epicondyle.

VALGUS EXTENSION OVERLOAD SYNDROME

Valgus extension overload can occur with an attenuated UCL or in a physiologic lax elbow with repetitive valgus stress from throwing. Athletes most commonly complain of posteromedial elbow pain during the extension (late acceleration) or follow-through phase of throwing.[128] During these phases, the elbow subluxates and increases force in the lateral and posterior compartments. Continued compressive and rotatory forces in the lateral compartment lead to synovitis and osteochondrosis of the radiocapitellar joint.[3,36] Posterior and posteromedial olecranon osteophytes that form from impingement may fracture and contribute to loose bodies along with osteochondral fragments from the radiocapitellar joint (Fig. 11). When athletes complain of locking or catching, loose bodies should be considered. Radiographs may demonstrate osteophytes or loose bodies. Cohen and colleagues[129] have found a typical pattern of valgus extension overload syndrome on MRI findings. All 9 throwing athletes had pathology at the articular surfaces of the posterior trochlea and the anterior, medial olecranon. The investigators also found that these MRI findings correlated with arthroscopic findings.

Nonoperative Treatment

Initial treatment should consist of active rest with cryotherapy, iontophoresis, and antiinflammatory medications to relieve pain. As symptoms subside and motion returns to baseline, rehabilitation should include dynamic stabilization and strengthening exercises with emphasis on eccentric strengthening of the elbow flexors to control rapid extension of the elbow. Manual resistance exercises of concentric and eccentric elbow flexion are performed prior to an interval throwing program.[130]

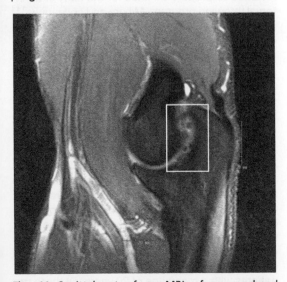

Fig. 11. Sagittal cut of an MRI of an overhead throwing athlete demonstrating multiple irregularities of the posterior articular surface of the olecranon (*square*).

Operative Treatment

Andrews and Timmerman[69] reported posteromedial olecranon impingement the most common diagnosis requiring surgery in baseball players (78%). Failure of nonoperative management for impingement-related pain is a surgical indication. Nonoperative treatment is deferred in overhead athletes with symptomatic posterior medial osteophytes or loose bodies. The treatment of choice in these instances is débridement and removal of the loose bodies. Arthroscopic treatment has become the mainstay of olecranon débridement and excision of loose bodies.[36,131] Arthroscopic evaluation also allows for débridement or drilling of osteochondral defects, resection of hypertropic synovium, and inspection for undersurface tears of the UCL.[132] Athletes must understand the risk of recurrence with continued throwing as well as risk of damage to the ulnar nerve with this technique.[69]

Reddy and colleagues[133] reported 187 arthroscopies done in 172 patients at the Kerlan-Jobe Orthopaedic Clinic. The most common diagnosis was posterior impingement (51%), followed by loose bodies (31%) and degenerative joint disease (22%). Laxity of the UCL was seen in 6% of cases. Although 68 patients were lost to follow-up, they reported 49% excellent, 36% good, 11% average, and 4% poor results, based on the modified Figgie score; 47 of the 55 professional athletes (85%) returned to their previous level of competition. There were 3 transient complications, 1 related to the ulnar nerve. Andrews and Timmerman[69] evaluated 56 professional baseball players who underwent arthroscopic olecranon osteophyte excision either as an isolated procedure or with concomitant ulnar nerve transposition or UCL reconstruction; 23 of 34 patients (68%) available for minimum 24-month follow-up returned to play at least 1 season. However, 14 (41%) required reoperation, including repeat débridement of olecranon osteophytes (6) and UCL reconstruction (5). The investigators cautioned against excessive olecranon excision. Resection of more than 3 mm of the posteromedial olecranon jeopardizes the function of the anterior bundle of the UCL because it exposes a potentially attenuated UCL to higher stresses.[134,135] Thus, it is recommended that only the osteophyte and no native olecranon be removed.

OLECRANON STRESS FRACTURE

Proximal olecranon stress fractures occur from the repetitive microtrauma, excessive tensile stress from the triceps tendon, and posterior impingement of the olecranon against the olecranon fossa associated with competitive overhead throwing.[136] Stress fractures can have posterolateral or posteromedial olecranon pain and tenderness during and after throwing.[137] There is typically no pain at rest and there is a gradual onset rather than a single event. Schickendantz and colleagues[137] state pain with percussion of the proximal ulna may indicate a stress fracture because it was a positive test in all 7 athletes with MRI-confirmed stress reactions. Stress fractures of the proximal olecranon should be differentiated from avulsion fractures of the tip of the olecranon and from a persistent olecranon apophysis, which may be treated differently. Standard radiographs as well as advanced imaging may be needed for diagnosis.

Nonoperative Treatment

Initial treatment includes rest, immobilization, and throwing cessation. Specifically, any valgus stress should be avoided for a minimum of 6 weeks. Full extension should also be avoided with the use of a splint or orthosis set to approximately 20° of extension for the first 4 weeks. At 4 weeks, full ROM is allowed and progressive resistance exercises of the elbow are initiated. At 6 weeks, sport-specific rehabilitation is initiated and an interval throwing program typically starts at approximately 8 weeks. Nuber and Diment[138] successfully treated 2 olecranon stress fractures in competitive pitchers with splinting and cessation of throwing. Both players had radiographic union and returned to pitching.

Operative Treatment

Complete olecranon stress fractures in competitive throwers often require surgical treatment with cannulated screws or plate osteosynthesis. The goal of surgical fixation is compression and rigid fixation across the fracture site. Paci and colleagues[139] have published the only report on surgical fixation of proximal olecranon stress fractures in baseball players. They performed percutaneous fixation of the proximal ulna stress fracture in 25 baseball players and had follow-up on 18 of the athletes. All 18 fractures went on to union, with 17 of 18 (94%) athletes able to return to preinjury level of play.

OSTEOCHONDRITIS DISSECANS OF THE CAPITELLUM

The radiocapitellar joint experiences compressive forces during valgus stress from overhead throwing motions. Repetitive compressive trauma, in addition to ischemia and genetics, has been implicated in the formation of OCD of the capitellum. The exact cause, however, remains unclear. A wide spectrum of injuries can result, including subchondral changes to secondary osteochondrosis of the radial head to loose bodies. Treatment depends on the severity and stability of the osteochondral lesion. Patients often complain of lateral elbow pain on palpation and valgus stress. There is frequently an associated loss of elbow extension, ranging from 5° to 20°. Athletes may also have swelling or effusion, tenderness over the lateral aspect of the elbow, and crepitance with motion.[140] Standard radiographs demonstrate classic findings of a subchondral cyst of the capitellum in early cases. In more advanced stages, flattening and irregularity of the capitellar articular surface may be seen.

Mihata and colleagues[141] performed a biomechanical cadaveric study and found that OCDs of the radiocapitellar joint increase elbow valgus laxity and contact pressure without increasing UCL strain. Natural history suggests that as many as 50% of patients experience some degeneration in the radiocapitellar joint.[142]

Nonoperative Treatment

Nonoperative management should be reserved for early lesions and consists of a minimum 6-week period of rest from throwing and valgus stress.[143] After pain resolves, a strengthening program is initiated with isometric exercises, followed by isotonic exercises. Aggressive high-speed, eccentric, and plyometric exercises are progressively included to prepare athletes for the start of an interval throwing program. Mihara and colleagues[144] reported on 39 baseball players with a mean age of 12.8 years with OCD lesions of the capitellum treated nonoperatively. At a mean follow-up of 14.4 months, 25 of 30 early lesions were healed compared with 1 of 9 advanced lesions. A majority of the lesions in patients with open physes healed (16 of 17) compared with only 11 of 22 patients with closed physes.

Operative Treatment

Surgical intervention is limited to patients who do not respond to a nonoperative course of treatment or those with advanced disease resulting in the development of loose fragments within the joint. Initially, surgical management consisted of open débridement and fragment excision. Bauer and colleagues[145] reported long-term outcomes in 31 patients with a mean age of 20 years. Of these patients, 22 had loose body excision and 1 had radial head excision, and most cases seemed to be advanced lesions (20 of 31). At average 23-year follow-up, there was a 40% recurrence of symptoms and loss of elbow extension, with greater than 60% of examined radiocapitellar joints demonstrating degenerative joint disease. In an initial study, Takahara and colleagues[142] reported 39 patients with an average age of 17.6 years treated with open fragment excision. At average 14.7 years' follow-up, 26% of patients reported good results, and 49% returned to full sports participation. Takahara and colleagues[146] followed their initial study with another study adding 16 patients to their original cohort. The investigators added that better results in terms of pain and radiographic findings were seen in patients with lesions measuring less than 50% of the capitellar articular width.

Arthroscopic débridement and abrasion chondroplasty have had promising results in numerous short and midterm follow-up studies, with pain relief and objective improvements in elbow ROM.[140,147–150] Byrd and Jones[148] examined 10 patients ages 11 to 16 years, 7 with advanced disease (grade IV or V lesions based on the American Sports Medicine Institute classification system of OCD lesions). At 4-year follow-up, although all 7 lesions healed, only 4 of 10 patients had returned to sport, and 2 demonstrated degenerative radiographic findings. The investigators found no correlation between grade of lesion and postoperative outcomes or return to sport. Ruch and colleagues[151] treated 12 patients, ages 11 to 17 years, with unstable elbow lesions (mean size 2.5 cm) for a mean of 3.2 years. Improved extension was seen postoperatively, mechanical symptoms resolved in 11 patients, and 11 of 12 patients were highly satisfied. Radiographs demonstrated capitellar remodeling in all elbows. Only 3 patients, however, returned to sport.

Fragment fixation has been attempted through a variety of techniques and implants.[146,152–155] Reliable results have been seen in advanced cases, but published data have been limited to small case series. Lateral closing wedge osteotomy has been used to unload the radiocapitellar joint. The procedure is technically challenging because ulnohumeral joint alignment must be maintained. Because the lesion is not directly addressed, this procedure is reserved for early lesions that are stable. Kiyoshige and colleagues[156] evaluated 7 baseball players ages 11 to 18 who underwent a lateral closing wedge osteotomy. At 7- to 12-year follow-up, 6 of 7 patients (86%) had complete relief of pain with return to sport.

Osteochondral autograft transplantation (OAT) is another technique to treat advanced OCD lesions of the capitellum. Contraindications include degenerative changes in the radiocapitellar compartment and radial head and capitellar deformity. Placement of grafts in the tight lateral compartment make congruent placement of the graft difficult.[157] Early results demonstrate reasonable outcomes with OAT but long-term follow-up in the throwing population is needed before definitive conclusions can be drawn.[158,159]

SUMMARY

Overhead throwing activities expose the elbow to tremendous valgus stress, making athletes vulnerable to a specific constellation of injuries. Although baseball players, in particular pitchers, are the athletes most commonly affected, overhead athletes in football, volleyball, tennis, and javelin throwing also are affected.

Increasing participation in overhead throwing sports has led to a sharp increase in injuries. Understanding the anatomy and function of the elbow, along with the biomechanical relationship between the two, remains vital to appropriate management. Advances in surgical technique to reconstruct the UCL have led to improved outcomes while multiple fixation devices and grafts have been evaluated.

REFERENCES

1. Nassab PF, Schickendantz MS. Evaluation and treatment of medial ulnar collateral ligament injuries in the throwing athlete. Sports Med Arthrosc 2006;14(4):221–31.
2. National Federation of State High School Associations. National Federation of State High School Associations 2012–2013 High school athletics participation survey. 2013.
3. Millor CD, Savoie FH 3rd. Valgus extension injuries of the elbow in the throwing athlete. J Am Acad Orthop Surg 1994;2(5):261–9.
4. Morrey BF, Tanaka S, An KN. Valgus stability of the elbow. A definition of primary and secondary constraints. Clin Orthop Relat Res 1991;(265):187–95.
5. Schwab GH, Bennett JB, Woods GW, et al. Biomechanics of elbow instability: the role of the medial collateral ligament. Clin Orthop Relat Res 1980;(146):42–52.
6. Morrey BF. Applied anatomy and biomechanics of the elbow joint. Instr Course Lect 1986;35:59–68.
7. Jobe FW, Kvitne RS. Elbow instability in the athlete. Instr Course Lect 1991;40:17–23.
8. Sojbjerg JO, Ovesen J, Nielsen S. Experimental elbow instability after transection of the medial collateral ligament. Clin Orthop Relat Res 1987;(218):186–90.
9. Regan WD, Korinek SL, Morrey BF, et al. Biomechanical study of ligaments around the elbow joint. Clin Orthop Relat Res 1991;(271):170–9.

10. Callaway GH, Field LD, Deng XH, et al. Biomechanical evaluation of the medial collateral ligament of the elbow. J Bone Joint Surg Am 1997; 79(8):1223–31.

11. Davidson PA, Pink M, Perry J, et al. Functional anatomy of the flexor pronator muscle group in relation to the medial collateral ligament of the elbow. Am J Sports Med 1995;23(2):245–50.

12. Jobe FW, Moynes DR, Tibone JE, et al. An EMG analysis of the shoulder in pitching. A second report. Am J Sports Med 1984;12(3):218–20.

13. Hamilton CD, Glousman RE, Jobe FW, et al. Dynamic stability of the elbow: electromyographic analysis of the flexor pronator group and the extensor group in pitchers with valgus instability. J Shoulder Elbow Surg 1996;5(5):347–54.

14. Glousman RE, Barron J, Jobe FW, et al. An electromyographic analysis of the elbow in normal and injured pitchers with medial collateral ligament insufficiency. Am J Sports Med 1992;20(3):311–7.

15. Digiovine NM, Jobe FW, Pink M, et al. An electromyographic analysis of the upper extremity in pitching. J Shoulder Elbow Surg 1992;1(1):15–25.

16. Sisto DJ, Jobe FW, Moynes DR, et al. An electromyographic analysis of the elbow in pitching. Am J Sports Med 1987;15(3):260–3.

17. MacWilliams BA, Choi T, Perezous MK, et al. Characteristic ground-reaction forces in baseball pitching. Am J Sports Med 1998;26(1):66–71.

18. Watkins RG, Dennis S, Dillin WH, et al. Dynamic EMG analysis of torque transfer in professional baseball pitchers. Spine 1989;14(4):404–8.

19. Pappas AM, Zawacki RM, Sullivan TJ. Biomechanics of baseball pitching. A preliminary report. Am J Sports Med 1985;13(4):216–22.

20. Fleisig GS, Andrews JR, Dillman CJ, et al. Kinetics of baseball pitching with implications about injury mechanisms. Am J Sports Med 1995;23(2): 233–9.

21. Dines JS, Frank JB, Akerman M, et al. Glenohumeral internal rotation deficits in baseball players with ulnar collateral ligament insufficiency. Am J Sports Med 2009;37(3):566–70.

22. Garrison JC, Cole MA, Conway JE, et al. Shoulder range of motion deficits in baseball players with an ulnar collateral ligament tear. Am J Sports Med 2012;40(11):2597–603.

23. Meister K, Day T, Horodyski M, et al. Rotational motion changes in the glenohumeral joint of the adolescent/Little League baseball player. Am J Sports Med 2005;33(5):693–8.

24. Crockett HC, Gross LB, Wilk KE, et al. Osseous adaptation and range of motion at the glenohumeral joint in professional baseball pitchers. Am J Sports Med 2002;30(1):20–6.

25. Borsa PA, Wilk KE, Jacobson JA, et al. Correlation of range of motion and glenohumeral translation in professional baseball pitchers. Am J Sports Med 2005;33(9):1392–9.

26. Mihata T, Lee Y, McGarry MH, et al. Excessive humeral external rotation results in increased shoulder laxity. Am J Sports Med 2004;32(5):1278–85.

27. Polster JM, Bullen J, Obuchowski NA, et al. Relationship between humeral torsion and injury in professional baseball pitchers. Am J Sports Med 2013;41(9):2015–21.

28. Burkhart SS, Morgan CD, Kibler WB. The disabled throwing shoulder: spectrum of pathology Part I: pathoanatomy and biomechanics. Arthroscopy 2003;19(4):404–20.

29. Hang DW, Chao CM, Hang YS. A clinical and roentgenographic study of Little League elbow. Am J Sports Med 2004;32(1):79–84.

30. Limpisvasti O, ElAttrache NS, Jobe FW. Understanding shoulder and elbow injuries in baseball. J Am Acad Orthop Surg 2007;15(3):139–47.

31. Kooima CL, Anderson K, Craig JV, et al. Evidence of subclinical medial collateral ligament injury and posteromedial impingement in professional baseball players. Am J Sports Med 2004;32(7):1602–6.

32. Nazarian LN, McShane JM, Ciccotti MG, et al. Dynamic US of the anterior band of the ulnar collateral ligament of the elbow in asymptomatic major league baseball pitchers. Radiology 2003;227(1): 149–54.

33. Ellenbecker TS, Mattalino AJ, Elam EA, et al. Medial elbow joint laxity in professional baseball pitchers. A bilateral comparison using stress radiography. Am J Sports Med 1998;26(3):420–4.

34. Mair SD, Uhl TL, Robbe RG, et al. Physeal changes and range-of-motion differences in the dominant shoulders of skeletally immature baseball players. J Shoulder Elbow Surg 2004;13(5):487–91.

35. King JW, Brelsford HJ, Tullos HS. Analysis of the pitching arm of the professional baseball pitcher. Clin Orthop Relat Res 1969;67:116–23.

36. Wilson FD, Andrews JR, Blackburn TA, et al. Valgus extension overload in the pitching elbow. Am J Sports Med 1983;11(2):83–8.

37. Yocum LA. The diagnosis and nonoperative treatment of elbow problems in the athlete. Clin Sports Med 1989;8(3):439–51.

38. Conway JE, Jobe FW, Glousman RE, et al. Medial instability of the elbow in throwing athletes. Treatment by repair or reconstruction of the ulnar collateral ligament. J Bone Joint Surg Am 1992;74(1):67–83.

39. Beals RK. The normal carrying angle of the elbow. A radiographic study of 422 patients. Clin Orthop Relat Res 1976;(119):194–6.

40. Childress HM. Recurrent ulnar-nerve dislocation at the elbow. Clin Orthop Relat Res 1975;(108):168–73.

41. Del Pizzo W, Jobe FW, Norwood L. Ulnar nerve entrapment syndrome in baseball players. Am J Sports Med 1977;5(5):182–5.

42. Morrey BF, An KN. Functional anatomy of the ligaments of the elbow. Clin Orthop Relat Res 1985;(201):84–90.

43. Morrey BF, An KN. Articular and ligamentous contributions to the stability of the elbow joint. Am J Sports Med 1983;11(5):315–9.

44. Boatright JR, D'Alessandro DF. Nerve entrapment syndromes at the elbow. Operative techniques in upper extremity sports injuries. St Louis (MO): Mosby-Year; 1996. p. 518–37.

45. Azar FM, Andrews JR, Wilk KE, et al. Operative treatment of ulnar collateral ligament injuries of the elbow in athletes. Am J Sports Med 2000; 28(1):16–23.

46. Greaney RB, Gerber FH, Laughlin RL, et al. Distribution and natural history of stress fractures in U.S. Marine recruits. Radiology 1983;146(2):339–46.

47. Nielsen MB, Hansen K, Holmer P, et al. Tibial periosteal reactions in soldiers. A scintigraphic study of 29 cases of lower leg pain. Acta Orthop Scand 1991;62(6):531–4.

48. Zwas ST, Elkanovitch R, Frank G. Interpretation and classification of bone scintigraphic findings in stress fractures. J Nucl Med 1987;28(4):452–7.

49. Wilcox JR Jr, Moniot AL, Green JP. Bone scanning in the evaluation of exercise-related stress injuries. Radiology 1977;123(3):699–703.

50. Geslien GE, Thrall JH, Espinosa JL, et al. Early detection of stress fractures using 99mTc-polyphosphate. Radiology 1976;121(3):683–7.

51. Prather JL, Nusynowitz ML, Snowdy HA, et al. Scintigraphic findings in stress fractures. J Bone Joint Surg Am 1977;59(7):869–74.

52. Ammann W, Matheson GO. Radionuclide bone imaging in the detection of stress fractures. Clin J Sport Med 1991;1(2):115–22.

53. Roub LW, Gumerman LW, Hanley EN Jr, et al. Bone stress: a radionuclide imaging perspective. Radiology 1979;132(2):431–8.

54. Matheson GO, Clement DB, McKenzie DC, et al. Stress fractures in athletes. A study of 320 cases. Am J Sports Med 1987;15(1):46–58.

55. Nakanishi K, Masatomi T, Ochi T, et al. MR arthrography of elbow: evaluation of the ulnar collateral ligament of elbow. Skeletal Radiol 1996;25(7):629–34.

56. Schwartz ML, al-Zahrani S, Morwessel RM, et al. Ulnar collateral ligament injury in the throwing athlete: evaluation with saline-enhanced MR arthrography. Radiology 1995;197(1):297–9.

57. Gaary EA, Potter HG, Altchek DW. Medial elbow pain in the throwing athlete: MR imaging evaluation. AJR Am J Roentgenol 1997;168(3):795–800.

58. Potter HG. Imaging of posttraumatic and soft tissue dysfunction of the elbow. Clin Orthop Relat Res 2000;(370):9–18.

59. Timmerman LA, Schwartz ML, Andrews JR. Preoperative evaluation of the ulnar collateral ligament by magnetic resonance imaging and computed tomography arthrography. Evaluation in 25 baseball players with surgical confirmation. Am J Sports Med 1994;22(1):26–31 [discussion: 32].

60. Kenter K, Behr CT, Warren RF, et al. Acute elbow injuries in the National Football League. J Shoulder Elbow Surg 2000;9(1):1–5.

61. Arendt EA, editor. Orthopaedic knowledge update sports medicine. Rosemont (IL): AAOS; 1999.

62. Rettig AC, Sherrill C, Snead DS, et al. Nonoperative treatment of ulnar collateral ligament injuries in throwing athletes. Am J Sports Med 2001;29(1): 15–7.

63. Podesta L, Crow SA, Volkmer D, et al. Treatment of partial ulnar collateral ligament tears in the elbow with platelet-rich plasma. Am J Sports Med 2013; 41(7):1689–94.

64. Jobe FW, Stark H, Lombardo SJ. Reconstruction of the ulnar collateral ligament in athletes. J Bone Joint Surg Am 1986;68(8):1158–63.

65. Norwood LA, Shook JA, Andrews JR. Acute medial elbow ruptures. Am J Sports Med 1981;9(1):16–9.

66. Morrey BF, Regan WD. Throwing injuries. In: DeLee JC, Drez D Jr, editors. Orthopaedic sports medicine: principles and practice. Philadelphia: WB Saunders; 1994. p. 882–9.

67. Cain EL Jr, Andrews JR, Dugas JR, et al. Outcome of ulnar collateral ligament reconstruction of the elbow in 1281 athletes: results in 743 athletes with minimum 2-year follow-up. Am J Sports Med 2010;38(12):2426–34.

68. Savoie FH 3rd, Trenhaile SW, Roberts J, et al. Primary repair of ulnar collateral ligament injuries of the elbow in young athletes: a case series of injuries to the proximal and distal ends of the ligament. Am J Sports Med 2008;36(6):1066–72.

69. Andrews JR, Timmerman LA. Outcome of elbow surgery in professional baseball players. Am J Sports Med 1995;23(4):407–13.

70. Savoie FH 3rd, Morgan C, Yaste J, et al. Medial ulnar collateral ligament reconstruction using hamstring allograft in overhead throwing athletes. J Bone Joint Surg Am 2013;95(12):1062–6.

71. Smith GR, Altchek DW, Pagnani MJ, et al. A muscle-splitting approach to the ulnar collateral ligament of the elbow. Neuroanatomy and operative technique. Am J Sports Med 1996;24(5): 575–80.

72. Thompson WH, Jobe FW, Yocum LA, et al. Ulnar collateral ligament reconstruction in athletes: muscle-splitting approach without transposition of the ulnar nerve. J Shoulder Elbow Surg 2001; 10(2):152–7.

73. Langer P, Fadale P, Hulstyn M. Evolution of the treatment options of ulnar collateral ligament injuries of the elbow. Br J Sports Med 2006;40(6): 499–506.

74. Armstrong AD, Dunning CE, Ferreira LM, et al. A biomechanical comparison of four reconstruction techniques for the medial collateral ligament-deficient elbow. J Shoulder Elbow Surg 2005; 14(2):207–15.

75. Ahmad CS, Lee TQ, ElAttrache NS. Biomechanical evaluation of a new ulnar collateral ligament reconstruction technique with interference screw fixation. Am J Sports Med 2003;31(3):332–7.

76. Ciccotti MG, Siegler S, Kuri JA 2nd, et al. Murphy DJt. Comparison of the biomechanical profile of the intact ulnar collateral ligament with the modified Jobe and the Docking reconstructed elbow: an in vitro study. Am J Sports Med 2009;37(5):974–81.

77. Dodson CC, Thomas A, Dines JS, et al. Medial ulnar collateral ligament reconstruction of the elbow in throwing athletes. Am J Sports Med 2006; 34(12):1926–32.

78. Hurbanek JG, Anderson K, Crabtree S, et al. Biomechanical comparison of the docking technique with and without humeral bioabsorbable interference screw fixation. Am J Sports Med 2009;37(3):526–33.

79. Large TM, Coley ER, Peindl RD, et al. A biomechanical comparison of 2 ulnar collateral ligament reconstruction techniques. Arthroscopy 2007;23(2):141–50.

80. McAdams TR, Lee AT, Centeno J, et al. Two ulnar collateral ligament reconstruction methods: the docking technique versus bioabsorbable interference screw fixation–a biomechanical evaluation with cyclic loading. J Shoulder Elbow Surg 2007; 16(2):224–8.

81. Morgan RJ, Starman JS, Habet NA, et al. A biomechanical evaluation of ulnar collateral ligament reconstruction using a novel technique for ulnar-sided fixation. Am J Sports Med 2010;38(7): 1448–55.

82. Nissen CW. Effectiveness of interference screw fixation in ulnar collateral ligament reconstruction. Orthopedics 2008;31(7):646.

83. Paletta GA Jr, Klepps SJ, Difelice GS, et al. Biomechanical evaluation of 2 techniques for ulnar collateral ligament reconstruction of the elbow. Am J Sports Med 2006;34(10):1599–603.

84. Paletta GA Jr, Wright RW. The modified docking procedure for elbow ulnar collateral ligament reconstruction: 2-year follow-up in elite throwers. Am J Sports Med 2006;34(10):1594–8.

85. Shah RP, Lindsey DP, Sungar GW, et al. An analysis of four ulnar collateral ligament reconstruction procedures with cyclic valgus loading. J Shoulder Elbow Surg 2009;18(1):58–63.

86. Rohrbough JT, Altchek DW, Hyman J, et al. Medial collateral ligament reconstruction of the elbow using the docking technique. Am J Sports Med 2002;30(4):541–8.

87. Starman JS, Morgan RJ, Fleischli JE, et al. Ulnar collateral ligament reconstruction using the Toggle-Loc with ZipLoop for ulnar side fixation. Orthopedics 2010;33(5):312–6.

88. Bowers AL, Dines JS, Dines DM, et al. Elbow medial ulnar collateral ligament reconstruction: clinical relevance and the docking technique. J Shoulder Elbow Surg 2010;19(Suppl 2):110–7.

89. Koh JL, Schafer MF, Keuter G, et al. Ulnar collateral ligament reconstruction in elite throwing athletes. Arthroscopy 2006;22(11):1187–91.

90. Watson JN, McQueen P, Hutchinson MR. A systematic review of ulnar collateral ligament reconstruction techniques. Am J Sports Med 2013. [Epub ahead of print].

91. Dines JS, ElAttrache NS, Conway JE, et al. Clinical outcomes of the DANE TJ technique to treat ulnar collateral ligament insufficiency of the elbow. Am J Sports Med 2007;35(12):2039–44.

92. Domb BG, Davis JT, Alberta FG, et al. Clinical follow-up of professional baseball players undergoing ulnar collateral ligament reconstruction using the new Kerlan-Jobe Orthopaedic Clinic overhead athlete shoulder and elbow score (KJOC Score). Am J Sports Med 2010;38(8):1558–63.

93. Vitale MA, Ahmad CS. The outcome of elbow ulnar collateral ligament reconstruction in overhead athletes: a systematic review. Am J Sports Med 2008;36(6):1193–205.

94. Petty DH, Andrews JR, Fleisig GS, et al. Ulnar collateral ligament reconstruction in high school baseball players: clinical results and injury risk factors. Am J Sports Med 2004;32(5):1158–64.

95. Lee GH, Limpisvasti O, Park MC, et al. Revision ulnar collateral ligament reconstruction using a suspension button fixation technique. Am J Sports Med 2010;38(3):575–80.

96. Dines JS, Yocum LA, Frank JB, et al. Revision surgery for failed elbow medial collateral ligament reconstruction. Am J Sports Med 2008;36(6): 1061–5.

97. Schickendantz MS. Diagnosis and treatment of elbow disorders in the overhead athlete. Hand Clin 2002;18(1):65–75.

98. Li X, Dines JS, Gorman M, et al. Anconeus epitrochlearis as a source of medial elbow pain in baseball pitchers. Orthopedics 2012;35(7): e1129–32.

99. Aoki M, Kanaya K, Aiki H, et al. Cubital tunnel syndrome in adolescent baseball players: a report of six cases with 3- to 5-year follow-up. Arthroscopy 2005;21(6):758.

100. Bradshaw DY, Shefner JM. Ulnar neuropathy at the elbow. Neurol Clin 1999;17(3):447–61, v–vi.

101. Huang JH, Samadani U, Zager EL. Ulnar nerve entrapment neuropathy at the elbow: simple decompression. Neurosurgery 2004;55(5):1150–3.

102. Rokito AS, Iviciviahon PJ, Jobe FW. Cubital tunnel syndrome. Oper Tech Sports Med 1996;4(1): 15–20.

103. Glousman RE. Ulnar nerve problems in the athlete's elbow. Clin Sports Med 1990;9(2):365–77.

104. Gabel GT, Morrey BF. Operative treatment of medical epicondylitis. Influence of concomitant ulnar neuropathy at the elbow. J Bone Joint Surg Am 1995;77(7):1065–9.

105. Griffin LY. Orthopaedic knowledge update sports medicine. Rosemont (IL): AAOS; 1994. p. 179–90.

106. Pechan J, Julis I. The pressure measurement in the ulnar nerve. A contribution to the pathophysiology of the cubital tunnel syndrome. J Biomech 1975; 8(1):75–9.

107. Chen FS, Rokito AS, Jobe FW. Medial elbow problems in the overhead-throwing athlete. J Am Acad Orthop Surg 2001;9(2):99–113.

108. Wei SH, Jong YJ, Chang YJ. Ulnar nerve conduction velocity in injured baseball pitchers. Arch Phys Med Rehabil 2005;86(1):21–5 [quiz: 180].

109. Cain EL Jr, Dugas JR, Wolf RS, et al. Elbow injuries in throwing athletes: a current concepts review. Am J Sports Med 2003;31(4):621–35.

110. Rettig AC, Ebben JR. Anterior subcutaneous transfer of the ulnar nerve in the athlete. Am J Sports Med 1993;21(6):836–9 [discussion: 839–40].

111. Zlowodzki M, Chan S, Bhandari M, et al. Anterior transposition compared with simple decompression for treatment of cubital tunnel syndrome. A meta-analysis of randomized, controlled trials. J Bone Joint Surg Am 2007;89(12):2591–8.

112. Macadam SA, Gandhi R, Bezuhly M, et al. Simple decompression versus anterior subcutaneous and submuscular transposition of the ulnar nerve for cubital tunnel syndrome: a meta-analysis. J Hand Surg 2008;33(8):1314.e1–2.

113. Larson RL, Singer KM, Bergstrom R, et al. Little league survey: the Eugene study. Am J Sports Med 1976;4(5):201–9.

114. Gugenheim JJ Jr, Stanley RF, Woods GW, et al. Little League survey: the Houston study. Am J Sports Med 1976;4(5):189–200.

115. Grana WA, Rashkin A. Pitcher's elbow in adolescents. Am J Sports Med 1980;8(5):333–6.

116. Benjamin HJ, Briner WW Jr. Little league elbow. Clin J Sport Med 2005;15(1):37–40.

117. Lyman S, Fleisig GS, Andrews JR, et al. Effect of pitch type, pitch count, and pitching mechanics on risk of elbow and shoulder pain in youth baseball pitchers. Am J Sports Med 2002;30(4):463–8.

118. Lyman S, Fleisig GS, Waterbor JW, et al. Longitudinal study of elbow and shoulder pain in youth baseball pitchers. Med Sci Sports Exerc 2001; 33(11):1803–10.

119. Fleisig GS, Barrentine SW, Zheng N, et al. Kinematic and kinetic comparison of baseball pitching among various levels of development. J Biomech 1999;32(12):1371–5.

120. Bennett GE. Elbow and shoulder lesions of baseball players. Am J Surg 1959;98:484–92.

121. Wei AS, Khana S, Limpisvasti O, et al. Clinical and magnetic resonance imaging findings associated with Little League elbow. J Pediatr Orthop 2010; 30(7):715–9.

122. Harada M, Takahara M, Hirayama T, et al. Outcome of nonoperative treatment for humeral medial epicondylar fragmentation before epiphyseal closure in young baseball players. Am J Sports Med 2012;40(7):1583–90.

123. Torg JS. The little league pitcher. Am Fam Physician 1972;6(2):71–6.

124. Woods GW, Tullos HS. Elbow instability and medial epicondyle fractures. Am J Sports Med 1977;5(1): 23–30.

125. Hines RF, Herndon WA, Evans JP. Operative treatment of medial epicondyle fractures in children. Clin Orthop Relat Res 1987;(223):170–4.

126. Ireland ML, Andrews JR. Shoulder and elbow injuries in the young athlete. Clin Sports Med 1988; 7(3):473–94.

127. Lawrence JT, Patel NM, Macknin J, et al. Return to competitive sports after medial epicondyle fractures in adolescent athletes: results of operative and nonoperative treatment. Am J Sports Med 2013;41(5):1152–7.

128. Loftice J, Fleisig GS, Zheng N, et al. Biomechanics of the elbow in sports. Clin Sports Med 2004;23(4): 519–30, vii–viii.

129. Cohen SB, Valko C, Zoga A, et al. Posteromedial elbow impingement: magnetic resonance imaging findings in overhead throwing athletes and results of arthroscopic treatment. Arthroscopy 2011; 27(10):1364–70.

130. Wilk KE, Macrina LC, Cain EL, et al. Rehabilitation of the Overhead Athlete's Elbow. Sports Health 2012;4(5):404–14.

131. Andrews JR, St Pierre RK, Carson WG Jr. Arthroscopy of the elbow. Clin Sports Med 1986;5(4): 653–62.

132. Timmerman LA, Andrews JR. Undersurface tear of the ulnar collateral ligament in baseball players. A newly recognized lesion. Am J Sports Med 1994; 22(1):33–6.

133. Reddy AS, Kvitne RS, Yocum LA, et al. Arthroscopy of the elbow: a long-term clinical review. Arthroscopy 2000;16(6):588–94.

134. Kamineni S, ElAttrache NS, O'Driscoll SW, et al. Medial collateral ligament strain with partial posteromedial olecranon resection. A biomechanical study. J Bone Joint Surg Am 2004;86A(11): 2424–30.

135. Ahmad CS, Park MC, Elattrache NS. Elbow medial ulnar collateral ligament insufficiency alters

posteromedial olecranon contact. Am J Sports Med 2004;32(7):1607–12.

136. Griggs SM, Weiss AP. Bony injuries of the wrist, forearm, and elbow. Clin Sports Med 1996;15(2): 373–400.

137. Schickendantz MS, Ho CP, Koh J. Stress injury of the proximal ulna in professional baseball players. Am J Sports Med 2002;30(5):737–41.

138. Nuber GW, Diment MT. Olecranon stress fractures in throwers. A report of two cases and a review of the literature. Clin Orthop Relat Res 1992;(278): 58–61.

139. Paci JM, Dugas JR, Guy JA, et al. Cannulated screw fixation of refractory olecranon stress fractures with and without associated injuries allows a return to baseball. Am J Sports Med 2013;41(2): 306–12.

140. Ruchelsman DE, Hall MP, Youm T. Osteochondritis dissecans of the capitellum: current concepts. J Am Acad Orthop Surg 2010;18(9):557–67.

141. Mihata T, Quigley R, Robicheaux G, et al. Biomechanical characteristics of osteochondral defects of the humeral capitellum. Am J Sports Med 2013;41(8):1909–14.

142. Takahara M, Ogino T, Sasaki I, et al. Long term outcome of osteochondritis dissecans of the humeral capitellum. Clin Orthop Relat Res 1999;(363):108–15.

143. Takahara M, Ogino T, Fukushima S, et al. Nonoperative treatment of osteochondritis dissecans of the humeral capitellum. Am J Sports Med 1999;27(6): 728–32.

144. Mihara K, Tsutsui H, Nishinaka N, et al. Nonoperative treatment for osteochondritis dissecans of the capitellum. Am J Sports Med 2009;37(2):298–304.

145. Bauer M, Jonsson K, Josefsson PO, et al. Osteochondritis dissecans of the elbow: a long-term follow-up study. Clin Orthop Relat Res 1992;284: 156–60.

146. Takahara M, Mura N, Sasaki J, et al. Classification, treatment, and outcome of osteochondritis dissecans of the humeral capitellum. J Bone Joint Surg Am 2007;89(6):1205–14.

147. Baumgarten TE, Andrews JR, Satterwhite YE. The arthroscopic classification and treatment of osteochondritis dissecans of the capitellum. Am J Sports Med 1998;26(4):520–3.

148. Byrd JW, Jones KS. Arthroscopic surgery for isolated capitellar osteochondritis dissecans in

adolescent baseball players: minimum three-year follow-up. Am J Sports Med 2002;30(4):474–8.

149. Brownlow HC, O'Connor-Read LM, Perko M. Arthroscopic treatment of osteochondritis dissecans of the capitellum. Knee Surg Sports Traumatol Arthrosc 2006;14(2):198–202.

150. Rahusen FT, Brinkman JM, Eygendaal D. Results of arthroscopic debridement for osteochondritis dissecans of the elbow. Br J Sports Med 2006; 40(12):966–9.

151. Ruch DS, Cory JW, Poehling GG. The arthroscopic management of osteochondritis dissecans of the adolescent elbow. Arthroscopy 1998;14(8):797–803.

152. Yadao MA, Field LD, Savoie FH 3rd. Osteochondritis dissecans of the elbow. Instr Course Lect 2004; 53:599–606.

153. Harada M, Ogino T, Takahara M, et al. Fragment fixation with a bone graft and dynamic staples for osteochondritis dissecans of the humeral capitellum. J Shoulder Elbow Surg 2002;11(4):368–72.

154. Takeda H, Watarai K, Matsushita T, et al. A surgical treatment for unstable osteochondritis dissecans lesions of the humeral capitellum in adolescent baseball players. Am J Sports Med 2002;30(5): 713–7.

155. Kuwahata Y, Inoue G. Osteochondritis dissecans of the elbow managed by Herbert screw fixation. Orthopedics 1998;21(4):449–51.

156. Kiyoshige Y, Takagi M, Yuasa K, et al. Closed-Wedge osteotomy for osteochondritis dissecans of the capitellum. A 7- to 12-year follow-up. Am J Sports Med 2000;28(4):534–7.

157. Miyamoto W, Yamamoto S, Kii R, et al. Oblique osteochondral plugs transplantation technique for osteochondritis dissecans of the elbow joint. Knee Surg Sports Traumatol Arthrosc 2009;17(2):204–8.

158. Iwasaki N, Kato H, Ishikawa J, et al. Autologous osteochondral mosaicplasty for osteochondritis dissecans of the elbow in teenage athletes. J Bone Joint Surg Am 2009;91(10):2359–66.

159. Shimada K, Yoshida T, Nakata K, et al. Reconstruction with an osteochondral autograft for advanced osteochondritis dissecans of the elbow. Clin Orthop Relat Res 2005;(435):140–7.

160. Farrow LD, Mahoney AJ, Stefancin JJ, et al. Quantitative analysis of the medial ulnar collateral ligament ulnar footprint and its relationship to the ulnar sublime tubercle. Am J Sports Med 2011; 39(9):1936–41.

Shoulder Instability in Older Patients

E. Scott Paxton, MD[a],*, Christopher C. Dodson, MD[b], Mark D. Lazarus, MD[b]

KEYWORDS

- Shoulder instability • Elderly • Rotator cuff tear • Locked dislocation • Hill-Sachs • Bankart

KEY POINTS

- Shoulder instability in the older patient has a lower recurrence rate (0%–31%) compared with high recurrence rates in younger patients.
- Shoulder dislocations in older patients are more likely to be associated with fractures, neurovascular injuries, and rotator cuff tears.
- An older patient with inability to lift the arm after an anterior shoulder dislocation likely has a rotator cuff tear, as opposed to a nerve injury.
- Treatment of posterior shoulder instability in the older patient often presents as a chronic dislocation and depends more on length of time from injury and amount of humeral bone loss.

INCIDENCE

The Incidence of shoulder instability in older patients (age >60 years) has been estimated to be as high as 20% of acute anterior dislocations.[1] The lowest rates of shoulder dislocations are in those 50 to 59 years old, with increasing incidence with increasing age after age 59 years. Women also had a higher incidence compared with men in the elderly, as opposed to a higher incidence in men in the younger population. Incidence in women 80 to 89 years of age is 38.8/100,000 person-years at risk.[2]

RECURRENCE

The low recurrence rate of instability in older patients is one of the biggest differences from shoulder instability in younger patients, which has been reported to be as high as 100%.[3] Recurrence rates in various reports are listed here:

- Rowe[4] J Bone Joint Surg Am 1956
  - 94% in ages younger than 20 years
  - 74% in ages 20 to 40 years
  - 14% in ages older than 40 years
- Simonet and colleagues[5] Am J Sports Med 1984
  - 0% in 41 shoulder dislocations (>40 years old)
- Penvy and colleagues[6] Arthroscopy 1998
  - 4% in 125 patients in ages older than 40 years
- Wenner[7] Orthopedics 1985
  - 17% in ages older than 40 years
- Gumina and Postacchini[1] J Bone Joint Surg Am 1997
  - 22% recurrence in ages older than 60 years
  - 50% of those only had 1 recurrent dislocation
- Rapariz and colleagues[8] Int J Shoulder Surg 2010
  - 31% recurrence in ages older than 60 years
- Stayner and colleagues[9] Orthop Clinic North Am 2000
  - 10.5% in ages older than 40 years
- Davy and Drew[10] Injury 2002
  - 6% in age older than 40 years

[a] Division of Shoulder and Elbow Surgery, Warren Alpert Medical School of Brown University, 2 Dudley Street, Suite 200, Providence, RI 02905, USA; [b] Department of Orthopedics, Rothman Institute, Thomas Jefferson University, 925 Chestnut Street, 5th Floor, Philadelphia, PA 19107, USA
* Corresponding author.
E-mail address: escottpaxton@gmail.com

Orthop Clin N Am 45 (2014) 377–385
http://dx.doi.org/10.1016/j.ocl.2014.04.002
0030-5898/14/$ – see front matter © 2014 Elsevier Inc. All rights reserved.

MECHANISM OF SHOULDER INSTABILITY

An acute dislocation is usually the result of some traumatic event to the involved shoulder. The injury needs to impart enough energy to the glenohumeral joint to overcome either the soft tissue restraints or osseous restraints. The anterior soft tissue restraints generally include the anterior capsule, the anterior glenohumeral ligaments (specifically the anterior inferior glenohumeral ligament), the anterior labrum, and the subscapularis. The posterior soft tissue restraints to anterior instability generally include the superior and posterior rotator cuff. General teaching is that either the anterior or posterior supporting structures need to be disrupted for an anterior dislocation to occur.[11]

Anterior Mechanism for Anterior Instability

The lesion most associated with anterior shoulder instability is the Bankart lesion.[12] This is a tear of the labrum and capsuloligamentous structures off the anterior inferior glenoid. This is the most common finding in younger patients with shoulder instability as a result of the theory that the attachment site of the capsule and labrum to the glenoid is the weakest of the anterior elements in the younger patient.

Reeves[13] evaluated 110 cadavers within 25 hours of death in regard to the strength of the different supporting structures of the anterior shoulder with relation to age. This investigator found that during the first 3 decades of life, the attachment of the labrum was weaker than the subscapularis tendon and its attachment as well as the anterior capsule. In older patients, the anterior capsule and subscapularis were weaker than the labral attachment site (which maintained a relatively constant strength throughout the remainder of life), and failure more commonly occurred with capsular rupture than labral avulsion from the labrum.

In addition, it is believed that because the labrum and capsuloligamentous structures are static restraints to the shoulder joint, their disruption more likely leads to recurrence. This belief provides 1 proposed theory behind the higher rate of recurrence in younger patients.[11] Araghi and colleagues[14] found that only 11 of 265 patients (4.1%) requiring open anterior stabilization for recurrent instability were older than 40 years. However, in the low percentage of older patients with recurrent instability, a high rate of anterior capsulolabral injury necessitating repair has been reported.[14,15]

Posterior Mechanism for Anterior Instability

As humans age, the rotator cuff weakens and is more prone to tearing.[16,17] So, in the older patient with preexisting degenerative weakening of the rotator cuff, it is more likely that the posterior structures fail rather than the anterior structures. Shin and colleagues[18] reported on 67 patients older than 60 years with a primary shoulder dislocation, finding 33 rotator cuff tears (RCTs) and only 3 isolated Bankart lesions. Because the rotator cuff is a dynamic structure, this might be an explanation for the lower recurrence rate in the older patient after a dislocation.[19]

Hsu and colleagues[20] showed that in a cadaver model, RCTs could result in abnormal glenohumeral translations. Small tears resulted in anteroinferior translation, and larger tears resulted in more direct anterior translation. This abnormal translation has recently been shown to correct with posterior rotator cuff reconstruction using a latissimus transfer.[21]

Pouliart and Gagey[22] showed that the humeral head dislocates in the presence of less extensive capsuloligamentous lesions when rotator cuff lesions are present. Also, the passive stabilization provided by the rotator cuff appeared more easily disrupted when associated with ligamentous lesions on the humeral side than with lesions on the glenoid side. The investigators postulated that this situation may be because interdigitation of the cuff tendons with each other and with the capsule through the rotator cable is maintained with glenoid-sided lesions. It is also possible that the higher prevalence of preexisting rotator cuff disease in the older patient may lead to abnormal glenohumeral motion and predispose an older individual to shoulder instability with a low-energy trauma.[20,23]

ASSOCIATED INJURIES
RCT

Reported incidence after anterior shoulder dislocation ranges from 35% to 86% in patients aged 40 years or older.[1,6,15,24,25] Rotator cuff pathology can range from small tears to massive posterosuperior tears to anterosuperior tears. Neviaser and Neviaser[26] reported that all patients older than 40 years with recurrent anterior instability had a subscapularis tear and anterior capsule tear.

Anteroinferior Labral (eg, Bankart) Lesions

- Interpretation of labral tears seen radiographically in this age group is difficult because tears may be degenerative or preexisting before dislocation.

Humeral Fractures

- Large Hill-Sachs lesions: osteoporotic bone more at risk

- Two-part, 3-part, and 4-part fracture dislocations
- Head-split fractures
- Isolated greater tuberosity (GT) fracture
  - Incidence increases exponentially with age, with an average age of 69.3 years[18]
  - Less risk of recurrence if fracture heals than without fracture, because the rotator cuff is typically not torn with GT fracture[24,27]

Glenoid Fractures

- Osseous Bankart lesions
- Complex glenoid fractures

Neurologic Injuries

Neurologic injuries are more common with shoulder dislocations in the elderly and are also more severe. Rates as high as 50% to 65% have been reported after dislocation in older patients.[28] Toolanen and colleagues[25] looked at patients older than 40 years using electromyography after an anterior shoulder dislocation and found that 36 of 55 cases had electromyographically verified axillary nerve or brachial plexus injury. Robinson and colleagues[29] reported on 3633 shoulder dislocations and found that the most common neurologic injury after an anterior dislocation was an isolated axillary nerve injury. This neurologic injury occurs in a similar distribution to an isolated anterior dislocation (bimodal age distribution, sex, mechanism of injury). However, patients suffering from multiple nerve lesions or diffuse brachial plexus injuries were typically older than 60 years and more likely to be female.

The primary mechanism is likely stretching of the infraclavicular brachial plexus, causing neurapraxia. Literature on infraclavicular neurapraxia reports complete resolution in 4 to 6 months in 80% of cases.[30] However, most of the patients examined were young. Toolanen and colleagues found that 14 of 27 patients older than 40 years with a moderate to total axillary nerve injury were still symptomatic at 3 years, as were 3 of the 6 patients with more diffuse plexus injuries. The nerve recovery in the older patient is likely not as reliable as in the younger patient.

Combined Neurologic Injury and RCT

The patient older than 40 years who cannot raise their arm after an anterior shoulder dislocation provides a diagnostic challenge. Older individuals are at a higher risk for nerve injury after a dislocation[31] but also at a higher risk for a RCT. The management of these 2 entities is different, because an acute RCT might be better managed with early surgical repair.[32] Therefore, it is detrimental to attribute a lack of shoulder function to a neurologic injury without confirming the integrity of the rotator cuff, because delay may make a massive tear more difficult or impossible to repair.[26] In a study of 31 such patients with an average age of 57.5 years, 29 were believed to be unable to lift their arm secondary to an axillary nerve lesion. However, all were found to have RCTs, and only 4 were found to have an axillary nerve lesion with further testing. In addition, the presence of a neurologic injury does not rule out a rotator cuff lesion. Robinson and colleagues[29] found many patients with combined injuries.

Vascular Injuries

The axillary artery in elderly patients is less elastic and more sclerotic and, therefore, is more prone to tearing. Most reported axillary artery injuries occur when chronic dislocations are reduced but can occur with acute dislocations. Calvet and Lacroix[33] reported on the largest series of arterial injuries associated with shoulder instability, with 64 axillary artery ruptures occurring after closed reduction of 91 chronically dislocated shoulders. These investigators reported 50% mortality, with the remaining patients losing their upper extremity or having a functionless limb.

The third part of the axillary artery (lateral to the pectoralis minor) is most commonly injured, but the second part (behind the pectoralis minor) can also be injured with avulsion of the thoracoacromial trunk. The third part of the axillary artery is fairly fixed and tethered by the subscapular and circumflex humeral arteries. With abduction and external rotation, the artery becomes taut and the pectoralis minor may act as a fulcrum to injure the vessel when the shoulder is dislocated anteriorly.

The presentation of this injury has been described as having a pathognomonic triad, consisting of an anterior shoulder dislocation, an expanding axillary hematoma, and a diminished peripheral pulse.[34] This injury is associated with a brachial plexus injury in 60% of cases, which can be a large determinate of functional outcome.[35] The presence of signals in the distal vessels that can be noted with Doppler does not exclude an axillary artery injury, because those signals may be secondary to collateral blood flow, and if the clinical picture is consistent with an arterial injury, an angiographic study should be obtained. There is also some thought that in the presence of an axillary artery lesion and brachial plexus injury, the brachial plexus should be explored at the time of vascular repair to reconnect any transected nerves.[36]

Acute Anterior Dislocation

Initial treatment

- Gentle closed reduction if diagnosed early
- Consider closed reduction under general anesthesia for:
  - ○ Dislocation more than a few days old
  - ○ Severe osteoporosis

Elderly patients can often have humeral head fractures during dislocation, and therefore, reduction techniques need to be gentle. General anesthesia should be considered sooner than with a younger patient. It is also imperative to be aware of the presence of a nondisplaced surgical neck fracture before reduction, especially if there is a GT fracture, because the reduction technique may displace the fracture.

Thorough radiographic evaluation is critical. Radiographs should include at least a true scapular anteroposterior (AP) and an axillary view. Internal rotation, external rotation, and scapular Y views are often helpful for identifying and evaluating tuberosity fractures. In addition, signs of chronic RCTs such as undersurface acromial changes or proximal humeral head migration should be recognized, because these may help to determine the chronicity of a RCT if one is found radiographically.

Two-dimensional and especially three-dimensional computed tomography (CT) scans can be helpful for evaluation of osseous irregularities. A CT scan should be ordered for any of the following:

- Any radiographic evidence of glenoid fracture
- Any suspicion of head-split humeral fracture
- To adequately assess the size of any Hill-Sachs lesion
- Persistent (chronic) dislocation

Magnetic resonance imaging, ultrasonography, or CT arthrography should be used to evaluate the rotator cuff of any patient older than 40 years who presents with continued symptoms consistent with a RCT for 4 weeks after a dislocation (abduction weakness, external rotation weakness, positive provocative testing, positive testing for subscapularis weakness). This procedure should be carried out regardless of the presence or absence of a suspected neurologic injury.

Definitive treatment

- Nonoperative management is appropriate for:
  - ○ First-time dislocation
  - ○ No or nondisplaced fracture
  - ○ No or chronic appearing RCT with quick return of cuff function
  - ○ Subscapularis intact
  - ○ Stable arc after closed reduction
- Sling immobilization for 7 to 10 days, then begin range of motion exercises and proceed to strengthening as tolerated

Surgical Treatment

Instability in the elderly often results from a combination of diseases including: soft tissue injury, RCT, Bankart tear, capsular tear (**Fig. 1**), glenoid fracture, and humeral fracture. Failure to address all of the disease surgically leads to a higher incidence of recurrence. Preoperative planning is

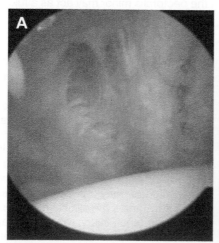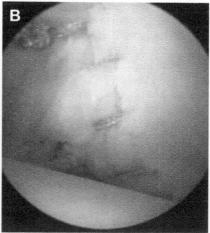

Fig. 1. (*A*) A 67-year-old man with capsular tear suffered after acute anterior dislocation (*B*) treated with a suture repair.

critical, and deciding which combination of diseases to address leads to the best approach to use. For a posterosuperior RCT and Bankart repair, an arthroscopic technique is likely better. For a subscapularis avulsion and a Bankart repair with a Hill-Sachs lesion, an open anterior approach is likely more suitable, depending on the degree of subscapularis tear and amount of the bony deficiency.

Overall, the appropriate treatment necessary is likely more aggressive than the traditional teaching.[37] Addressing all of the disease surgically may lead to a higher incidence of stiffness. Therefore, there is likely no surgical procedure that works 100% of the time in this difficult patient population.

Rotator cuff repairs (RCRs) should be performed for large or massive acute or chronic RCT, specifically if there is persistent loss of function or there is an associated neuropraxic injury to the axillary nerve. Often, these patients have an associated Hill-Sachs lesion, so posterosuperior cuff tears can be repaired into the lesion, which medializes the repair, accomplishing 2 goals: less tension on the repair and performing essentially a remplissage procedure (rendering the lesion extra-articular). In addition, early surgery should be considered when there is a reparable subscapularis tear. Neviaser and colleagues[26] found that 100% of patients in their series with recurrence had a subscapularis tear with disruption of the anterior capsule.

However, an RCR is not always the answer. Classic teaching is to perform an RCR, leaving the Bankart lesion alone in the elderly population.[6] Our indications for Bankart repair with RCR are recurrent instability without osseous injury and cuff tear size that does not account for degree of instability. Combined Bankart repair and RCR repair, if both present at time of surgery, has been reported, typically in the case of recurrent instability.[1,15]

In the elderly, deficiency of the anterior glenoid rim is a major contributing factor to recurrence and should always be addressed in the setting of surgery for recurrent instability. An open repair may be best to address this disease if there is poor bone quality, comminution, or an associated but isolated subscapularis avulsion. Fixation options for glenoid disease include screw fixation (3.5 or 4.0 mm), minifragment T-plates, or suture fixation if the bone is of poor quality or comminuted.

Glenoid Osseous Deficiency

- Consider the same reconstructive options for glenoid deficiency that are performed in a younger patient
  - Bankart repair for defects less than 15% to 20%
  - Latarjet
    - Hart and colleagues[38] reported 0% recurrence in patients with an average age of 65 years, with only mild loss of forward flexion at 4 years
  - Autograft or allograft glenoid reconstruction

Humeral Fractures

- GT
  - Does not eliminate possibility of concurrent RCT[6]
  - Repair if displaced more than 5 to 10 mm superior, displaced superior to articular surface, or displaced posterior greater than 10 mm
  - Can be repaired open or arthroscopically, but arthroscopic treatment gives improved visualization of reduction, decreased risk of postoperative adhesions, and ability to address other disease. Repair techniques include percutaneous placement of 4.0-mm cannulated screws or double-row suture bridge type RCR, compressing the tuberosity into its bed.
- Hill-Sachs lesion
  - In the young, a significant lesion is one that engages on the anterior glenoid during abduction and external rotation (ABD/ER); no clear definition of a significant lesion for the elderly

There are arthroscopic treatment options for Hill-Sachs lesions that are found to be the cause of recurrent instability, including osteochondral allograft plugs and remplissage. In the elderly, an arthroscopic procedure is ideal for patients with combined RCT and Hill-Sachs lesion, as discussed earlier. This procedure can result in motion loss, particularly for larger lesions. Open options include large osteochondral allografts (**Fig. 2**), partial resurfacing arthroplasty and hemiarthroplasty, and total shoulder arthroplasty.

- Osteochondral allograft
  - Can be performed through an anterior approach
  - Can be performed while you are addressing anterior disease
  - By fashioning a wedged graft, you can completely fill the defect
  - Risk of late collapse
- Partial resurfacing
  - Probably the easiest and fastest technique
  - May be the best option for the elderly

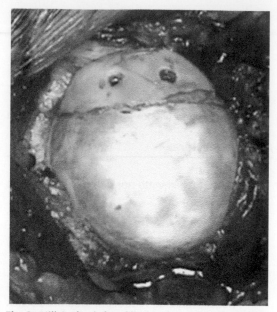

Fig. 2. Hill-Sachs defect filled with osteochondral allograft from a femoral head.

- Can be performed through an anterior approach by dislocating and ER
- Can be performed while you are addressing anterior disease
- Fitting a circle into a wedge leaves gaps that can be significant
- Hemiarthroplasty
  - Head-split fracture
  - Three-part or 4-part fracture: dislocation age older than 75 years
  - Hill-Sachs lesion greater than 45% of humeral head[39]
  - Locked dislocation greater than 6 months
- Total shoulder arthroplasty

- Same indications for hemiarthroplasty with underlying glenohumeral degenerative joint disease
- Rotator cuff must be intact for standard total shoulder arthroplasty

The reverse ball and socket replacement may be best suited for patients with an irreparable RCT with persistent pseudoparalysis, unreconstructable humeral and glenoid osseous defects, 3-part or 4-part fracture, dislocation age older than 75 years, or salvage of failed surgery (**Fig. 3**).

- Treatment options that are probably not likely to work for recurrent anterior instability in the elderly:
  - Muscle transfer operations
    - Pectoralis major for anterosuperior cuff deficiency
    - Latissimus for posterosuperior cuff deficiency
  - Subscapularis or capsular tightening operations

Posterior Instability

The mechanism is typically a fall on to (axial load) a forward flexed, adducted, internally rotated arm. If no trauma is reported, the patient must be evaluated for seizure. Fracture into the surgical neck may occur in up to 50%, and approximately 15% present bilaterally (**Fig. 4**).[40]

The evaluation of the patient is paramount, because up to 50% of posterior dislocations are initially missed.[39,41,42] Radiographs in orthogonal planes must be obtained (ideally, a true scapular AP and an axillary view). Some physical examination findings consistent with a missed posterior

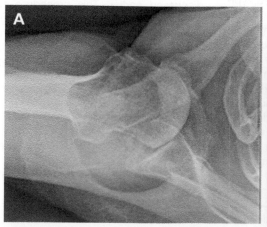
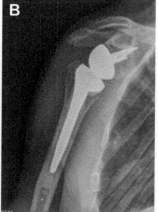

Fig. 3. (*A*) An 82-year-old man with recurrent anterior instability with subscapularis deficiency, Hill-Sachs defect, and glenoid deficiency. (*B*) The patient was treated with a reverse shoulder arthroplasty.

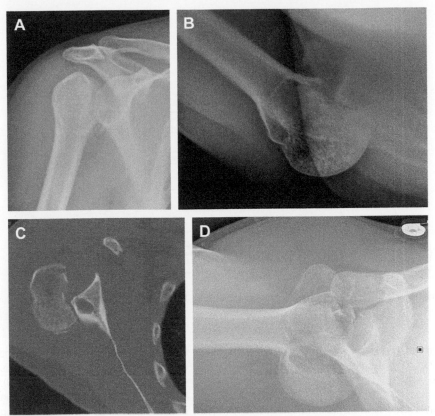

Fig. 4. (*A, B*) AP and axillary view of a posteriorly dislocated shoulder with lesser tuberosity fracture (*C*) CT scan shows evidence of chronic dislocation with cystic changes in the glenoid (*D*) after closed reduction with sedation only, resulting in fracture through the surgical neck.

dislocation are a prominent coracoid process and locked internal rotation contracture.

Gentle closed reduction is advised if the condition is diagnosed early, but consider closed reduction under general anesthesia for:

- Dislocation more than a few days old
- Severe osteoporosis
- Large, engaged reverse Hill-Sachs lesion (>20%)

CT before reduction should be obtained for:

- Any radiographic evidence of posterior glenoid fracture
- Any suspicion of head-split humeral fracture
- To adequately assess the size of the reverse Hill-Sachs lesion (anterior humeral head defect)

In the young patient, the primary condition is posterior labral disease, capsular laxity, and posterior glenoid rim fractures. Although these conditions are often seen in the elderly as well, they rarely require treatment. Treatment in the elderly

is based on the size of the reverse Hill-Sachs lesion and the length of time of dislocation (**Fig. 5**).

Chronic Anterior Dislocation

Chronic anterior dislocation is more common in the elderly and more difficult to reconstruct than either recurrent anterior instability or posterior instability. There are often osseous deficiencies on both the humeral and glenoid sides. Also, capsular contracture is typically present and usually severe for chronic anterior dislocation. Rotator cuff deficiencies are not uncommon either. This condition requires extensive anterior release (including the pectoralis major) to gain a reduction. This procedure can pose significant risk to the patient if the axillary artery is more likely to be scarred to the anterior structures and can be encountered in nonanatomic positions or injured during reduction.

Arthroplasty should be considered for severe glenoid or humeral deficiency or degenerative chondral changes. If the subscapularis can be mobilized, an anatomic total shoulder arthroplasty

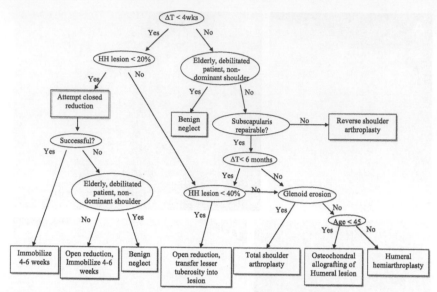

Fig. 5. Treatment algorithm for posterior shoulder instability. HH, humeral head.

is indicated; if not, then a reverse total shoulder arthroplasty should be considered. If bone deficiencies are severe, a reverse total shoulder arthroplasty may be more beneficial, because grafting rarely works in chronic cases, especially if glenoid grafting is required. However, the extensive releases needed pose an instability risk.

SUMMARY

Although recurrence of instability occurs less frequently in the elderly, when it does occur, it can be a challenging problem. For the very unstable patient, it is best to be aggressive in addressing all of the disease, recognizing that you are likely trading motion for stability.

REFERENCES

1. Gumina S, Postacchini F. Anterior dislocation of the shoulder in elderly patients. J Bone Joint Surg Br 1997;79:540–3.
2. Zacchilli MA, Owens BD. Epidemiology of shoulder dislocations presenting to emergency departments in the United States. J Bone Joint Surg Am 2010; 92(3):542–9.
3. Marans HJ, Angel KR, Schemitsch EH, et al. The fate of traumatic anterior dislocation of the shoulder in children. J Bone Joint Surg Am 1992;74(8):1242–4.
4. Rowe CR. Prognosis in dislocations of the shoulder. J Bone Joint Surg Am 1956;38A(5):957–77.
5. Simonet WT, Melton LJ, Cofield RH, et al. Incidence of anterior shoulder dislocation in Olmsted County, Minnesota. Clin Orthop Relat Res 1984;186:186–91.

6. Pevny T, Hunter RE, Freeman JR. Primary traumatic anterior shoulder dislocation in patients 40 years of age and older. Arthroscopy 1998;14(3):289–94.
7. Wenner SM. Anterior dislocation of the shoulder in patients over 50 years of age. Orthopedics 1985; 8(9):1155–7.
8. Rapariz JM, Martin-Martin S, Pareja-Bezares A, et al. Shoulder dislocation in patients older than 60 years of age. Int J Shoulder Surg 2010;4(4):88–92.
9. Stayner LR, Cummings J, Andersen J, et al. Shoulder dislocations in patients older than 40 years of age. Orthop Clin North Am 2000;31(2):231–9.
10. Davy AR, Drew SJ. Management of shoulder dislocation–are we doing enough to reduce the risk of recurrence? Injury 2002;33(9):775–9.
11. McLaughlin H. Injuries of the shoulder and arm. Philadelphia: WB Saunders; 1959.
12. Bankart AS. Recurrent or habitual dislocation of the shoulder-joint. Br Med J 1923;2(3285):1132–3.
13. Reeves B. Experiments on the tensile strength of the anterior capsular structures of the shoulder in man. J Bone Joint Surg Br 1968;50(4):858–65.
14. Araghi A, Prasarn M, St Clair S, et al. Recurrent anterior glenohumeral instability with onset after forty years of age: the role of the anterior mechanism. Bull Hosp Jt Dis 2005;62(3–4):99–101.
15. Hawkins RJ, Bell RH, Hawkins RH, et al. Anterior dislocation of the shoulder in the older patient. Clin Orthop Relat Res 1986;(206):192–5.
16. Yamaguchi K, Ditsios K, Middleton WD, et al. The demographic and morphological features of rotator cuff disease. A comparison of asymptomatic and symptomatic shoulders. J Bone Joint Surg Am 2006;88(8):1699–704.

17. Yamaguchi K, Tetro AM, Blam O, et al. Natural history of asymptomatic rotator cuff tears: a longitudinal analysis of asymptomatic tears detected sonographically. J Shoulder Elbow Surg 2001;10(3): 199–203.

18. Shin SJ, Yun YH, Kim DJ, et al. Treatment of traumatic anterior shoulder dislocation in patients older than 60 years. Am J Sports Med 2012;40(4):822–7.

19. McLaughlin HL, MacLellan DI. Recurrent anterior dislocation of the shoulder. II. A comparative study. J Trauma 1967;7(2):191–201.

20. Hsu HC, Luo ZP, Cofield RH, et al. Influence of rotator cuff tearing on glenohumeral stability. J Shoulder Elbow Surg 1997;6(5):413–22.

21. Oh JH, Tilan J, Chen YJ, et al. Biomechanical effect of latissimus dorsi tendon transfer for irreparable massive cuff tear. J Shoulder Elbow Surg 2013; 22(2):150–7.

22. Pouliart N, Gagey O. Concomitant rotator cuff and capsuloligamentous lesions of the shoulder: a cadaver study. Arthroscopy 2006;22(7):728–35.

23. Loehr JF, Helmig P, Sojbjerg JO, et al. Shoulder instability caused by rotator cuff lesions. An in vitro study. Clin Orthop Relat Res 1994;(304):84–90.

24. Sonnabend DH. Treatment of primary anterior shoulder dislocation in patients older than 40 years of age: conservative versus operative. Clin Orthop Relat Res 1994;304:74–7.

25. Toolanen G, Hildingsson C, Hedlund T, et al. Early complications after anterior dislocation of the shoulder in patients over 40 years. An ultrasonographic and electromyographic study. Acta Orthop Scand 1993;64(5):549–52.

26. Neviaser RJ, Neviaser TJ, Neviaser JS. Concurrent rupture of the rotator cuff and anterior dislocation of the shoulder in the older patient. J Bone Joint Surg Am 1988;70(9):1308–11.

27. Hovelius L, Eriksson K, Fredin H, et al. Recurrences after initial dislocation of the shoulder. Results of a prospective study of treatment. J Bone Joint Surg Am 1983;65(3):343–9.

28. Bumbasirevic M, Lesic A, Vidakovic A, et al. Nerve lesions after acute anterior dislocation of the humeroscapular joint–electrodiagnostic study. Med Pregl 1993;46(5–6):191–3 [in Croatian].

29. Robinson CM, Shur N, Sharpe T, et al. Injuries associated with traumatic anterior glenohumeral dislocations. J Bone Joint Surg Am 2012;94(1):18–26.

30. Alnot JY. Traumatic brachial plexus palsy in the adult: retro- and infraclavicular lesions. Clin Orthop Relat Res 1988;(237):9–16.

31. de Laat EA, Visser CP, Coene LN, et al. Nerve lesions in primary shoulder dislocations and humeral neck fractures. A prospective clinical and EMG study. J Bone Joint Surg Br 1994;76(3): 381–3.

32. Bassett RW, Cofield RH. Acute tears of the rotator cuff. The timing of surgical repair. Clin Orthop Relat Res 1983;(175):18–24.

33. Calvet J, Leroy M, Lacroix L. Luxations de l'epaule et lesions vasculaires. J Chir 1942;58:337–46 [in French].

34. Kelley SP, Hinsche AF, Hossain JF. Axillary artery transection following anterior shoulder dislocation: classical presentation and current concepts. Injury 2004;35(11):1128–32.

35. Johnson SF, Johnson SB, Strodel WE, et al. Brachial plexus injury: association with subclavian and axillary vascular trauma. J Trauma 1991;31(11): 1546–50.

36. Nichols JS, Lillehei KO. Nerve injury associated with acute vascular trauma. Surg Clin North Am 1988; 68(4):837–52.

37. Porcellini G, Paladini P, Campi F, et al. Shoulder instability and related rotator cuff tears: arthroscopic findings and treatment in patients aged 40 to 60 years. Arthroscopy 2006;22(3):270–6.

38. Hart R, Sváb P, Krejzla J. Modified Latarjet procedure for recurrent shoulder dislocation in elderly patients. Acta Chir Orthop Traumatol Cech 2010;77: 105–11.

39. Hawkins RJ, Neer CS 2nd, Pianta RM, et al. Locked posterior dislocation of the shoulder. J Bone Joint Surg Am 1987;69(1):9–18.

40. Loebenberg MI, Cuomo F. The treatment of chronic anterior and posterior dislocations of the glenohumeral joint and associated articular surface defects. Orthop Clin North Am 2000;31(1):23–34.

41. Heller KD, Forst J, Forst R. Differential therapy of traumatically-induced persistent posterior shoulder dislocation. Review of the literature. Unfallchirurg 1995;98(1):6–12 [in German].

42. Michos IB, Michaelides DP. Reduction of missed posterior dislocation of the shoulder. Report of 2 cases, 1 of them bilateral. Acta Orthop Scand 1993;64(5):599–600.

The Thrower's Shoulder

Stuart D. Kinsella, BA, MD, MTR[a], Stephen J. Thomas, PhD, ATC[b],
G. Russell Huffman, MD, MPH[c], John D. Kelly IV, MD[c],*

KEYWORDS

- Labrum • Rotator cuff • Humeral retroversion • GIRD

KEY POINTS

- Injuries specific to throwers most commonly involve the labrum and the undersurface of the rotator cuff.
- The act of throwing has been described as occurring in several distinct phases. Of particular importance are the late-cocking, ball release and follow-through phases. These portions of the throwing motion produce the largest forces about the glenohumeral joint, and therefore, the highest injury risk.
- In late-cocking, the anterior capsule is under significant strain in an effort to prevent anterior translation of the humerus. Tensile failure and attenuation of the anterior capsule is thought to occur from repetitive 'hard throwing'.
- During the follow through phase, the posterior capsule and posterior cuff undergo tremendous eccentric loads - up to 108% of body weight - in order to decelerate the rapidly internally rotating arm and to restrain the significant distractive forces seen at the posterior shoulder joint.
- The thrower's shoulder is prone to injury secondary to the convergence of the following factors: attenuation of the anterior capsular constraints, acquisition of a posterior capsular contracture, development of scapula dyskinesis, breakdown of the kinetic chain and repetitive contact of the posterior superior labrum and greater tuberosity.

INTRODUCTION

Throwers, or athletes who engage in repetitive overhead motions, are a unique subset of athletes who experience distinct shoulder injuries. For purposes of clarity, this article focuses on athletes engaged in baseball, because this patient population comprises most patients seeking orthopedic care for throwing-related injuries. Baseball remains one of America's favorite pastimes, and children often participate in the sport by the age of 5 or 6 years. The common participation in overhead throwing by today's youth increases the likelihood of orthopedic surgeons encountering patients with throwing-related shoulder pathology.

Injuries peculiar to throwers most commonly involve the labrum and the undersurface of the rotator cuff. In addition, tissue changes in both the anterior and posterior glenohumeral capsule are common with repetitive overhead motions. These capsular changes alter shoulder kinematics and subsequently contribute to both labral and cuff injury. Furthermore, the glenohumeral joint and the scapula are inextricably linked. In fact, scapular issues may herald the development of tissue breakdown in the shoulder. This article examines the pathomechanics of injuries to throwers, elaborates means of diagnoses of cuff and labral injury, and discusses recent advances in both nonoperative and operative interventions, including preventative principles.

---

[a] Department of Orthopaedic Surgery, Massachusetts General Hospital, 55 Fruit Street, Boston, MA 02114, USA; [b] Division of Nursing and Health Sciences, Neumann University, 1 Neumann Drive, Aston, PA 19104, USA; [c] Department of Orthopaedic Surgery, Hospital of the University of Pennsylvania, 34th and Spruce Street, Philadelphia, PA 19104, USA
* Corresponding author.
E-mail address: John.Kelly@uphs.upenn.edu

Orthop Clin N Am 45 (2014) 387–401
http://dx.doi.org/10.1016/j.ocl.2014.04.003
0030-5898/14/$ – see front matter © 2014 Elsevier Inc. All rights reserved.

orthopedic.theclinics.com

THE ACT OF THROWING

Throwing a baseball more than 90 mph generates great demands on the shoulder girdle. Humeral angular velocities have been estimated to exceed 7000° per second,[1] with estimated external rotation (ER) torques as high as 67 Nm.[2] The act of throwing has been elegantly described as occurring in several distinct phases. Of particular importance are the late-cocking, ball release, and follow-through phases. These portions of the throwing motion produce the largest forces about the glenohumeral joint and, therefore, the highest injury risk.

In late cocking, the anterior capsule is under significant strain in an effort to prevent anterior translation of the humerus. Tensile failure and attenuation of the anterior capsule is thought to occur from repetitive hard throwing. Throwers demonstrate increased passive ER in the abducted and externally rotated (ABER) position compared with controls.[3] Furthermore, stretching of the coracohumeral ligament (CHL) may also occur during forced ER and explain the rotator interval laxity commonly seen in overhead athletes.[4]

During the follow-through phase, the posterior capsule and posterior cuff undergo tremendous eccentric loads, up to 108% of body weight,[5] to decelerate the rapidly internally rotating arm and to restrain the significant distractive forces seen at the posterior shoulder joint. In time, the continual strains across the posterior cuff may lead to muscular fatigue and thereby a much larger transfer of stress to the posterior capsule.[6,7] Chronic attritional tearing of the posterior capsule may result in a fibroblastic healing response, increased collagen deposition, and loss of tissue compliance. All these elements converge and are thought to give the overhead thrower a stiff posterior cuff and capsule.[7]

To obtain the great arm velocity required to pitch effectively, throwers must attain increased degrees of ER.[8] The greater the arm can externally rotate, the more time the arm has to accelerate before ball release. Pitchers who are able to pitch at great velocities possess not only great muscle strength and fast twitch muscle capability but also inordinate degrees of ER ability.[9]

HUMERAL RETROVERSION

Fetal humeri demonstrate significantly greater degrees of retroversion compared with adult humeri, along the order of 78°.[10] During development and growth, retroversion slowly decreases until the adult average of roughly 30° is attained (**Fig. 1**).[10] Immature throwers, on the other hand, by virtue

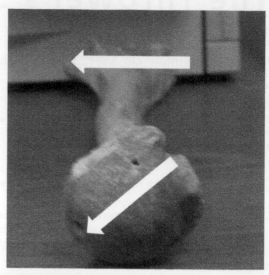

Fig. 1. Humeral retroversion (HRT). HRT is measured as the angle formed by an arrow drawn through the center of the longitudinal axis of the humeral head and neck meeting an arrow drawn along the transverse axis of the condyles, when looking proximal to distal along the humerus.

of Wolf's law, impose stresses across the proximal humeral physis, which impedes the loss of retroversion.[11] It is not unusual for a thrower, who began pitching in Little League, to present with more than 45° of retroversion in adulthood. There is also a particular asymmetry of the throwing and nonthrowing shoulders. A study in pitchers demonstrated that a the dominant shoulder exhibited increased humeral retroversion (HRT), glenoid retroversion (GRV), ER at 90°, ER in the scapular plane, and decreased internal rotation (IR) relative to their nondominant shoulder. In another study of professional baseball pitchers, the HRT to GRV ratio was found to be 2.3:1 for throwing shoulders and 7:1 for nonthrowing shoulders. The adaptive morphologic changes of increased proximal HRT and GRV in throwing shoulders are thought to be at least initially adaptive.[12] On the contrary, nonthrowing individuals do not display this discrepancy between their dominant and nondominant shoulders.[13]

Increased retroversion resets the clock in terms of the arc of motion for the thrower, in which ER is gained with a symmetric loss of IR. This increased retroversion allows a greater amount of ER to occur before the greater tuberosity abuts the posterior superior labrum in the ABER position. This contact between the greater tuberosity and posterior superior labrum, sustained repetitively, can lead to posterior cuff and labral injury in many throwers. Although this contact, known as internal impingement, has been shown to occur normally in overhead athletes,[14] contact pressures between the posterior cuff and labrum are less than in those throwers endowed with increased retroversion. Those who embrace throwing after skeletal maturity, by virtue of lessened retroversion, may be more susceptible to impingement type injury than a lifetime thrower. However, Thomas and colleagues[15] have posited the increased retroversion may predispose the thrower to increased posterior capsular thickness, which is thought to increase the risk of injury. These investigators found a correlation between posterior capsular thickness and retroversion. That is, the same retroversion thought to be beneficial to throwing velocity and avoidance of cuff and labral impingement may predispose the athlete to posterior capsular contracture, or glenohumeral internal rotation deficit (GIRD). The potential negative effects of GIRD on shoulder kinematics are discussed in more detail.

PATHOMECHANICS

The thrower's shoulder is prone to injury secondary to the convergence of the following factors: attenuation of the anterior capsular constraints, acquisition of a posterior capsular contracture, development of scapula dyskinesis, breakdown of the kinetic chain, and repetitive contact of the posterior superior labrum and greater tuberosity. Each of these factors has been examined, and strategies have been suggested to prevent injury.

Anterior Capsule

Biomechanical studies demonstrate that the anterior capsule, particularly the anterior band of the inferior glenohumeral ligament, is the primary restraint to anterior translation of the humerus when the arm is ABER.[16–18] Thus, repetitive stress to this area and the thrower's unconscious desire to attain extreme ER (the slot) conceivably leads to anterior capsular laxity or attrition. Although the attributed causes are somewhat controversial, throwers do indeed demonstrate more passive ER than in the contralateral arm.[19,20] If this excessive rotation exceeds that which is expected to occur from increased retroversion, that is, excessive ER gain is greater than IR loss, then the soft-tissue restraint is lax. In support of this notion is the work of Jobe and colleagues,[21] which describes tensioning of the anterior capsule (anterolabral capsular reconstruction) as a means of returning pitchers to throwing. Although this open procedure was successful for many, violation of the subscapularis and excessive tightening potentially explain why not all patients were able to throw at preinjury levels of performance after reconstruction. In a study investigating patients who underwent labral repair, Levitz and colleagues[22] reported that those who underwent subtle thermal shrinkage of the anterior capsule, in addition to superior labral repair, enjoyed greater success than those who had superior labral repairs alone. As anterior laxity evolves, ER increases and further increases contact of the posterior cuff and labrum, thereby facilitating injury.[23] Rizio and colleagues[24] demonstrated increased superior labral strain in cadaveric shoulders placed in the ABER position after surgically creating subtle anterior laxity. These studies lend support to the notion of anterior capsular laxity as one contributing factor to shoulder pathology in the thrower and that HRT is beneficial against anterior capsular attenuation.

In addition, because the CHL is a primary restraint to ER, stretching of the CHL and superior glenohumeral ligament (SGHL) may ensue with repetitive throwing. The thrower may present with increased passive ER with the arm adducted, as well as a positive sulcus sign, inferior shoulder laxity that persists in ER. On arthroscopic examination, interval laxity manifests as a capacious biceps sling, the enclosure of the intra-articular biceps comprising the SGHL, CHL, and supraspinatus insertion. Morgan has posited that interval laxity must be addressed during concomitant labral surgery to increase the likelihood of successful return to throwing (Craig D. Morgan, personal communication, 2013) (Fig. 2). In addition, because the CHL inserts into the deep fibers of the supraspinatus, injury to this structure may be intimately associated with the undersurface supraspinatus tears commonly seen with overhead athletes. Habermeyer and colleagues[25] found lesions of the CHL accompanied by undersurface supraspinatus lesions in 73% of subjects studied.

Posterior Capsular Contracture

With time, throwers demonstrate decreased IR, especially when measured in the abducted position. This diminished IR is thought to occur for 2 reasons. First, as mentioned previously, increases in HRT observed in throwers manifests as a loss of IR. This loss, due to boney remodeling, however, is accompanied by a symmetric gain of ER. This resetting the clock of rotation usually accounts for no more than 10° to 17° of rotational loss.[13,26,27] The second means of IR loss is ascribed to a posterior capsular/cuff contracture. This GIRD is thought to occur, as stated previously, as a healing response to chronic distractive forces applied to the posterior capsule during

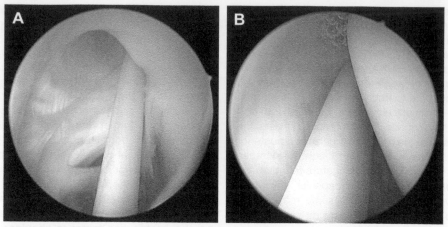

Fig. 2. Interval laxity and widening, preinterval (*A*) and postinterval (*B*) tightening with suture closure. Tightening of the posterior biceps pulley improves enclosure of the long head of the biceps and may increase the likelihood of a return to throwing. (*Courtesy of* C.D. Morgan, MD, Wilmington, DE.)

follow-through. Rotational loss due to capsular contracture is evident when GIRD exceeds that which can be explained by boney remodeling alone (more than 12°) and when the internal rotational loss exceeds the external rotational gain as compared with the contralateral shoulder. For example, a young thrower who presents with GIRD of 35° surely has more than increased retroversion to account for internal rotational loss. In a study investigating change in passive range of motion (ROM) and development of GIRD in professional pitching shoulders between spring training in consecutive years, Shanley and colleagues[28] found that even accounting for HRT, ROM was significantly altered between seasons of pitching secondary to soft-tissue adaptations. The finding suggests that some changes in the pitching shoulder may be transient and amenable to modulation. Furthermore, many throwers, particularly less mature athletes, often demonstrate dramatic increases in IR after a dedicated stretching regime.[29] Boney restraints would not respond to stretching programs. In a study investigating the effects of a stretching protocol on passive IR in the throwing shoulders of collegiate baseball players, Aldridge and colleagues[30] found that the posterior capsule stretching program was effective in increasing passive IR, and total ROM, but not on ER in the throwing shoulder. The stretching program had no effect on nonthrowing arm IR, ER, or total ROM.

Biomechanical Consequences of GIRD

Recent clinical and biomechanical studies lend credence to the notion that GIRD may be the sentinel event in the pathologic cascade that many throwers experience. Burkhart and colleagues[31] noted that professional throwers who presented to preseason with GIRD values less than 25°, as compared with the contralateral shoulder, experienced less shoulder difficulties during the ensuing season. Others have noted that throwers who present with superior labral injuries invariably exhibit GIRD generally greater than 25° to 30°. Even small degrees of GIRD place the thrower at increased risk for injury, as evidenced by a study by Wilk and colleagues,[32] which found that pitchers with as little as 5° of GIRD were at higher risk for injury and shoulder surgery.

Cadaveric studies have helped elucidate the association between GIRD and labral or cuff injuries. Clabbers and colleagues[33] imbricated the posterior capsule of cadaveric shoulders and placed them in the late-cocking position. They observed a tendency (nonsignificant) for posterior capsule tightening to encourage relative posterior/superior migration of the humeral head.[34] Grossman and colleagues[35] and Huffman and colleagues[36] elegantly demonstrated the same phenomenon and introduced anterior laxity, in addition to posterior capsular tightness, to a compressively loaded joint, which more closely mimicked the in vivo condition. All 3 studies suggested that posterior capsular tightness, with or without anterior capsular laxity, promoted a relative shift of the humeral head contact point on the glenoid in the ABER position. In another cadaveric model, Gates and colleagues[37] further found that decreases in posterior and inferior translation of the humeral head could be observed with as little as 5% GIRD, further highlighting the importance of the finding.

This shift in contact theoretically brings the humeral head closer to the superior labrum in late cocking, promoting increased contact between the 2 structures. Furthermore, Laudner and colleagues[38] showed that throwers with internal impingement present with significantly more GIRD than asymptomatic throwers. In addition, a more posterior vector could conceivably increase the posterior force on the labrum in late cocking. This increased peel back force may result in a higher incidence of posterior labral injury. Kuhn and colleagues[4] have shown that the posterior labrum is more prone to failure in the late cocking rather than in the follow-through phase of throwing.

The posterior superior shift that occurs with GIRD is thought to result from the inferior tether that posterior/inferior capsular contractures produce. A contracted posterior/inferior capsule does not permit full ER of the humerus. In an effort to find the slot, the thrower begins to rotate around a new instant center of rotation, one that is more posterior and proximal. In essence, a tightened posterior inferior capsule drives the humerus more proximally and posteriorly. Burkhart and colleagues[39] liken this to a yo-yo on a string. In support of this tethering phenomenon, the investigators have noted several pitchers who have presented with both posterior-superior and posterior-inferior labral tears, confirming the notion that GIRD increases both the capsular tether inferiorly and labral shear posterior-superiorly. With the concomitant posterior shift in humeral head contact, an obligatory anterior laxity is thought to occur, owing to the cam-shaped structure of the humerus. Burkhart and Lo[40] describe this as pseudolaxity and has shown that posterior shift in contact point does indeed introduce laxity of the anterior capsule. The same laxity allows the thrower to hyperrotate, promoting even more contact between the posterior labrum and cuff. In addition, hyper ER may introduce excessive strain on the rotator cuff. Hyper twist of cuff fibers may lead to eccentric fiber failure and undersurface tearing.

Scapular Dyskinesis

An abnormality of either the static or dynamic position of the scapula is termed scapular dyskinesis (**Fig. 3**). The scapula normally accommodates the proximal humerus closely so that a stable platform (the glenoid) and concavity compression of the cuff is optimally attained.[41] Kibler and McMullen[42] likened this relationship to a seal balancing a ball on its nose. With time, throwers may develop

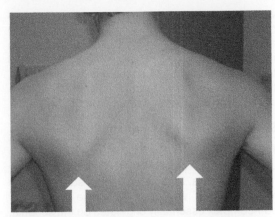

Fig. 3. Scapular dyskinesis. An abnormality in the static or dynamic position of the scapula. The right scapula of the patient indicated by the white *arrow* is protracted and anteriorly tilted compared to the left scapula, deviating away from the midline, anterior to the frontal plane.

scapula dyskinesis, which may, in turn, potentiate further cuff or labral injury.

Origins of Dyskinesis

Muscles commonly respond to proximate joint afflictions with atrophy or contracture. For example, quad atrophy often accompanies knee pain and hamstring tightness often accompanies low-back discomfort. Shoulder pain commonly results in inhibition of the lower trapezius and serratus anterior,[42–45] as well as tightening of the upper trapezius and pectoralis minor. The net effect of this muscular imbalance is a protracted and anterior tilted scapula, one that deviates away from the midline and anterior to the frontal plane. Because the thorax is ellipsoid, a protracted scapula essentially follows the contour of the rib cage and rests in a relative internally rotated and inferior position.[46,47] Myers and colleagues[48] noted that throwers who suffer from internal impingement demonstrate increased scapular protraction during humeral elevation. Pink and colleagues[49] has advanced the concept of scapula windup (secondary to GIRD) as a means to increasing scapular protraction. In essence, throwers with loss of capsular IR rely more on scapular IR as a means of attaining follow-through. In time, as the scapula winds up and over the ellipsoid thorax, it loosens its static restraints and perhaps overwhelms dynamic stabilizers. The net effect is a scapula that is deviated from the midline and anteriorly tilted.

Thomas and colleagues[50,51] have studied adolescent and collegiate pitchers and have noted a temporal relationship between GIRD and dyskinesis. Less mature pitchers developed GIRD without scapular dyskinesis, whereas more mature throwers tended to develop more GIRD and began to manifest scapular changes in the throwing shoulder. GIRD more than 15° seemed to herald the onset of scapular changes. Thus, there seems to be a dose response of GIRD leading to scapular abnormalities.

Effects of Excessive Protraction

There are numerous biomechanical consequences of a protracted or excessively internally rotated scapula. First, a protracted scapula leads to rotator cuff weakness. Because the rotator cuff complex essentially originates on the scapula, a dyskinetic or protracted scapula serves as an unstable platform and does not afford optimal length-tension relationships to the cuff muscles. Kibler's scapular retraction test affirms the importance of scapula position in optimizing cuff strength. To perform the test, an examiner checks supraspinatus strength, testing both with and without manual stabilization of the medial border of the scapula against the thorax. Patients with dyskinesis of the scapula demonstrate increases (often striking) in strength on affixing the medial border of the scapula to the thorax.[52] Second, increased protraction anteverts the glenoid, virtually uncovering the humeral head anteriorly and thereby leading to anterior destabilization and increased strain on the anterior ligaments.[53] Excessive protraction also increases the degree of impingement between the posterior superior glenoid and posterior rotator cuff by positioning the posterior glenoid closer to the greater tuberosity during ER and horizontal abduction.[31] Increased pinching or contact of the posterior superior glenoid and posterior supraspinatus occurs more readily in an anteverted glenoid. Supporting this fact, Laudner and colleagues[38] demonstrated that throwers with pathologic internal impingement exhibit a more protracted scapula. This internal impingement can result in posterior shoulder pain and potentiate posterior labral or cuff injury.

KINETIC CHAIN BREAKDOWN

Rubin describes a kinetic chain as a series of links, acting sequentially, to generate a force.[54] The image of cracking the whip illustrates how proximal links (the handle and base of the whip), when acting in unison with more distal aspects or segments of the whip, can produce a great force distally. Similarly, throwers generate great velocities by linking force generated by the lower extremity and core muscles funneled via the shoulder to the arm.[55] The lower extremities generate more than 50% of the kinetic energy of the throw.

Any break in the chain, from feet to fingers, results in loss of velocity and catch up demand in more distal links. For example, weak hip abductors on the stance leg or, more commonly, the stride leg of throwing creates an unstable base from which to throw. A recent kinematic and kinetic investigation of collegiate and professional pitchers found that increased time in lower extremity and trunk phases of the throwing motion not only decreased the magnitude of upper extremity kinetics linked to overuse injuries but also correlated with decreased ball speed.[9] In accordance with the distal catch up principle to maintain velocity, increased demand is placed on the more distal shoulder and elbow segments. Similarly, loss of IR of the shoulder promotes increased reliance on the more distal elbow and wrist links to produce the long axis IR necessary to complete a throw. Suzuki and colleagues[56] have demonstrated that scapula fatigue results in increased elbow demand in the act of throwing. The hip has also received more recent attention, as it pertains to throwing. Femoracetabular impingement of the hip necessarily diminishes IR of both lead leg and trail legs for a thrower. It has been posited that such deficits in motion translate to increased distal kinetic chain breakdown. Byrd[57] has described the positive effects of hip arthroscopy on restoring throwing ability in athletes.

It is imperative for the examiner to discern subtle breakdowns of the kinetic chain. The following often unnoticed kinetic chain abnormalities have been called to attention: ankle stiffness or instability, loss of IR of the lead leg, lumbar spine inflexibility, psoas tightness, and hip abductor weakness.[58] Spinal inflexibility, especially accentuated lumbar lordosis, may force the torso to become positioned anterior to the arm during late cocking. This, throwing out of the scapular plane, as mentioned previously, potentiates posterior cuff and labral contact.

DIAGNOSIS OF CUFF AND LABRAL INJURY IN THE THROWER
History

Throwers usually present with chief complaints of pain, loss of velocity or control, or mechanical symptoms of clicking or locking. These symptoms suggest cuff and/or labral injury. Tenderness is usually seen posteriorly and may reflect posterior labral tear or posterior cuff irritation. Anterior pain on palpation (less common) may indicate an anterior labral disruption or leading edge of the supraspinatus lesion. Anterior/medial pain, coursing in the subpectoral region, is more consistent with biceps tendon pathology.[59] Night pain,[60] especially pain lying on the ipsilateral shoulder, usually reflects rotator cuff involvement.

The loss of zip or an inability to find the slot during throwing may be due to labral or cuff damage, with subsequent abnormal mechanics. Kinetic chain breakdown may cause errant control. For example, loss of IR of the lead leg may cause the athlete to open up prematurely during late cocking and thereby generate a loss of pitch accuracy.

Often, the thrower relays a history of an event, or single pitch after which their throwing was never the same. The event may be described as a sudden dead arm during late cocking or merely one pitch, which elicited an inordinate amount of pain. These abrupt changes in symptoms may indicate a slap event and often indicate mechanical tissue failure.

Examination

Physical examination of the thrower must include all aspects of the kinetic chain and evaluation of scapula position.[61]

Because proper conditioning of the trunk and lower extremity musculature is essential for the transfer of energy from the lower extremity to the upper extremity during the pitching motion, pathology involving the spine, trunk, and lower extremities can ultimately affect the upper extremity and predispose the athlete to injury. A comprehensive shoulder examination, therefore, begins with a brief trunk and lower extremity examination. While standing, the athlete is examined for spinal mobility by asking him or her to touch their toes with knees straight and to perform side bends. Hip abductor strength is assessed by asking the athlete to perform multiple single-leg squats on the stance leg and stride leg. Dipping of the pelvis or knee valgus during this maneuver indicates gluteus medius weakness and a significant proximal kinetic chain breakdown.[62]

No shoulder examination is complete without a scapular examination, and the athlete is asked to remove the shirt if man or don a tank top if woman for optimal inspection. Kibler's scapular slide is useful in noting scapula position both at rest and under provocation. The posterior shoulder can be effectively examined with the athlete's hands at sides[42] and with resisted arm forward flexion, to elicit serratus anterior weakness. Any asymmetry of scapular position of the left versus the right shoulder indicates dyskinesis of the scapula. Although Kibler and colleagues[63] espoused a 4-part classification for scapular dyskinesis, it is only moderately reliable in symptomatic patients and was shown to have low reliability in healthy patients.[64] Regardless, care must be taken to carefully examine the scapula position, as the presence of scapular dyskinesis frequently indicates a kinetic chain abnormality, a continued painful stimulus, or persistent anatomic lesion (ie, labral/cuff injury).[65] True scapular pathology must be associated with pain or dysfunction. As Tate and colleagues[66] have indicated, the relief of symptoms with scapular assistance or relocation denotes true scapular dysfunction. Milder degrees of scapular asymmetry may, in fact, be adaptive responses to the thrower's demands and should not necessarily be treated in the absence of pain of dysfunction.

The examination continues with the athlete sitting, whereby tenderness of the joint, anterior cuff, bicipital groove, acromioclavicular joint, and coracoid may be noted. Rotator cuff strength, especially that of the supraspinatus, is elicited.

Although the specific utility of many special shoulder tests is often controversial, several must be highlighted in the physical examination of the thrower's shoulder. The empty can test, which involves resisted downward pressure of the forward-flexed arm in the scapular plane, is effective in assessing general supraspinatus strength. The Whipple test,[67] which involves resisted downward pressure of the adducted, forward-flexed arm allows for assessment of the anterior edge of the supraspinatus tendon. The scapula retraction test[52] indicates whether or not cuff weakness may be secondary to a malpositioned, protracted scapula. To perform this test, the examiner manually affixes the medial scapular wall to the thorax and notes if suprasinatus weakness and/or internal impingement pain of the ABER position is corrected with improved scapula position. The apposition of the scapula against the chest wall literally corrects scapula protraction and restores the stable platform necessary for cuff strength. Furthermore, less protraction moves the posterior labral/cuff complex away from the greater tuberosity in ABER.

Several physical examination maneuvers are also useful in assessing the integrity of the thrower's labrum. The O'Brien test, which involves resisted downward pressure to the 90° forward-flexed, slightly adducted, and internally rotated arm, may be useful in the detection of anterior labrum tears. Anterior joint line tenderness may denote an anterior labral lesion, while posterior joint line tenderness may indicate posterior labral injury or irritation of the posterior cuff. Anterior joint line tenderness similarly may denote an anterior labral lesion. The examination continues with the Mayo shear test,[68] whereby the abducted, externally rotated arm is hyperextended and brought down to adduction. This position may literally shear the posterior labrum in the presence of GIRD and/or anterior laxity. The presence of significant pain during this maneuver, especially at or near 100° of abduction, may indicate posterior labral injury.

The examination continues with the patient in the supine position, whereupon the presence of IR deficit is discerned by stabilizing the scapula in abduction and internally rotating the humerus. Differences between affected and unaffected sides are noted. A discrepancy of more than 20° may indicate a shoulder at risk.[69] Passive ER ROM in both adduction and abduction may indicate subtle interval and anterior capsular laxity, respectively. The relocation test is performed with the patient in the ABER position with humeral extension. Posterior pain relieved with a posteriorly directed force can indicate a posterior Superior Labrum Anterior to Posterior (SLAP) tear, internal impingement, or anterior capsular laxity.

The final sequence of the examination is conducted with the patient in the lateral decubitus position, where a variation of the load shift test is performed.[70] The examiner grasps the wrist with one hand and positions the arm in roughly 20° of forward flexion and 45° of abduction. With the other hand, he or she levers the humeral head anterior/inferiorly with the thumb so that the head rides over the glenoid rim. Next, the examiner abducts and externally rotates the arm, while maintaining pressure with the other thumb, and determines if the humeral head relocates. Failure to relocate in ABER, or the presence of a significant click or clunk, may indicate capsular or labral incompetency. The examination is repeated for the middle glenohumeral ligament (MGHL) by levering the humerus anteriorly and recruiting the MGHL by abducting the arm to 45° with ER. This examination is difficult to master but may reward the examiner with helpful information regarding the competency of the anterior capsular-labral tissues. Kim's test and the jerk test[71] can also be performed to assess the competency of the posterior inferior and posterior labrum, respectively. A variation of the jerk test, with the arm in lesser degrees of abduction, may sometimes also detect subtle posterior/superior labral lesions. Finally, the newly described passive compression test by Kim for superior labral tears uses the peel back phenomenon to elicit pain.[72] The arm is abducted to approximately 30°, and maximal ER is applied. As the arm is extended, the humerus is forcibly pushed superiorly to further strain the superior labral/glenoid junction.

The panoply of labral tests available to the orthopedist can certainly cause confusion as to determining which test is the most useful. A systematic review with meta-analysis found that no single shoulder physical examination test could be relied on to make a pathognomonic diagnosis.[73] Furthermore, not one of the 8 physical examination maneuvers examined revealed a sensitivity that would allow a physician to rule out an SLAP lesion after a negative test. That being said, other groups have shown success in combining physical examination maneuvers to improve diagnostic sensitivity. For example, a sensitivity analysis of physical examination and magnetic resonance imaging (MRI) findings found that, although the sensitivity of O'Brien test was 90%, the Mayo shear test was 80%, and Jobe relocation test was 76%; the sensitivity of a physical examination with any 1 of these 3 SLAP provocative tests being positive was 100%.[74] This point is critical, as it emphasizes the importance of a complete physical examination, even if individual tests may fail the examiner.

Imaging

Critical to obtaining a complete picture of a thrower's shoulder pathology is, of course, diagnostic imaging. Routine radiographs, including a true anteroposterior, axillary, and outlet views, are usually unremarkable; however, the presence of greater tuberosity cystic changes or, more reliably, a greater tuberosity notch has been associated with articular-sided rotator cuff tears.[75] The most useful imaging study is the magnetic resonance arthrogram, with most investigators indicating superior detection of subtle cuff and labral injuries over standard MRI.[76] The addition of the ABER view adds important information regarding the status of the supraspinatus tendon and the integrity of its deep surface.[77]

Despite advances in imaging, arthroscopic evaluation remains the gold standard in diagnosis of superior labral and subtle cuff injury. Furthermore, although physical examination and imaging are usually accurate in delineating labral pathology, combined tears are often only discovered intraoperatively.[78]

Nonoperative Treatment

Treatment of the thrower's shoulder begins with conservative measures. Overt mechanical, labral symptoms, such as locking, catching, or grinding indicates the need for arthroscopic evaluation.

Posterior capsular contracture and rotator cuff tightness must be addressed and are best relieved with a dedicated posterior shoulder stretching and mobilization program. Stretches must isolate the glenohumeral joint so that scapular compensation is minimized. The sleeper stretch, whereby the patient lies on the affected shoulder to stabilize the scapula and internally rotates the abducted arm until resistance is felt is particularly effective.[79]

Performance of the stretch in 60°, 90°, and 120° of abduction is recommended, and exercises should be performed at least twice daily. Joint mobilizations can be performed by athletic trainers or physical therapists in a posterior or posterior/inferior direction to target the contracted portion of the capsule.

Kinetic chain evaluation is essential, and subtleties such as lumbopelvic stiffness, hip flexor tightness, hip abductor weakness, and lead leg loss of IR must be investigated. Once each of the above-mentioned areas demonstrate improvements, lower extremity and upper extremity exercises should be incorporated together to stimulate functional movement patterns.

Scapular dyskinesis, usually present, can often be treated with exercises to help restore scapular ER and posterior tilt. The first step in scapular rehabilitation should focus on neuromuscular reeducation of the scapular stabilizing muscles. Strengthening should not be the primary focus until proper muscular control and firing patterns are reestablished. Serratus anterior strengthening can be achieved with push-ups with a plus and low rows (**Fig. 4**).[80] Lower trapezius strengthening can be attained with prone horizontal abduction and side lying forward flexion and ER.[81] Other scapula retraction exercises, such as close grip rowing, can help maintain the medial scapula affixed to the thorax. A recent cadaveric study demonstrated that the greatest changes in pectoralis minor length were observed with scapular retraction and 30° of flexion.[82] Pectoralis minor stretches, best performed supine, can further help reposition the scapula into a more physiologic position. Because of the triceps originating on the inferior glenoid neck, it often becomes tight in throwers. Therefore, stretching into forward flexion with the scapular stabilized is often required.

Rotator cuff strengthening, especially that of the infraspinatus through resisted ER, helps restore muscle imbalance about the shoulder, protects the cuff from injury, and stress shields the supraspinatus.[83] Rotator cuff exercises should be initiated with scapular retraction before ER to reinforce correct motor patterns.

Surgery

Indications for surgery include overt mechanical symptoms and/or failure of conservative treatment. The presence of shoulder soreness alone warrants at least 3 to 4 months of dedicated physical therapy before the decision for surgery is reached. Therapy can be extended longer than this if the athlete demonstrates improvement over each successive evaluation. The decision for surgery must be undertaken with great reverence. The vast majority of throwers, especially less mature ones, are able to recover once the biomechanical perturbations of GIRD and scapular dyskinesis are resolved. Obviously, no amount of exercise will correct mechanical manifestations such as locking and catching. Such symptoms can only be remedied with arthroscopic intervention.

Resolution of symptoms and recovery to tissue homeostasis is heralded by the return of the scapula to a normal position. Scapular dyskinesis has been described as a nonspecific response to painful shoulder pathology, rather than a specific response to particular conditions.[84] Scapula position is a good barometer of active pain or biomechanical dysfunction. Thus, resolution of scapular dyskinesis usually indicates a safe return to throwing.

Principles of Surgery

Shoulder arthroscopy is performed in either the beach chair or the lateral decubitus position. A standard posterior portal is usually used along with an anterior superior portal, located just off the anterolateral acromion. Routine standard evaluation of the joint must incorporate inspection of the entire labrum, including the posterior inferior aspect. Subtle labral injuries of the posterior quadrant (Kim lesions[85]) are often seen in throwers, in addition to the expected superior labral injuries. The posterior inferior labral tears may be a result of the significant tensile stress imparted to the posterior inferior labrum during ABER in the presence of GIRD.

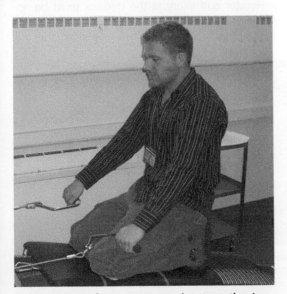

Fig. 4. Low row for serratus anterior strengthening.

The cuff is inspected carefully, especially at the leading edge of the supraspinatus and at the junction of the supraspinatus and infraspinatus, the most common site of internal impingement (**Fig. 5**). The superior labrum is probed and inspected for signs of fissuring, cracking, bleeding, or separation. Care must be undertaken to avoid mistaking a normal variant of the superior labrum, such as a meniscoid variant (with a peripheral attachment), a sublabral foramen, or a Buford complex (absent anterior labrum, cordlike MGHL), for a tear[86] for pathology. These variants are important to note, as they may render the remaining normal stabilizing structures more vulnerable to injury.[87–89] Taking the extremity out of traction and placing the arm in ABER changes the force vector of the biceps to a more posterior and medial direction. This position may elicit a peel back of the labrum off the posterior superior glenoid, thus confirming an incompetent superior labral attachment.[90] The degree of peel back was demonstrated in a cadaver study to correlate with the degree of posterior superior labral injury.[91] The discernment of pathologic versus normal variant superior labral tissue is often difficult, especially when abortive healing is present. Additional clues to labral incompetency include chondromalacial changes of the adjacent articular cartilage, a resting convex posture to the labrum, and easy separation of labral tissue from the glenoid with a semiblunt elevator.

Once the labrum is determined to be torn, the glenoid adjacent to the labrum is prepared with a shaver (not a burr, to conserve bone) until raw bony edges are attained. Percutaneous anchor placement, approaching the lesion obliquely approximately 40° to the glenoid surface, is acomplished with newer low-profile anchor systems. The Port of Wilmington (1 cm lateral and 1 cm anterior to the posterior lateral corner of the acromion), described by Morgan, may be useful to approach the type 2 posterior SLAP tear.[92] Cannulas in the posterior superior glenoid region are discouraged because the threat of cuff injury is significant. Percutaneous anchor insertion and percutaneous suture shuttling techniques avert supraspinatus/infraspinatus injury.[93] Shuttling suture limbs and tying to an anterior portal are readily accomplished without the need for an additional posterior cannula placement. Suture anchors are generally regarded to resist strain better than tacks and also obviate the concern for tack erosion or breakage.[94] A single-suture anchor placed just posterior to the biceps successfully eliminates peel back.[91] In addition, Yoo and colleagues[95] demonstrated that a single posterior anchor worked as well as 2 in a load to failure cadaver study. Furthermore, techniques using either 2 single-loaded suture anchors in a simple suture configuration or 1 double-loaded suture anchor in a V-shaped simple suture configuration were shown to result in significantly larger pressurized contact areas between the biceps-labrum complex and glenoid rim than a method using 1 double-loaded suture anchor with a hybrid simple and mattress suture configuration in another cadaveric study of SLAP repairs.[96]

In the presence of significant rotator interval laxity, gentle shortening of the course of the CHL should be considered with absorbable suture. This should be performed with the arm in ER so as not to overconstrain ER. McHale and colleagues[97] have demonstrated the arthroscopic localization of the CHL and its angular relationship to the biceps tendon to allow for such management.

Rotator cuff injury in the thrower must be approached with a conservative mind-set, and the temptation to anatomically reconstruct the cuff

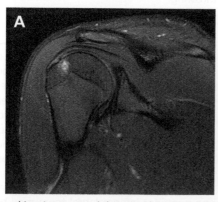
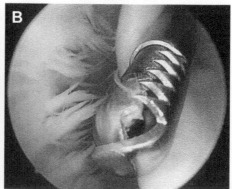

Fig. 5. Internal impingement. (*A*) Internal impingement with edema in the posterior lateral humeral head on coronal T2-weighted MRI. (*B*) Internal impingement noted arthroscopically with fraying at the junction of the supraspinatus and infraspinatus. Internal impingement is an important cause of posterior shoulder pain that may potentiate posterior cuff and labrum injury.

must be resisted. The excessive stiffness that footprint restoration engenders often prohibits the athlete from finding the slot, prevents throwing with any gainful velocity,[98] and therefore full return of preinjury level of function. Although there is no consensus on the surgical approach to partial-thickness rotator cuff tears of debridement or repair, a systematic review found data to support the notion that tears involving less than 50% of the tendon can be treated successfully with debridement (with or without acromioplasty), whereas tears involving greater than 50% of the tendon have been successfully managed with repair.[99] However, when debridement is sufficient, without the need for fixation, side-to-side suture or coaptation of intrasubstance tearing may be beneficial. There is no real role for acromioplasty in a young thrower. The coracoacromial arch confers some anterior stability to the glenohumeral joint. Furthermore, a review of the literature on the role of acromioplasty in the management of rotator cuff pathology failed to find additional benefits, and thus its routine use was not recommended.[100]

Anterior capsular laxity can be effectively addressed with a subtle plication of the anterior inferior capsule. A study in a cadaveric model further demonstrated that suture anchor capsulorrhaphy provided biomechanical advantages to labral-based suture capsulorrhaphy.[101] However, this is an area of great controversy, as others have found superior results when labral repair was accompanied by gentle thermal shrinkage of the anterior capsule.[22,102]

If persistent posterior capsular tightness is present, especially in more mature throwers, a posterior inferior capsulotomy may be performed.[103,104] This procedure is readily performed with a high anterior viewing portal and a standard posterior inferior working portal. Electrothermal devices create a bloodless field and may alert the surgeon to approximation to the axillary nerve as well. If the release is executed from the 6-o'clock to 9-o'clock position and close to the labrum, there is no significant threat of axillary nerve injury.[105]

Rehabilitation

Sling immobilization is generally recommended for 3 to 4 weeks after labral repair, with elbow motion and scapula retraction exercises encouraged immediately. Gentle forward flexion is permissible, but avoidance of abduction and ER is prudent to avoid peel back stress. If a concomitant posterior release was performed, sleeper stretches may be performed immediately without concern for disruption of the labral repair.

PREVENTION

Prevention of injury in the thrower is predicated on vigilance in monitoring for signs of the shoulder at risk. In particular, GIRD, scapular dyskinesis, kinetic chain breakdown, and cuff weakness must be recognized early before cuff or labral failure occurs. Proper pitching mechanics, especially encouragement of throwing in the scapular plane and maintenance of the raised elbow, may further protect the thrower from injury. Some of the biomechanical perturbations can be reversed quickly in the less mature athlete. As a result, many shoulders can be saved when the proper knowledge is applied in a timely fashion.

Adolescent pitchers are at particular risk for overuse injury, and some evidence suggests an increase in surgical rates for pitching-related injuries in immature throwers (**Fig. 6**).[106] In a 10-year follow-up study of shoulder injuries in young baseball pitchers, pitching more than 100 innings in a year significantly increased the risk of injury.[107] The use of breaking ball pitches as a risk factor for injury in youth is controversial, but many argue against their usage until age 13 years, because of improper mechanics. That being said, a recent biomechanical comparison of the fastball and curveball in adolescent pitchers actually found that kinematic and kinetic data indicated greater moments on the shoulder and elbow with fastballs, rather than curve balls.[108] The following recommendations for adolescent throwers have more consensus agreement: (1) avoid pitching with arm fatigue or pain, (2) avoid exceeding 80 pitches per game or 2500 pitches per year, (3) avoid competitive pitching more than 8 months a year,

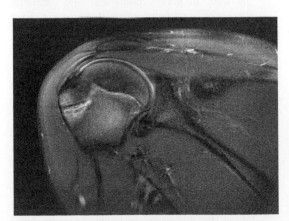

Fig. 6. Physeal edema in a young thrower. Adolescent pitchers are at particular risk for overuse injuries and are prone to unique pathology secondary to open physes. The coronal T2-weighted image demonstrates physeal edema in a young thrower that may be indirect evidence of physeal strain.

and (4) exercise caution and restraint in pitching showcases.[109] More recent recommendations from the Little League Baseball regulations committee include mandatory rest of up to 4 days, depending on the specific age and number of pitches thrown in a given day.[110]

The preponderance of throwing-related injuries can be prevented with vigilance of the shoulder at risk. Dedicated attention to maintaining the suppleness of the posterior capsule, awareness of kinetic chain breakdown, avoidance of overuse, and continual posterior rotator cuff strengthening may avert the development of rotator cuff and labral injuries.

REFERENCES

1. Kuhn JE, Lindholm SR, Huston LJ, et al. Failure of the biceps superior labral complex: a cadaveric biomechanical investigation comparing the late cocking and early deceleration positions of throwing. Arthroscopy 2003;19:373–9.
2. Fleisig GS, Andrews JR, Dillman CJ, et al. Kinetics of baseball pitching with implications about injury mechanisms. Am J Sports Med 1995;23:233–9.
3. Borsa PA, Laudner KG, Sauers EL. Mobility and stability adaptations in the shoulder of the overhead athlete: a theoretical and evidence-based perspective. Sports Med 2008;38:17–36.
4. Kuhn JE, Bey MJ, Huston LJ, et al. Ligamentous restraints to external rotation of the humerus in the late-cocking phase of throwing. A cadaveric biomechanical investigation. Am J Sports Med 2000;28:200–5.
5. Werner SL, Gill TJ, Murray TA, et al. Relationships between throwing mechanics and shoulder distraction in professional baseball pitchers. Am J Sports Med 2001;29:354–8.
6. Thomas SJ, Swanik CB, Higginson JS, et al. A bilateral comparison of posterior capsule thickness and its correlation with glenohumeral range of motion and scapular upward rotation in collegiate baseball players. J Shoulder Elbow Surg 2011;20:708–16.
7. Thomas SJ, Swanik CB, Higginson JS, et al. Neuromuscular and stiffness adaptations in division I collegiate baseball players. J Electromyogr Kinesiol 2013;23:102–9.
8. Reinold MM, Wilk KE, Macrina LC, et al. Changes in shoulder and elbow passive range of motion after pitching in professional baseball players. Am J Sports Med 2008;36:523–7.
9. Urbin MA, Fleisig GS, Abebe A, et al. Associations between timing in the baseball pitch and shoulder kinetics, elbow kinetics, and ball speed. Am J Sports Med 2013;41:336–42.

10. Edelson G. Variations in the retroversion of the humeral head. J Shoulder Elbow Surg 1999;8:142–5.
11. Sabick MB, Kim YK, Torry MR, et al. Biomechanics of the shoulder in youth baseball pitchers: implications for the development of proximal humeral epiphysiolysis and humeral retrotorsion. Am J Sports Med 2005;33:1716–22.
12. Wyland DJ, Pill SG, Shanley E, et al. Bony adaptation of the proximal humerus and glenoid correlate within the throwing shoulder of professional baseball pitchers. Am J Sports Med 2012;40:1858–62.
13. Crockett HC, Gross LB, Wilk KE, et al. Osseous adaptation and range of motion at the glenohumeral joint in professional baseball pitchers. Am J Sports Med 2002;30:20–6.
14. Halbrecht JL, Tirman P, Atkin D. Internal impingement of the shoulder: comparison of findings between the throwing and nonthrowing shoulders of college baseball players. Arthroscopy 1999;15:253–8.
15. Thomas SJ, Swanik CB, Kaminski TW, et al. Humeral retroversion and its association with posterior capsule thickness in collegiate baseball players. J Shoulder Elbow Surg 2012;21:910–6.
16. O'Connell PW, Nuber GW, Mileski RA, et al. The contribution of the glenohumeral ligaments to anterior stability of the shoulder joint. Am J Sports Med 1990;18:579–84.
17. O'Brien SJ, Schwartz RS, Warren RF, et al. Capsular restraints to anterior-posterior motion of the abducted shoulder: a biomechanical study. J Shoulder Elbow Surg 1995;4:298–308.
18. McMahon PJ, Tibone JE, Cawley PW, et al. The anterior band of the inferior glenohumeral ligament: biomechanical properties from tensile testing in the position of apprehension. J Shoulder Elbow Surg 1998;7:467–71.
19. Bigliani LU, Codd TP, Connor PM, et al. Shoulder motion and laxity in the professional baseball player. Am J Sports Med 1997;25:609–13.
20. Brown LP, Niehues SL, Harrah A, et al. Upper extremity range of motion and isokinetic strength of the internal and external shoulder rotators in major league baseball players. Am J Sports Med 1988;16:577–85.
21. Jobe FW, Giangarra CE, Kvitne RS, et al. Anterior capsulolabral reconstruction of the shoulder in athletes in overhand sports. Am J Sports Med 1991;19:428–34.
22. Levitz CL, Dugas J, Andrews JR. The use of arthroscopic thermal capsulorrhaphy to treat internal impingement in baseball players. Arthroscopy 2001;17:573–7.
23. Karduna AR, McClure PW, Michener LA, et al. Dynamic measurements of three-dimensional scapular kinematics: a validation study. J Biomech Eng 2001;123:184–90.

24. Rizio L, Garcia J, Renard R, et al. Anterior instability increases superior labral strain in the late cocking phase of throwing. Orthopedics 2007;30:544–50.

25. Habermeyer P, Krieter C, Tang KL, et al. A new arthroscopic classification of articular-sided supraspinatus footprint lesions: a prospective comparison with Snyder's and Ellman's classification. J Shoulder Elbow Surg 2008;17:909–13.

26. Meister K. Injuries to the shoulder in the throwing athlete. Part one: biomechanics/pathophysiology/classification of injury. Am J Sports Med 2000;28: 265–75.

27. Osbahr DC, Cannon DL, Speer KP. Retroversion of the humerus in the throwing shoulder of college baseball pitchers. Am J Sports Med 2002;30: 347–53.

28. Shanley E, Thigpen CA, Clark JC, et al. Changes in passive range of motion and development of glenohumeral internal rotation deficit (GIRD) in the professional pitching shoulder between spring training in two consecutive years. J Shoulder Elbow Surg 2012;21:1605–12.

29. Lintner D, Mayol M, Uzodinma O, et al. Glenohumeral internal rotation deficits in professional pitchers enrolled in an internal rotation stretching program. Am J Sports Med 2007;35:617–21.

30. Aldridge R, Stephen Guffey J, Whitehead MT, et al. The effects of a daily stretching protocol on passive glenohumeral internal rotation in overhead throwing collegiate athletes. Int J Sports Phys Ther 2012;7: 365–71.

31. Burkhart SS, Morgan CD, Kibler WB. Shoulder injuries in overhead athletes. The "dead arm" revisited. Clin Sports Med 2000;19:125–58.

32. Wilk KE, Macrina LC, Fleisig GS, et al. Correlation of glenohumeral internal rotation deficit and total rotational motion to shoulder injuries in professional baseball pitchers. Am J Sports Med 2011; 39:329–35.

33. Clabbers KM, Kelly JD, Bader D, et al. Effect of posterior capsule tightness on glenohumeral translation in the late-cocking phase of pitching. J Sport Rehabil 2007;16:41–9.

34. Koffler KM, Kelly JD. The effect of posterior capsular tightness on glenohumeral translation in the late-cocking phase of pitching: a cadaveric study, in Arthroscopy Association of North America Annual Meeting. Washington, DC, 2002.

35. Grossman MG, Tibone JE, McGarry MH, et al. A cadaveric model of the throwing shoulder: a possible etiology of superior labrum anterior-to-posterior lesions. J Bone Joint Surg Am 2005;87: 824–31.

36. Huffman GR, Tibone JE, McGarry MH, et al. Path of glenohumeral articulation throughout the rotational range of motion in a thrower's shoulder model. Am J Sports Med 2006;34:1662–9.

37. Gates JJ, Gupta A, McGarry MH, et al. The effect of glenohumeral internal rotation deficit due to posterior capsular contracture on passive glenohumeral joint motion. Am J Sports Med 2012;40: 2794–800.

38. Laudner KG, Myers JB, Pasquale MR, et al. Scapular dysfunction in throwers with pathologic internal impingement. J Orthop Sports Phys Ther 2006;36: 485–94.

39. Burkhart SS, Morgan CD, Kibler WB. The disabled throwing shoulder: spectrum of pathology. Part I: pathoanatomy and biomechanics. Arthroscopy 2003;19:404–20.

40. Burkhart SS, Lo IK. The cam effect of the proximal humerus: its role in the production of relative capsular redundancy of the shoulder. Arthroscopy 2007;23:241–6.

41. Lippitt SB, Vanderhooft JE, Harris SL, et al. Glenohumeral stability from concavity-compression: a quantitative analysis. J Shoulder Elbow Surg 1993;2:27–35.

42. Kibler WB, McMullen J. Scapular dyskinesis and its relation to shoulder pain. J Am Acad Orthop Surg 2003;11:142–51.

43. Pink MM, Perry J. Biomechanics of the shoulder. St Louis (MO): Mosby-Year Book; 1996.

44. McClure PW, Michener LA, Sennett BJ, et al. Direct 3-dimensional measurement of scapular kinematics during dynamic movements in vivo. J Shoulder Elbow Surg 2001;10:269–77.

45. McQuade KJ, Dawson J, Smidt GL. Scapulothoracic muscle fatigue associated with alterations in scapulohumeral rhythm kinematics during maximum resistive shoulder elevation. J Orthop Sports Phys Ther 1998;28:74–80.

46. Kibler WB, McMullen J, Uhl T. Shoulder rehabilitation strategies, guidelines, and practice. Orthop Clin North Am 2001;32:527–38.

47. Lukasiewicz AC, McClure P, Michener L, et al. Comparison of 3-dimensional scapular position and orientation between subjects with and without shoulder impingement. J Orthop Sports Phys Ther 1999;29:574–83 [discussion: 584–6].

48. Myers JB, Laudner KG, Pasquale MR, et al. Scapular position and orientation in throwing athletes. Am J Sports Med 2005;33:263–71.

49. Pink MM. Understanding the linkage system of the upper extremity. Sports Med Arthrosc Rev 2001; 9(1):52–60.

50. Thomas SJ, Swanik KA, Swanik CB, et al. The effect of GIRD on scapular upward rotation and protraction in competitive baseball players. Clin Orthop Relat Res 2009;468:1551–7.

51. Thomas SJ, Swanik KA, Swanik CB, et al. Internal rotation and scapular position differences: a comparison of collegiate and high school baseball players. J Athl Train 2010;45:44–50.

52. Kibler WB, Sciascia A, Dome D. Evaluation of apparent and absolute supraspinatus strength in patients with shoulder injury using the scapular retraction test. Am J Sports Med 2006;34:1643–7.

53. Weiser WM, Lee TQ, McMaster WC, et al. Effects of simulated scapular protraction on anterior glenohumeral stability. Am J Sports Med 1999;27:801–5.

54. Rubin BD, Kibler WB. Fundamental principles of shoulder rehabilitation: conservative to postoperative management. Arthroscopy 2002;18:29–39.

55. Sciascia A, Thigpen C, Namdari S, et al. Kinetic chain abnormalities in the athletic shoulder. Sports Med Arthrosc 2012;20:16–21.

56. Suzuki H, Huxel KC, Kelly JD IV, et al. Alterations in upper extremity motion after scapular-muscle fatigue. J Sport Rehabil 2006;15:71–88.

57. Byrd TJ. Hip arthroscopy in high level baseball players, in AANA Annual Meeting. San Antonio (TX), 2013.

58. Sciascia A, Cromwell R. Kinetic chain rehabilitation: a theoretical framework. Rehabil Res Pract 2012; 2012:853037.

59. Snyder GM, Mair SD, Lattermann C. Tendinopathy of the long head of the biceps. Med Sport Sci 2012; 57:76–89.

60. Xiao J, Cui GQ, Wang JQ. Diagnosis of bursal-side partial-thickness rotator cuff tears. Orthop Surg 2010;2:260–5.

61. Kelly JD IV, Thomas SJ. Identifying and managing scapular problems in overhead athletes. J Musculoskelet Med 2007;24:228–35.

62. Takacs J, Hunt MA. The effect of contralateral pelvic drop and trunk lean on frontal plane knee biomechanics during single limb standing. J Biomech 2012;45:2791–6.

63. Kibler WB, Uhl TL, Maddux JW, et al. Qualitative clinical evaluation of scapular dysfunction: a reliability study. J Shoulder Elbow Surg 2002;11: 550–6.

64. Ellenbecker TS, Kibler WB, Bailie DS, et al. Reliability of scapular classification in examination of professional baseball players. Clin Orthop Relat Res 2012;470:1540–4.

65. Kibler WB, Sciascia A, Wilkes T. Scapular dyskinesis and its relation to shoulder injury. J Am Acad Orthop Surg 2012;20:364–72.

66. Tate AR, McClure P, Kareha S, et al. A clinical method for identifying scapular dyskinesis, part 2: validity. J Athl Train 2009;44:165–73.

67. Savoie FH, Field LD, Atchinson S. Anterior superior instability with rotator cuff tearing: SLAC lesion. Oper Tech Sports Med 2000;8:221–4.

68. Kibler WB, Tambay NS. Shoulder inquiry encompasses kinetic chain structures. Biomechanics, 49–57, 2005.

69. Kibler WB, Sciascia A, Thomas SJ. Glenohumeral internal rotation deficit: pathogenesis and response to acute throwing. Sports Med Arthrosc 2012;20:34–8.

70. Silliman JF, Hawkins RJ. Classification and physical diagnosis of instability of the shoulder. Clin Orthop Relat Res 1993;(291):7–19.

71. Kim SH, Park JS, Jeong WK, et al. The Kim test: a novel test for posteroinferior labral lesion of the shoulder–a comparison to the jerk test. Am J Sports Med 2005;33:1188–92.

72. Kim YS, Kim JM, Ha KY, et al. The passive compression test: a new clinical test for superior labral tears of the shoulder. Am J Sports Med 2007;35:1489–94.

73. Hegedus EJ, Goode AP, Cook CE, et al. Which physical examination tests provide clinicians with the most value when examining the shoulder? Update of a systematic review with meta-analysis of individual tests. Br J Sports Med 2012;46:964–78.

74. Pandya NK, Colton A, Webner D, et al. Physical examination and magnetic resonance imaging in the diagnosis of superior labrum anterior-posterior lesions of the shoulder: a sensitivity analysis. Arthroscopy 2008;24:311–7.

75. Nakagawa S, Yoneda M, Hayashida K, et al. Greater tuberosity notch: an important indicator of articular-side partial rotator cuff tears in the shoulders of throwing athletes. Am J Sports Med 2001; 29:762–70.

76. Bencardino JT, Beltran J, Rosenberg ZS, et al. Superior labrum anterior-posterior lesions: diagnosis with MR arthrography of the shoulder. Radiology 2000;214:267–71.

77. Matava MJ, Purcell DB, Rudzki JR. Partial-thickness rotator cuff tears. Am J Sports Med 2005;33: 1405–17.

78. Dickens JF, Kilcoyne KG, Haniuk E, et al. Combined lesions of the glenoid labrum. Phys Sportsmed 2012;40:102–8.

79. Burkhart SS, Morgan CD, Kibler WB. The disabled throwing shoulder: spectrum of pathology. Part III: The SICK scapula, scapular dyskinesis, the kinetic chain, and rehabilitation. Arthroscopy 2003;19: 641–61.

80. Andersen CH, Zebis MK, Saervoll C, et al. Scapular muscle activity from selected strengthening exercises performed at low and high intensities. J Strength Cond Res 2012;26:2408–16.

81. Cools AM, Dewitte V, Lanszweert F, et al. Rehabilitation of scapular muscle balance: which exercises to prescribe? Am J Sports Med 2007;35:1744–51.

82. Muraki T, Aoki M, Izumi T, et al. Lengthening of the pectoralis minor muscle during passive shoulder motions and stretching techniques: a cadaveric biomechanical study. Phys Ther 2009;89:333–41.

83. Andarawis-Puri N, Kuntz AF, Ramsey ML, et al. Effect of glenohumeral abduction angle on the mechanical interaction between the supraspinatus

and infraspinatus tendons for the intact, partial-thickness torn, and repaired supraspinatus tendon conditions. J Orthop Res 2010;28:846–51.

84. Kibler WB, Sciascia A. Current concepts: scapular dyskinesis. Br J Sports Med 2010;44:300–5.

85. Kim SH, Ha KI, Yoo JC, et al. Kim's lesion: an incomplete and concealed avulsion of the posteroinferior labrum in posterior or multidirectional posteroinferior instability of the shoulder. Arthroscopy 2004;20:712–20.

86. Williams MM, Snyder SJ, Buford D Jr. The Buford complex–the "cord-like" middle glenohumeral ligament and absent anterosuperior labrum complex: a normal anatomic capsulolabral variant. Arthroscopy 1994;10:241–7.

87. Rao AG, Kim TK, Chronopoulos E, et al. Anatomical variants in the anterosuperior aspect of the glenoid labrum: a statistical analysis of seventy-three cases. J Bone Joint Surg Am 2003;85A:653–9.

88. Ilahi OA, Labbe MR, Cosculluela P. Variants of the anterosuperior glenoid labrum and associated pathology. Arthroscopy 2002;18:882–6.

89. Bents RT, Skeete KD. The correlation of the Buford complex and SLAP lesions. J Shoulder Elbow Surg 2005;14:565–9.

90. Burkhart SS, Morgan CD, Kibler WB. The disabled throwing shoulder: spectrum of pathology. Part II: evaluation and treatment of SLAP lesions in throwers. Arthroscopy 2003;19:531–9.

91. Seneviratne A, Montgomery K, Bevilacqua B, et al. Quantifying the extent of a type II SLAP lesion required to cause peel-back of the glenoid labrum–a cadaveric study. Arthroscopy 2006;22:1163.e1–6.

92. Morgan RJ, Kuremsky MA, Peindl RD, et al. A biomechanical comparison of two suture anchor configurations for the repair of type II SLAP lesions subjected to a peel-back mechanism of failure. Arthroscopy 2008;24:383–8.

93. Galano GJ, Ahmad CS, Bigliani L, et al. Percutaneous SLAP lesion repair technique is an effective alternative to portal of Wilmington. Orthopedics 2010;33:803.

94. McFarland EG, Park HB, Keyurapan E, et al. Suture anchors and tacks for shoulder surgery, part 1: biology and biomechanics. Am J Sports Med 2005;33:1918–23.

95. Yoo JC, Ahn JH, Lee SH, et al. A biomechanical comparison of repair techniques in posterior type II superior labral anterior and posterior (SLAP) lesions. J Shoulder Elbow Surg 2008;17:144–9.

96. Kim SJ, Kim SH, Lee SK, et al. Footprint contact restoration between the biceps-labrum complex and the glenoid rim in SLAP repair: a comparative cadaveric study using pressure-sensitive film. Arthroscopy 2013;29:1005–11.

97. McHale KP, Garcia G, Kelly J. Arthroscopic localization of the coracohumeral ligament, in AANA Annual Meeting. San Antonio (TX), 2013.

98. Mazoue CG, Andrews JR. Repair of full-thickness rotator cuff tears in professional baseball players. Am J Sports Med 2006;34:182–9.

99. Strauss EJ, Salata MJ, Kercher J, et al. Multimedia article. The arthroscopic management of partial-thickness rotator cuff tears: a systematic review of the literature. Arthroscopy 2011;27:568–80.

100. Shi LL, Edwards TB. The role of acromioplasty for management of rotator cuff problems: where is the evidence? Adv Orthop 2012;2012:467571.

101. Gillis RC, Donaldson CT, Kim H, et al. Arthroscopic suture anchor capsulorrhaphy versus labral-based suture capsulorrhaphy in a cadaveric model. Arthroscopy 2012;28:1615–21.

102. Jansen N, Van Riet RP, Meermans G, et al. Thermal capsulorrhaphy in internal shoulder impingement: a 7-year follow-up study. Acta Orthop Belg 2012;78:304–8.

103. Warner JJ, Ticker JB, Beim GM. Recognition and treatment of refractory capsular contracture of the shoulder. Arthroscopy 2000;16:673–4.

104. Ticker JB, Beim GM, Warner JJ. Recognition and treatment of refractory posterior capsular contracture of the shoulder. Arthroscopy 2000;16:27–34.

105. Yoneda M, Nakagawa S, Mizuno N, et al. Arthroscopic capsular release for painful throwing shoulder with posterior capsular tightness. Arthroscopy 2006;22:801.e1–5.

106. Fleisig GS, Kingsley DS, Loftice JW, et al. Kinetic comparison among the fastball, curveball, change-up, and slider in collegiate baseball pitchers. Am J Sports Med 2006;34:423–30.

107. Fleisig GS, Andrews JR, Cutter GR, et al. Risk of serious injury for young baseball pitchers: a 10-year prospective study. Am J Sports Med 2011;39:253–7.

108. Nissen CW, Westwell M, Ounpuu S, et al. A biomechanical comparison of the fastball and curveball in adolescent baseball pitchers. Am J Sports Med 2009;37:1492–8.

109. Olsen SJ 2nd, Fleisig GS, Dun S, et al. Risk factors for shoulder and elbow injuries in adolescent baseball pitchers. Am J Sports Med 2006;34:905–12.

110. Zarenski JL, Krabak BJ. Shoulder injuries in the skeletally immature baseball pitcher and recommendations for the prevention of injury. PM R 2012;4:509–16.

Oncology

Preface
Oncology

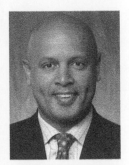

Felasfa M. Wodajo, MD
Editor

In the oncology section of this issue of *Orthopedic Clinics of North America*, we examine bisphosphonates, among the most widely used medications in orthopedics, and common polyostotic skeletal conditions.

In "Use of Bisphosphonates in Orthopaedic Surgery: Pearls and Pitfalls," Dr Santiago Lozano-Calderon and coauthors review the most common indications for these powerful anti-osteoclastic medications, including senile and glucocorticoid-mediated osteoporosis, metastatic carcinoma osteolysis in arthroplasty, and Paget disease. They also review the available evidence for bisphosphonate use in pediatric bone disorders.

Although increasing use has created more awareness of adverse effects, these drugs remain highly effective interventions and this review offers valuable insights for almost any orthopedic surgeon. Dr Lozano-Calderon recently completed fellowship in musculoskeletal oncology at Harvard University.

In "Five Polyostotic Conditions that General Orthopedic Surgeons Should Recognize (or Should Not Miss)," Dr Muthusamy and coauthors provide a well-organized description of multiple enchondromas and osteochondromas, polyostotic fibrous dysplasia, Paget disease, and skeletal metastases. While the radiographic diagnosis of bone tumors can sometimes be challenging for the non-oncologic orthopedist, the presence of multiple lesions markedly narrows the number of potential diagnoses–and thus familiarity with the most common polyostotic conditions can be very useful for the non-oncologic orthopedic surgeon.

Felasfa M. Wodajo, MD
Musculoskeletal Tumor Surgery
Virginia Hospital Center
Orthopedic Surgery
Georgetown University Hospital
VCU School of Medicine
Inova Campus
Arlington, VA 22205, USA

E-mail address:
wodajo@tumors.md

http://dx.doi.org/10.1016/j.ocl.2014.04.008
0030-5898/14/$ – see front matter

orthopedic.theclinics.com

Use of Bisphosphonates in Orthopedic Surgery
Pearls and Pitfalls

Santiago A. Lozano-Calderon, MD, PhD[a,b,c,*],
Matthew W. Colman, MD[a,b,c], Kevin A. Raskin, MD[a],
Francis J. Hornicek, MD, PhD[a], Mark Gebhardt, MD[b,c]

KEYWORDS

- Bisphosphonates • Osteoporosis • Osseous metastasis • Paget disease • Osteoclast
- Bone turnover • Pathologic fractures • Jaw osteonecrosis

KEY POINTS

- Bisphosphonates are the first line of therapy in most patients with osteoporosis.
- Bisphosphonates decrease the risk of fractures in the hip, the spine, and other nonvertebral sites in patients with osteoporosis.
- Bisphosphonates are cost-effective and effective in decreasing mortality and increasing survival in patients with osteoporosis.
- The protective effect of bisphosphonates continues with long-term therapy in patients with osteoporosis.
- The benefit of bisphosphonate use outweighs the risk of adverse effects, which are uncommon but are becoming more noticeable because of the current widespread use.
- Indications for the use of bisphosphonates are increasing because good results are being obtained when treating orthopedic conditions in which the common denominator is increased osteoclastic activity.

INTRODUCTION

There is a significant number of skeletal disorders affecting bone mineral density that are product of increased osteoclastic activity. Some of these are prevalent in the general population, such as osteoporosis and skeletal metastatic disease. Others are less frequent, such Paget disease and osteogenesis imperfecta (OI).

Bisphosphonates are the most clinically important and widely used antiresorptive medication for the treatment of conditions with increased bone resorption caused by osteoclastic activity, including osteoporosis, Paget disease, and metastatic bone disease.[1] These are synthetic, metabolically stable analogues of inorganic pyrophosphate in which the P-O-P bond has been replaced by a nonhydrolyzable P-C-P.[2] The diphosphate configuration of this molecule facilitates the binding of calcium molecules, which is thought to be the main biochemical reason for the high affinity to bone seen with these compounds. Because of this property they were initially used as bone scanning markers when combined with radioisotopes.[2]

Disclosures: None of the authors has any conflicts or disclosures related directly or indirectly to the work in this article.
[a] Department of Orthopedic Surgery, Massachusetts General Hospital, Boston, MA, USA; [b] Department of Orthopedic Surgery, Beth Israel Deaconess Medical Center, Boston, MA, USA; [c] Department of Orthopedic Surgery, Boston Children's Hospital, Boston, MA, USA
* Corresponding author. Massachusetts General Hospital, YAW 3B, 55 Fruit Street, Boston MA 02114.
E-mail address: slozanocalderon@mgh.harvard.edu

orthopedic.theclinics.com

In the last decade, this group of medications has been widely researched, especially in osteoporosis. Their efficacy has been proved by many investigations in fracture prevention.[3] Because bisphosphonates are cost-effective and safe to use, their current use is widespread: at least 4 million American women were prescribed bisphosphonates for the treatment of osteoporosis in 2008.[4]

Several bisphosphonates have been approved by the United States Food and Drug Administration (FDA) for the treatment of orthopedic conditions characterized by increased osteoclastic activity and/or decreased bone mineral density (**Table 1**).

Multiple investigations have shown good results with off-label use of these medications in a large and diverse spectrum of conditions. Orthopedic surgeons need to be familiar with the use of bisphosphonates and current indications. This article reviews of the use of bisphosphonates in orthopedic surgery.

MECHANISM OF ACTION

The general effect of bisphosphonates is to inhibit bone resorption.[5] Recent research has helped to clarify the molecular and cellular mechanisms through which this group of compounds works.

Bisphosphonates are classified into 2 major groups according to their chemical structure: nitrogen-containing (NC) and non–nitrogen-containing (NNC) bisphosphonates (**Fig. 1**).[5] The NNC group includes etidronate, clodronate, and tiludronate, which contain a simple nonnitrogen substitute group such as $-OH$, $-H$, or CH_3 that is metabolized into a toxic analogue of adenosine triphosphate (ATP). This analogue prompts inhibition of function and apoptosis in the osteoclast after intracellular accumulation.[6]

The NC group is a newer class in which the radical chain includes amino groups or molecules. These bisphosphonates are more potent (up to 1000-fold) in terms of antiresorptive effect. Bisphosphonates in this group include zoledronic acid, pamidronate, alendronate, and risedronate. Their main mechanism of action is inhibition of the enzyme farnesyl pyrophosphate synthase, an essential enzyme in the mevalonate pathway (**Fig. 2**) in the osteoclast.[7] This enzyme is key in the process known as protein prenylation (transferring of a lipid on to a cysteine residue of a protein). GTPase is an important signaling protein, the synthesis of which depends on prenylation.[8] The lack of GTPase causes osteoclast dysregulation, characterized by altered membrane trafficking, lack of cellular morphology control, disruption of integrin signaling, loss of membrane ruffling, and ultimately apoptosis.[1,6]

The NC bisphosphonates effect is not specific to the osteoclast. The mevalonate pathway is present in several cell types. It seems that, because the osteoclast is in intimate contact with the bone surface during resorption, it is exposed to

Table 1
Commonly used bisphosphonates and their indications

Generic Name	Commercial Name	Route of Administration	Potency	FDA Approval	FDA Approved Uses
Etidronate	Didronel	Oral	—	Yes	Osteoporosis
Clodronate	Multiple brands (Bonefos)	Oral Intravenous	1	Yes	Metastatic osteolysis
Tiludronate	Skelid	Oral	0.8	Yes	Paget disease
Alendronate	Fosamax	Oral	150	Yes	Osteoporosis Paget disease
Pamidronate	Aredia	Intravenous	20	Yes	Paget disease Hypercalcemia of malignancy Metastatic osteolysis
Risedronate	Actonel, Optinate	Oral	700	Yes	Osteoporosis Paget disease
Ibandronate	Bondronat Boniva	Oral Intravenous	860	Yes	Osteoporosis
Zoledronic acid	Zometa	Intravenous	>10,000	Yes	Hypercalcemia of Malignancy Metastatic Osteolysis

Potency reported as per Green and colleagues'[38] investigation. Comparisons made in relation to the medication's median inhibition of vitamin D–stimulated hyperkalemia in thyroid/parathyroidectomized rats.

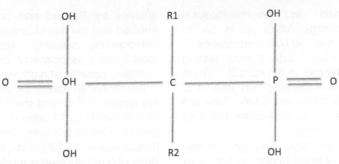

Fig. 1. Bisphosphonates skeleton.

higher concentration of bisphosphonates than other cells.[7-9] The clinical relevance of the bisphosphonate effect in other cellular groups still needs to be determined.

INDICATIONS

There are multiple conditions for which bisphosphonates are used; the common denominator of these is pathologic processes in which bone loss secondary to osteoclastic activity is characteristic.

Osteoporosis

Osteoporosis is one of the first indications for which bisphosphonates received FDA approval for use.[3,10] This common condition affects 75 million people in Europe, Japan, and the United States.[1] The World Health Organization has defined osteoporosis as a mineral bone density that is 2.5 standard deviations less than the peak of young adults of the same gender and race.[11]

This value is expressed as a T score. When the bone density value is compared with normal individuals of the same age and gender, it is expressed as the Z score. A Z score of less than −2, reflects the lowest 2.5%.

Osteoporosis is recognized as the primary independent risk factor for fractures in the elderly that can be treated and effectively risk reduced.[12,13] Multiple medications, including hormone replacement therapy, selective estrogen receptor modulators (Raloxifene), calcitonin therapy, and bisphosphonates, are available and have been used because of their antiresorptive effect. Bisphosphonates have become the most important antiresorptive because they are the only of such medications that have proved to reduce the risk of hip fracture in large, placebo-controlled, randomized trials (PCRTs).[14-20]

Most data regarding fracture reduction efficacy and safety of bisphosphonates come from prospective, randomized, placebo-controlled, phase

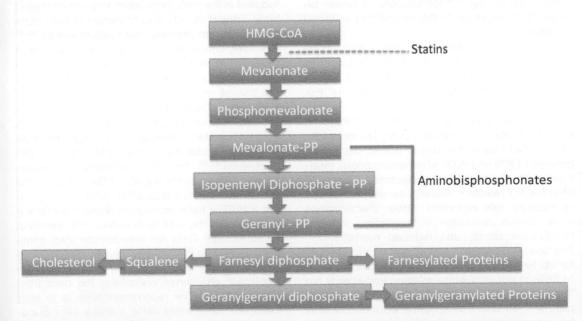

Fig. 2. Mevalonate pathway.

III regulatory trials in postmenopausal women.[10,14,16–23] Average follow-up is up to 3 years with fewer than 50,000 participants in terms of study samples.[10] Only 2 trials testing alendronate were extended to 10 years.[13,22] There are concerns in terms of the long-term effects of bisphosphonates (as discussed later). Data are scarce and there are no placebo-controlled data beyond the 5-year benchmark.[1,10]

There are 10 trials that have evaluated the efficacy of the antifracture effect of bisphosphonates in osteoporosis. **Table 2** presents a summary of these. The first landmark study is the Fracture Intervention Trial (FIT),[17] which was a multicenter prospective investigation in 3658 women at risk of osteoporotic fractures, who were randomized to receive alendronate or placebo for 3 to 4 years; patients and examiners were blinded to the intervention. The main end point was the presence of a vertebral fracture, defined as clinically evident vertebral fracture or the loss of more than 20% of the lateral radiograph view in a given vertebral body. Of the women treated with alendronate, only 8% presented radiographically evident vertebral fractures versus 15% in the placebo group. Other secondary end points showed a reduction in the risk of developing any type of fracture in the alendronate group (2.3% vs 5%). The overall number of hip and wrist fractures in the alendronate group decreased as well.[17]

The available data from these trials assessing the antifracture effect of bisphosphonates suggest that alendronate, risedronate, and zoledronic acid decrease fracture risk at the spine, nonvertebral sites, and the hip.[3,10] Ibandronate, a newer bisphosphonate, reduces the risk only in vertebral fractures.[3,10]

A general observation in all these investigations is that efficacy in fracture risk reduction depends on the patient's risk profile: patients with higher fracture risk presented a higher absolute risk reduction.

The benefit of bisphosphonates in patients with osteoporosis in the midterm is clear. The incidence of hip fractures in the United States decreased between 1996 and 2007 when osteoporosis treatment with bisphosphonates became widespread after the FIT results.[24] Benefits are also not limited to fracture risk reduction. Other investigations have shown reduction in morbidity, reduced health-care costs, and reduced mortality.[25–29] The use of bisphosphonates, oral or intravenous, for up to a 3-year period decreased mortality up to 28% in patients who sustained low-energy hip fractures.[20,30] The adjusted reduction risk of mortality in men and women using bisphosphonates for a period of 5 years is 27%.[29] A recent meta analysis by Bolland and colleagues in 2010[31] showed that the use of antiresorptive therapies in osteoporosis including bisphosphonates for at least 1 year is associated with decreased mortality in elderly patients at high risk of fracture.

As mentioned earlier, the data for long-term use are scarce.[13,22] One of the 2 studies is the extension of the FIT to 10 years of use.[13] This investigation showed an increase in mineral density in the lumbar spine (13.7%) and other skeletal sites. A dose of 5 mg showed a modest increase in bone mineral density. This investigation did not compare with placebo but with different dosages. The efficacy of alendronate in terms of fracture reduction risk did not seem to diminish with the 10 years of sustained therapy.[13] This investigation was also useful in showing that a 70-mg weekly dose is therapeutically as effective as 10 mg daily. This weekly dosage has become the standard therapy. This study also confirmed the direct relationship between alendronate use and increased bone mineral density because discontinuation of treatment caused gradual loss of bone density and increased N-telopeptide level.[13]

Osteoporosis in Men and Glucocorticoid Use

Although the disease is more prevalent in women, osteoporosis in men has recently become an area of research focus, because of an increase in hip fractures occurring in men.[1,32] The high prevalence of hip fractures in men (25%–30% of all hip fractures) is significant because the 1-year mortality doubles after a hip fracture.[32] Two trials focused in the male population showed increased bone mineral density and reduction in both bone turnover serum markers and fracture events.[33,34] However, difficulties still exist in the treatment of this population, because evidence is scarce and there is lack of agreement about the definition of the disease and the best time to start therapy.

Patients receiving therapy with glucocorticoids are also known to develop osteoporosis as a direct secondary effect of this therapy. Fracture incidence is also 1.3 to 2.6 times higher in this population.[35,36] The bisphosphonates alendronate and risedronate are also FDA approved for use in this clinical indication. Data are scarce but 2 PCRTs have proved risedronate's efficacy in these patients, with 70% reduction in vertebral fractures rate. Data for alendronate also come from 2 PCRTs.[35,36] However, increased bone mineral density and decreased fracture risk are significant only when combining the data from both studies.[37] The recommendation is to start treatment early when using therapy with glucocorticoids as a prevention plan, given that

Table 2
Effect of bisphosphonates (fracture reduction risk) in patients with osteoporosis

Medication	Trial	Follow-up (y)	Fracture Risk (Absolute Reduction)			Fracture Risk (Relative Risk)			Number of Patients to Treat to Prevent 1 Fracture			Reference
			Hip Fracture (%)	Vertebral Fracture (%)	Nonvertebral Fracture (%)	Hip Fracture (%)	Vertebral Fracture (%)	Nonvertebral Fracture (%)	Hip Fracture (%)	Vertebral Fracture (%)	Nonvertebral Fracture (%)	
Alendronate	FIT I	3	1.1	7.1	2.8	50.8	47.1	18.9	90	14	36	Black et al,[17] 1996
Alendronate	FIT II	3	0.2	1.7	1.5	20.7	44.3	11.1	447	60	68	Cummings et al,[14] 1998
Alendronate	MALE	2	N/A	5.0	N/A	N/A	62.0	N/A	N/A	9	N/A	Orwoll et al,[33] 2000
Ibandronate	BONE	3	N/A	4.9	−0.9	N/A	62.0	−11.0	N/A	20	N/A	Chesnut et al,[91] 2004
Risedronate	VERT NA	3	0.4	5.0	3.2	19.7	30.7	38.1	276	20	31	Harris et al,[19] 1999
Risedronate	VERT MN	3	0.5	10.9	5.1	18.2	37.6	31.9	203	9	20	Reginster et al,[21] 2000
Risedronate	HIP	3	1.1	N/A	1.8	28.2	N/A	16.1	91	N/A	56	McClung et al,[16] 2001
Risedronate	GIO	1	N/A	11.0	N/A	N/A	70.0	N/A	N/A	9	N/A	Wallach et al,[36] 2000
Zoledronic acid	HORIZON PFT	3	1.1	7.6	2.7	44.0	70.0	25.2	91	13	37	Black et al,[18] 2007
Zoledronic acid	HORIZON RFT	3	1.5	N/A	3.1	42.9	N/A	29.0	67	NA	32	Lyles et al,[20] 2007

Abbreviations: FIT, Fracture Intervention Trial; GIO, glucocorticoid-induced osteoporosis; HIP, Hip Intervention Program; N/A, not assessed; VERT, Vertebral Efficacy with Risedronate Therapy Study.

reduction in bone density occurs during the first months of treatment.[1]

METASTATIC DISEASE TO BONE

Despite progress in the treatment of primary cancers that metastasize to bone (breast, lung, kidney, prostate, and thyroid cancer), the burden of metastatic disease is significant because 40% to 90% of patients with carcinoma develop skeletal metastasis during the course of their disease.[38] Metastatic tumors are more common than primary bone tumors (25:1). After the lungs and the liver, the skeleton is the third most common place for metastasis. There is a wide spectrum of skeletal metastatic disease complications that include bone pain, pathologic fractures, cord compression in vertebral fractures, and hypercalcemia of malignancy.

At present, bisphosphonates are included in the standard of care in patients with cancers that include osseous metastasis. Several trials in patients with breast and lung cancer and other tumors with higher prevalence of skeletal metastatic disease have proved not only effectiveness in the inhibition of osteoclastic activity[39,40] but also reduction in the local release of growth factors.[41,42] This effect has been correlated with trends of increased survival.[38,41,42]

Pain and Pathologic Fractures in Oncologic Patients

There is a large number of publications evaluating the effect of bisphosphonates in patients with skeletal metastatic disease. Studies have focused on particular types of cancers but one that has been researched the most is breast cancer.

The Cochrane Brest Cancer Group reported their review in 2012. The investigators assessed the effect of bisphosphonates and other agents in terms of skeletal events, bone pain, quality of life, recurrence, and survival in women with breast cancer with bone metastasis, advanced breast cancer without clinical evidence of bone metastasis, and early breast cancer.[39] Thirty-four PCRTs comparing bisphosphonates with placebo, other bisphosphonates, and denosumab, and early versus delayed treatment in the scenarios described earlier were included. A total sample of 2865 patients with breast cancer with bone metastasis was available for analysis. Bisphosphonates reduced the risk of skeletal events by 15% compared with placebo (risk ratio, 0.85; 95% confidence interval, 0.77–0.94; $P<.01$). The benefit was most certain with intravenous zoledronic acid, intravenous pamidronate, and intravenous ibandronate. Bisphosphonates reduced the

number of skeletal events in 12 studies (median reduction, 28%), this difference being significant in 10 of the studies. Patients with metastatic disease treated with bisphosphonates had a longer period of time without skeletal events. Compared with placebo and other medications different than bisphosphonates, patients with treatment had a significant improvement in terms of bone pain (6 11 studies). Improvement in terms of quality of life was seen in 2 studies, both with ibandronate. In addition, the investigators found no data supporting bisphosphonates decreasing the incidence of metastasis and no evidence of bisphosphonates improving survival.[39]

The multiple myeloma group from the Cochrane Foundation did a similar review but in patients with multiple myeloma.[43] Using 20 trials enrolling 6692 patients, they found that bisphosphonates reduce the risk of vertebral fracture and bone pain in patients with multiple myeloma. Zoledronate proved to be better than etidronate and placebo, but not superior to pamidronate or clodronate, for survival increase or any other outcomes including vertebral and nonvertebral fractures.[43]

The American Society of Clinical Oncology publishes evidence-based guidelines for a variety of cancer treatments.[44] Their last recommendations, published in 2011 for breast cancer, state that "Bone-modifying agent therapy is only recommended for patients with breast cancer with evidence of bone metastases; denosumab 120 mg subcutaneously every 4 weeks, intravenous pamidronate 90 mg over no less than 2 hours, or zoledronic acid 4 mg over no less than 15 minutes every 3 to 4 weeks is recommended. There is insufficient evidence to demonstrate greater efficacy of one bone-modifying agent over another." Biochemical markers are not as reliable as radiographs for monitoring clinical response and adjusting therapy.[44]

Current recommendations do not support the use of bisphosphonates in patients without metastatic disease at any stage of their cancerous disease. Nevertheless there is new evidence from trials using clodronate in patients with lymph node–positive disease or positive involvement of bone marrow. Two of these trials reported satisfactory results characterized by reduction in skeletal and nonskeletal metastasis, prolongation of disease-free periods, and overall survival increase.[45]

Despite these guidelines and the body of literature for metastatic breast cancer and multiple myeloma, benefit in other primary tumors that metastasize to bone is assumed, because potential benefit can be expected given the similar pathophysiology in these clinical scenarios. Several recent publications have reported the benefit of using bisphosphonates in patients with tumors that metastasize to bone (prostate, thyroid, and kidney).[46,47] This benefit can be summarized as increased bone density, fracture risk reduction, and decreased bone pain. These effects vary according to the tumor and the medication being used but more data should soon become available to better define the role of bisphosphonates in patients with skeletal metastatic disease with tumors other than breast, lung, or multiple myeloma.

Neoplastic Hypercalcemia

The most common metabolic complication of advanced cancer is hypercalcemia of malignancy. It affects up to 20% of patients, but the incidence is variable and depends on the cancer type. It is most commonly observed in patients with multiple myeloma and in patients with metastatic carcinoma of the lung, breast, and kidney.[38] The main mediators of this process are molecules such as the parathyroid-related hormone-related peptide (PTHrP) and cytokines produced by tumor cells. Molecules such as these increase the production of receptor activator of nuclear factor kappa-B (RANK) ligand in osteoblasts. This ligand molecule attaches to the RANK receptor of the osteoclasts, which activates the c-Fos and the TRAF6 cascades, which trigger osteoclastic activity and subsequent bone resorption. Osteoblasts produce osteoprotegerin (OPG), which inhibits RANK receptor activation by binding to the RANK ligand. This regulation system is affected because malignant cells overstimulate osteoblasts (PTHrP) with subsequent RANK ligand production. Osteoblasts cannot keep producing enough OPG and the result is an increase in osteoclastic activity.

Bisphosphonates are the most effective therapy in the management of hypercalcemia of malignancy.[48] Two prospective randomized trials showed pamidronate (90 mg, 2-hour infusion) and zoledronic acid (4 or 8 mg, 5-minute infusion) to be effective and safe.[48] There is a trend to use more zoledronic acid because administration is more convenient to patients.

PAGET DISEASE

Osteitis deformans or Paget disease is a rare condition with an approximate incidence of 3.3% in patients older than 40 years.[49] The cause of this disorder is unknown. However, this disease is thought to have a strong family history because more than 40% of affected patients have a first-degree relative with the disease.[50,51] In the study of a single large family in which the pattern of transmission was autosomal dominant, a region on chromosome 18 was found to be strongly

associated with Paget disease.[51] Viral infection has been suggested as a cause, and paramyxo-virus-like nuclear inclusions have been identified in osteoclasts of patients with the disease.[52,53] This disorder is characterized by localized and accelerated bone resorption followed by ineffective and random dense bone matrix deposition. Symptoms include bone pain, headaches, and neurologic symptoms secondary to peripheral and central nerve compression. When patients with this condition require surgical treatment, the treating orthopedic surgeon should be aware that this is a hypervascular disorder with increased perioperative blood loss. Elective surgical prophylaxis is required to decrease perioperative bleeding.

Calcitonin and bisphosphonates have been used with success in the treatment of Paget disease. Bisphosphonates include oral etidronate, alendronate, tiludronate and risedronate, and intravenous pamidronate. Sustained remission and normalization in serum alkaline phosphatase can be obtained with the most potent medications: pamidronate, alendronate, and risedronate. Intravenous pamidronate is preferred because it allows the dose to be titrated according to the severity of the disease. Optimal dosage and treatment regimen remain controversial. Mild disease may normalize after a 60-mg infusion over 3 to 4 hours. Patients with moderate to severe disease usually need weekly or biweekly 60-mg infusions with cumulative doses up to 400 mg.[54] The oral regimen is with alendronate 40 mg daily for 6 months with subsequent clinical evaluation and measurement of serum alkaline phosphatase. Investigations have shown normalization of serum alkaline phosphatase in more than 60% of patients using these protocols.[55] Similar findings have been reported with the use of risedronate and tiludronate.[56,57]

OI

This is a syndromic condition that affects type I collagen. Common denominator symptoms include osteopenia, low-energy fractures, progressive deformity, loss of mobility, and chronic bone pain. The severity and combination of symptoms and signs depend on the subtype. Four subtypes were traditionally distinguished according to their clinical presentation, genetics, and severity (**Table 3**).

Types V to VII have been added to the traditional system. These types do not have a collagen type I mutation but present a similar phenotype. In the past, treatment has focus on pain control and surgical management of deformities.

Recent published literature has shown bisphosphonates to be effective in the treatment of

Table 3
Silence classification for OI

Type	Severity	Inheritance	Sclerae	Dentinogenesis	Features
Type I	Mild	Autosomal dominant	Blue	Divided into type A and B based on tooth involvement	Mildest form. Presents at preschool age (tarda). Hearing deficit in 50%
Type II	Severe (lethal)	Autosomal recessive	Blue	N/A	Lethal in perinatal period
Type III	Severe (survivable)	Autosomal recessive	Normal	N/A	Fractures at birth. Progressively short stature
Type IV	Moderate	Autosomal dominant	Normal	Divided into type A and B based on tooth involvement	Bowing bones and vertebral fractures are common
Type V	Moderate	Variable	Variable	Variable	Hypertrophic callus after fracture. Ossification of IOM between radius and ulna and tibia and fibula
Type VI	Moderate	Variable	Variable	Similar to type IV	Similar to type IV
Type VII	Moderate	Variable	Variable	Variable	Associated with rhizomelia and coxa vara

Modifications adding types V to VII that present phenotypical characteristics similar to OI but are not caused by mutations in collagen type I.

OI.[58] A landmark study by Glorieux and colleagues[58] in 1998 was an uncontrolled observational investigation in 30 children aged 3 to 16 years that showed intravenous pamidronate to be effective in maintaining sustained reduction in serum alkaline phosphatase concentrations and showed increased bone mineral density, increased thickness in cortical bone visible in radiographs, decreased fracture rates and pain, and improved walking. Recommended dosage of intravenous pamidronate ranges from 0.5 to 1.5 mg/kg.

This and other subsequent investigations have shown the benefit of bisphosphonates in patients with OI independently of age and clinical presentation. The benefits seem to be significant despite most of these investigations having been observational and having compared patients with historical controls.

Some of these patients require osteotomies for the treatment of associated deformities in the extremities or the spine. A retrospective investigation by Munns and colleagues[59] in patients with moderate to severe OI evaluated factors influencing fracture and osteotomy site healing. The use of pamidronate delayed osteotomy healing but not fracture healing. Additional independent factors of osteotomy-delayed healing included older age and osteotomies at the tibia.[59]

Bisphosphonates are not curative because they do not alter or modify the genetic defect in OI but provide significant impact in terms of symptomatic treatment. Optimal doses and regimens remain unclear. Current investigations are assessing the effect of other bisphosphonates, comparing their efficacy with pamidronate.

OSTEOLYSIS IN ARTHROPLASTY

As the number of total joint replacements and the average lifespan continue to increase, complications related to loosening and periprosthetic fractures are becoming more prevalent. Failure of components is usually secondary to bone loss after implant insertion. Mechanisms that cause bone loss include wear-debris osteolysis, stress-shielding forces, and immobilization. Research has established that macrophages that absorb small particles of wear debris activate osteoclasts to start bone resorption.[60] This process is mediated through the RANK/RANK ligand system.

Use of bisphosphonates in this setting has been shown to stop this cycle, at least in preliminary results, although the clinical outcome of this intervention has not been clearly defined.[61,62] In a PCRT, Skoldenberg and colleagues[63] reported their findings in 2011. Seventy-three patients between the ages of 40 and 70 years were randomized to receive 35 mg of risedronate or placebo. Their primary end point was the change of bone mineral density in the Gruen femoral zones 1 to 7. Patients were evaluated at 2 days and at 3, 6,

12, and 24 months. Secondary end points included stem migration and clinical outcomes. The investigators found higher mineral bone density at 6 months (7.2%) and at 1 year (9.2%) in zones 1 and 7 in patients taking bisphosphonates. However, migration of the femoral stem and clinical outcome did not differ between groups.[63]

Two other PCRTs showed similar findings. One showed increased bone mineral density at 1 year in the distal femur and proximal tibia and reduction in bone loss during the immediate postoperative period in patients with total knee arthroplasty who received 10 mg of alendronate during a 1-year period.[61] The other showed increased bone mineral density in patients who received a single dose of intravenous pamidronate (90 mg) 5 days after total hip arthroplasty.[64] Reduction of markers of bone turnover in urine and serum, including bone-specific alkaline phosphatase, osteocalcin, and the N-terminal propeptide of type I collagen, was observed in this investigation.[64]

All these data suggest some benefit, although clinical relevance is not clear or understood. Effective inhibition of wear debris–induced osteolysis has been observed only in animal models, not in human trials.[65] At this point, it seems that the use of bisphosphonates in this clinical scenario is safe, even in uncemented prostheses,[66] but there are insufficient data to support their use to prevent progression of osteolysis around implants once it is identified.

PEDIATRIC DISORDERS

The use of bisphosphonates in the pediatric population is controversial. Published literature in this area mainly reflects sporadic and limited experience: case reports, case series, and retrospective studies.

Prospective studies are scarce. Only a few PCRTs have proved the efficacy of bisphosphonates in nonambulatory patients with quadriparetic cerebral palsy.[67] Patients receiving bisphosphonates had improved bone mineral density without any symptomatic adverse effects.

In recent years, the off-label use of bisphosphonates has increased in the pediatric population for the treatment of conditions in which osteopenia and/or osteolysis are part of the pathophysiology.

Concerns regarding its use include the possibility of detrimental effects in skeletal development and function, and the potential for teratogenic effect.[68]

Prolonged use of bisphosphonates has been associated with brittle bones.[15,68] A report by Whyte and colleagues[69] in 2003 presented the case of a pediatric male patient who developed what was termed secondary osteopetrosis caused by the use of bisphosphonates. This patient received treatment with 60 mg of pamidronate every 3 weeks for a period of 2.5 years. Increased bone density and defective remodeling persisted for more than 18 months after treatment was discontinued.[69]

Bisphosphonates should be used carefully in children. Reservations concerning long-term effect should not preclude their use in pediatrics but should stimulate new controlled studies that use close follow-up using biochemical markers in serum for close monitoring. Multiple pediatric conditions with subjacent osteopenia and/or osteoclastic activity may benefit from treatment with bisphosphonates. Guidelines of treatment based on safe and well-monitored clinical studies are needed in this area. The current status of pediatric disorders that may benefit from bisphosphonates is discussed later.

Osteoporosis in Children

Primary osteoporosis in children is uncommon. However, secondary osteoporosis is increasing in incidence and prevalence. As in adults, this process is characterized by loss of bone mass and changes in microarchitectural integrity that result in bone fragility and a higher risk of fracture. This condition may arise from intrinsic genetic abnormalities or extrinsic factors such as the use of medications (steroids), nutritional deficiencies (vitamin D, C, and K; calcium), or chronic medical conditions associated with chronic inflammation or organ failure (liver, kidney).[68]

Idiopathic juvenile osteoporosis is a classic example of primary osteoporosis. This disorder occurs sporadically in prepubertal children with no history of bone disease. This diagnosis is one of exclusion. It is characterized clinically by recurrent low-energy fractures in the vertebral bodies or the metaphysis in long bones. There is formation of new osteoporotic bone without callus formation. There is typically gradual remission after the onset of puberty.[70]

Children may experience recurrent fractures, bone pain, and kyphosis, and in severe cases the fractures may lead to permanent skeletal damage. Bisphosphonates in pediatric patients with symptomatic disease are beneficial in terms of bone pain control, reduction of fractures, and increase in bone mineral density.[71] Benefits are irrespective of the bisphosphonate used. Available literature supporting these findings does not provide comparisons with controls and therefore is limited.[70–72]

Based on their unpublished observational study in 2012, Sebestyen and colleagues[68] reported their experience treating children with idiopathic juvenile osteoporosis associated with vertebral collapse fractures that depended on multiple narcotic medication and spine brace immobilization. Therapy with intravenous zoledronic acid was successful in discontinuing all narcotic medication and spinal brace use without affecting the healing of the fractures.

Secondary osteoporosis as a consequence of another pathologic process is more prevalent. Glucocorticoid-induced osteoporosis is in this category. Steroid therapy inhibits osteoblastic activity, increases osteoclastogenesis, reduces intestinal calcium resorption, and increases renal tubular calcium excretion.[68] Bone loss typically occurs in the first 6 to 12 months of corticosteroid use.[73,74] Vertebral fractures are the most common form of this disorder.

A 2-year follow-up by Reyes and colleagues[75] in 2007 in 55 children with glucocorticoid-induced osteoporosis showed a higher risk of osteoporosis among nonambulatory, growth-retarded patients, and in those with long-term methotrexate therapy and family history of osteoporosis. Two years of treatment with alendronate in patient from this cohort who had vertebral fractures improved bone mineral density from 2.69 to −1.39 (Z score).[75]

Osteoporosis associated with immobilization is also in this category. It develops in patients with cerebral palsy and other neurologic conditions that confine children to bed or a wheelchair. Osteoporosis in this scenario is secondary to impaired weight-bearing ambulation, lack of muscular forces on bone, inadequate nutrition, low calcium and vitamin D intake, and/or the use of anticonvulsant therapy.

Long-term follow-up studies of up to 10 years observed reduced rates of fractures at 1 year in nonambulatory patients with cerebral palsy. This reduction was maintained for up to 4 years.[76] A subset of patients sustained fractures after discontinuation of bisphosphonates.[76] Additional, smaller, noncomparative investigations found improvement in bone density, decreased fracture rate, and reduction in pain in children with cerebral palsy treated with bisphosphonates.[76,77]

Similar findings have been observed in patients with other disabling chronic neurologic disorders[78,79] and in patients with acute immobilization (spinal cord injury[80]) who have been treated with bisphosphonates.

Secondary osteoporosis can also be seen in patients with gastrointestinal disorders such as inflammatory bowel disease, celiac disorder, or liver diseases. In these conditions there is loss of bone mineral density secondary to decreased absorption of calcium and fat-soluble vitamins in the gastrointestinal tract. This condition is cause by the direct effect of cytokines and chronic glucocorticoid use.[68] In a small, randomized study of 13 adolescents with Crohn disease, patients were randomized either to saline infusion or zoledronic acid (1 dose of 0.066 mg/kg).[81] At the 6-month follow-up, the investigators found a significant increase in lumbar spine bone mineral density in the bisphosphonates group (Z scores of 0.7 vs 0.1). This effect was still present at 12 months with associated decreased urinary C telopeptide excretion indicating reduced bone resorption in the intervention group.[81]

Fibrous Dysplasia and McCune-Albright Syndrome

Fibrous dysplasia is a disorder in which there is production of fibrous tissue and woven bone at sites where normal bone should develop. The lesions are osteolytic and affect the ribs and the craniofacial and long bones. The abnormal bone leaves the skeleton weak and prone to fractures. The characteristic defect is a somatic mutation in the gene coding for the alpha subunit of the G protein that stimulates production of cAMP. Overproduction of cAMP generates c-fos gene overexpression, which is an important regulator in osteoblastic/osteoclastic proliferation and differentiation. The excessive osteoclastic activity in this disorder has been targeted with bisphosphonates.[82]

Bisphosphonates in this setting have been examined in several clinical trials.[82–87] All clinical series evaluated intravenous pamidronate with the exception of an investigation that initially used intravenous pamidronate and subsequently replaced the intervention for oral etidronate.[88] Results consistently showed improvement in pain, and increased N-telopeptide values. Cortical thickening and progressive ossification were seen on radiographs of skeletally mature patients. Results in children are less consistent, with most patients not showing radiographic improvement.

Legg-Calvé-Perthes

This is the infantile form of osteonecrosis of the femoral head. The incidence varies from 8.5 to 21 cases per100,000 children per year.[89] The most serious sequela of this disorder is femoral head deformity secondary to subchondral collapse, which leads to early degenerative arthritis. It is thought that osteoclastic activity mediates the subchondral collapse, therefore it is plausible that inhibition of this activity with bisphosphonates may attenuate or prevent the progression of the disease.

Literature is scarce in this area, with only 3 level IV studies evaluating the effect of bisphosphonates in clinical trials. Only 1 study used the bisphosphonates in the precollapse stage. Prevention of femoral head deformity was obtained in 9 of 17 patients.[90]

Despite lack of data, the small body of literature in this disease is promising and further investigations are assessing the impact of bisphosphonates in pediatric patients with this condition.

SUMMARY

The use of bisphosphonates in orthopedic conditions has increased considerably in the last decade. The results in treating conditions characterized by increased osteoclastic activity and decreased bone mineral density are promising, expanding the therapeutic horizon of this group of medications.

This article presets and summarizes the most common indications and applications of therapy with bisphosphonates. Widespread use has raised concerns in terms of adverse effects, especially with long-term exposure. In osteoporosis, there is enough evidence in the published literature that the benefit outweighs the risk when using bisphosphonates.

REFERENCES

1. Morris CD, Einhorn TA. Bisphosphonates in orthopaedic surgery. J Bone Joint Surg Am 2005; 87(7):1609–18.
2. Bisaz S, Jung A, Fleisch H. Uptake by bone of pyrophosphate, diphosphonates and their technetium derivatives. Clin Sci Mol Med 1978;54(3): 265–72.
3. Schmidt GA, Horner KE, McDanel DL, et al. Risks and benefits of long-term bisphosphonate therapy. Am J Health Syst Pharm 2010;67(12):994–1001.
4. Siris ES, Pasquale MK, Wang Y, et al. Estimating bisphosphonate use and fracture reduction among US women aged 45 years and older, 2001-2008. J Bone Miner Res 2011;26(1):3–11.
5. Russell RG, Watts NB, Ebetino FH, et al. Mechanisms of action of bisphosphonates: similarities and differences and their potential influence on clinical efficacy. Osteoporos Int 2008;19(6): 733–59.
6. Amin D, Cornell SA, Gustafson SK, et al. Bisphosphonates used for the treatment of bone disorders inhibit squalene synthase and cholesterol biosynthesis. J Lipid Res 1992;33(11):1657–63.
7. Luckman SP, Hughes DE, Coxon FP, et al. Nitrogen-containing bisphosphonates inhibit the mevalonate pathway and prevent post-translational

prenylation of GTP-binding proteins, including Ras. J Bone Miner Res 1998;13(4):581–9.
8. Fisher JE, Rogers MJ, Halasy JM, et al. Alendronate mechanism of action: geranylgeraniol, an intermediate in the mevalonate pathway, prevents inhibition of osteoclast formation, bone resorption, and kinase activation in vitro. Proc Natl Acad Sci U S A 1999;96(1):133–8.
9. Zhang D, Udagawa N, Nakamura I, et al. The small GTP-binding protein, rho p21, is involved in bone resorption by regulating cytoskeletal organization in osteoclasts. J Cell Sci 1995;108(Pt 6):2285–92.
10. McClung M, Harris ST, Miller PD, et al. Bisphosphonate therapy for osteoporosis: benefits, risks, and drug holiday. Am J Med 2013;126(1):13–20.
11. Kanis JA, Melton LJ 3rd, Christiansen C, et al. The diagnosis of osteoporosis. J Bone Miner Res 1994; 9(8):1137–41.
12. Bonnick SL, Shulman L. Monitoring osteoporosis therapy: bone mineral density, bone turnover markers, or both? Am J Med 2006;119(4 Suppl 1): S25–31.
13. Bone HG, Hosking D, Devogelaer JP, et al. Ten years' experience with alendronate for osteoporosis in postmenopausal women. N Engl J Med 2004;350(12):1189–99.
14. Cummings SR, Black DM, Thompson DE, et al. Effect of alendronate on risk of fracture in women with low bone density but without vertebral fractures: results from the Fracture Intervention Trial. JAMA 1998;280(24):2077–82.
15. Marini JC. Do bisphosphonates make children's bones better or brittle? N Engl J Med 2003; 349(5):423–6.
16. McClung MR, Geusens P, Miller PD, et al. Effect of risedronate on the risk of hip fracture in elderly women. Hip Intervention Program Study Group. N Engl J Med 2001;344(5):333–40.
17. Black DM, Cummings SR, Karpf DB, et al. Randomised trial of effect of alendronate on risk of fracture in women with existing vertebral fractures. Fracture Intervention Trial Research Group. Lancet 1996;348(9041):1535–41.
18. Black DM, Delmas PD, Eastell R, et al. Once-yearly zoledronic acid for treatment of postmenopausal osteoporosis. N Engl J Med 2007;356(18): 1809–22.
19. Harris ST, Watts NB, Genant HK, et al. Effects of risedronate treatment on vertebral and nonvertebral fractures in women with postmenopausal osteoporosis: a randomized controlled trial. Vertebral Efficacy With Risedronate Therapy (VERT) Study Group. JAMA 1999;282(14):1344–52.
20. Lyles KW, Colon-Emeric CS, Magaziner JS, et al. Zoledronic acid and clinical fractures and mortality after hip fracture. N Engl J Med 2007;357(18): 1799–809.

21. Reginster J, Minne HW, Sorensen OH, et al. Randomized trial of the effects of risedronate on vertebral fractures in women with established postmenopausal osteoporosis. Vertebral Efficacy with Risedronate Therapy (VERT) Study Group. Osteoporos Int 2000;11(1):83–91.

22. Black DM, Schwartz AV, Ensrud KE, et al. Effects of continuing or stopping alendronate after 5 years of treatment: the Fracture Intervention Trial Long-term Extension (FLEX): a randomized trial. JAMA 2006; 296(24):2927–38.

23. Ensrud KE, Barrett-Connor EL, Schwartz A, et al. Randomized trial of effect of alendronate continuation versus discontinuation in women with low BMD: results from the Fracture Intervention Trial long-term extension. J Bone Miner Res 2004; 19(8):1259–69.

24. Wang Z, Bhattacharyya T. Trends in incidence of subtrochanteric fragility fractures and bisphosphonate use among the US elderly, 1996-2007. J Bone Miner Res 2011;26(3):553–60.

25. Center JR, Bliuc D, Nguyen ND, et al. Osteoporosis medication and reduced mortality risk in elderly women and men. J Clin Endocrinol Metab 2011; 96(4):1006–14.

26. Dell R, Greene D. Is osteoporosis disease management cost effective? Curr Osteoporos Rep 2010; 8(1):49–55.

27. Nevitt MC, Thompson DE, Black DM, et al. Effect of alendronate on limited-activity days and bed-disability days caused by back pain in postmenopausal women with existing vertebral fractures. Fracture Intervention Trial Research Group. Arch Intern Med 2000;160(1):77–85.

28. Newman ED, Ayoub WT, Starkey RH, et al. Osteoporosis disease management in a rural health care population: hip fracture reduction and reduced costs in postmenopausal women after 5 years. Osteoporos Int 2003;14(2):146–51.

29. Sambrook PN, Cameron ID, Chen JS, et al. Oral bisphosphonates are associated with reduced mortality in frail older people: a prospective five-year study. Osteoporos Int 2011;22(9): 2551–6.

30. Beaupre LA, Morrish DW, Hanley DA, et al. Oral bisphosphonates are associated with reduced mortality after hip fracture. Osteoporos Int 2011;22(3): 983–91.

31. Bolland MJ, Grey AB, Gamble GD, et al. Effect of osteoporosis treatment on mortality: a meta-analysis. J Clin Endocrinol Metab 2010;95(3):1174–81.

32. Cooper C, Campion G, Melton LJ 3rd. Hip fractures in the elderly: a world-wide projection. Osteoporos Int 1992;2(6):285–9.

33. Orwoll E, Ettinger M, Weiss S, et al. Alendronate for the treatment of osteoporosis in men. N Engl J Med 2000;343(9):604–10.

34. Ringe JD, Orwoll E, Daifotis A, et al. Treatment of male osteoporosis: recent advances with alendronate. Osteoporos Int 2002;13(3):195–9.

35. Reid DM, Adami S, Devogelaer JP, et al. Risedronate increases bone density and reduces vertebral fracture risk within one year in men on corticosteroid therapy. Calcif Tissue Int 2001;69(4):242–7.

36. Wallach S, Cohen S, Reid DM, et al. Effects of risedronate treatment on bone density and vertebral fracture in patients on corticosteroid therapy. Calcif Tissue Int 2000;67(4):277–85.

37. Saag KG, Emkey R, Schnitzer TJ, et al. Alendronate for the prevention and treatment of glucocorticoid-induced osteoporosis. Glucocorticoid-Induced Osteoporosis Intervention Study Group. N Engl J Med 1998;339(5):292–9.

38. Green JR. Antitumor effects of bisphosphonates. Cancer 2003;97(Suppl 3):840–7.

39. Wong MH, Stockler MR, Pavlakis N. Bisphosphonates and other bone agents for breast cancer. Cochrane Database Syst Rev 2012;(2):CD003474.

40. Pavlakis N, Schmidt R, Stockler M. Bisphosphonates for breast cancer. Cochrane Database Syst Rev 2005;(3):CD003474.

41. Clezardin P. The antitumor potential of bisphosphonates. Semin Oncol 2002;29(6 Suppl 21):33–42.

42. Lee MV, Fong EM, Singer FR, et al. Bisphosphonate treatment inhibits the growth of prostate cancer cells. Cancer Res 2001;61(6):2602–8.

43. Mhaskar R, Redzepovic J, Wheatley K, et al. Bisphosphonates in multiple myeloma: a network meta-analysis. Cochrane Database Syst Rev 2012;(5):CD003188.

44. Hillner BE, Ingle JN, Berenson JR, et al. American Society of Clinical Oncology guideline on the role of bisphosphonates in breast cancer. American Society of Clinical Oncology Bisphosphonates Expert Panel. J Clin Oncol 2000;18(6):1378–91.

45. Powles T, Paterson S, Kanis JA, et al. Randomized, placebo-controlled trial of clodronate in patients with primary operable breast cancer. J Clin Oncol 2002;20(15):3219–24.

46. Rosen HN, Moses AC, Garber J, et al. Randomized trial of pamidronate in patients with thyroid cancer: bone density is not reduced by suppressive doses of thyroxine, but is increased by cyclic intravenous pamidronate. J Clin Endocrinol Metab 1998;83(7): 2324–30.

47. Smith MR, McGovern FJ, Zietman AL, et al. Pamidronate to prevent bone loss during androgen-deprivation therapy for prostate cancer. N Engl J Med 2001;345(13):948–55.

48. Major P, Lortholary A, Hon J, et al. Zoledronic acid is superior to pamidronate in the treatment of hypercalcemia of malignancy: a pooled analysis of two randomized, controlled clinical trials. J Clin Oncol 2001;19(2):558–67.

49. Siris ES. Paget's disease of bone. J Bone Miner Res 1998;13(7):1061–5.

50. Morales-Piga AA, Rey-Rey JS, Corres-Gonzalez J, et al. Frequency and characteristics of familial aggregation of Paget's disease of bone. J Bone Miner Res 1995;10(4):663–70.

51. Siris ES, Ottman R, Flaster E, et al. Familial aggregation of Paget's disease of bone. J Bone Miner Res 1991;6(5):495–500.

52. Mills BG, Singer FR, Weiner LP, et al. Evidence for both respiratory syncytial virus and measles virus antigens in the osteoclasts of patients with Paget's disease of bone. Clin Orthop Relat Res 1984;(183):303–11.

53. Rebel A, Malkani K, Basle M, et al. Is Paget's disease of bone a viral infection? Calcif Tissue Res 1977;22(Suppl):283–6.

54. Siris ES. Perspectives: a practical guide to the use of pamidronate in the treatment of Paget's disease. J Bone Miner Res 1994;9(3):303–4.

55. Siris E, Weinstein RS, Altman R, et al. Comparative study of alendronate versus etidronate for the treatment of Paget's disease of bone. J Clin Endocrinol Metab 1996;81(3):961–7.

56. McClung MR, Tou CK, Goldstein NH, et al. Tiludronate therapy for Paget's disease of bone. Bone 1995;17(Suppl 5):493S–6S.

57. Siris ES, Chines AA, Altman RD, et al. Risedronate in the treatment of Paget's disease of bone: an open label, multicenter study. J Bone Miner Res 1998;13(6):1032–8.

58. Glorieux FH, Bishop NJ, Plotkin H, et al. Cyclic administration of pamidronate in children with severe osteogenesis imperfecta. N Engl J Med 1998;339(14):947–52.

59. Munns CF, Rauch F, Zeitlin L, et al. Delayed osteotomy but not fracture healing in pediatric osteogenesis imperfecta patients receiving pamidronate. J Bone Miner Res 2004;19(11):1779–86.

60. Kim KJ, Hijikata H, Itoh T, et al. Joint fluid from patients with failed total hip arthroplasty stimulates pit formation by mouse osteoclasts on dentin slices. J Biomed Mater Res 1998;43(3):234–40.

61. Soininvaara TA, Jurvelin JS, Miettinen HJ, et al. Effect of alendronate on periprosthetic bone loss after total knee arthroplasty: a one-year, randomized, controlled trial of 19 patients. Calcif Tissue Int 2002;71(6):472–7.

62. Wang CJ, Wang JW, Weng LH, et al. The effect of alendronate on bone mineral density in the distal part of the femur and proximal part of the tibia after total knee arthroplasty. J Bone Joint Surg Am 2003;85(11):2121–6.

63. Skoldenberg OG, Salemyr MO, Boden HS, et al. The effect of weekly risedronate on periprosthetic bone resorption following total hip arthroplasty: a randomized, double-blind, placebo-controlled trial. J Bone Joint Surg Am 2011;93(20):1857–64.

64. Wilkinson JM, Stockley I, Peel NF, et al. Effect of pamidronate in preventing local bone loss after total hip arthroplasty: a randomized, double-blind, controlled trial. J Bone Miner Res 2001;16(3):556–64.

65. Shanbhag AS, Hasselman CT, Rubash HE. The John Charnley Award. Inhibition of wear debris mediated osteolysis in a canine total hip arthroplasty model. Clin Orthop Relat Res 1997;(344):33–43.

66. Mochida Y, Bauer TW, Akisue T, et al. Alendronate does not inhibit early bone apposition to hydroxyapatite-coated total joint implants: a preliminary study. J Bone Joint Surg Am 2002;84-A(2):226–35.

67. Henderson RC, Lark RK, Kecskemethy HH, et al. Bisphosphonates to treat osteopenia in children with quadriplegic cerebral palsy: a randomized, placebo-controlled clinical trial. J Pediatr 2002;141(5):644–51.

68. Sebestyen JF, Srivastava T, Alon US. Bisphosphonates use in children. Clin Pediatr 2012;51(11):1011–24.

69. Whyte MP, Wenkert D, Clements KL, et al. Bisphosphonate-induced osteopetrosis. N Engl J Med 2003;349(5):457–63.

70. Kauffman RP, Overton TH, Shiflett M, et al. Osteoporosis in children and adolescent girls: case report of idiopathic juvenile osteoporosis and review of the literature. Obstet Gynecol Surv 2001;56(8):492–504.

71. Melchior R, Zabel B, Spranger J, et al. Effective parenteral clodronate treatment of a child with severe juvenile idiopathic osteoporosis. Eur J Pediatr 2005;164(1):22–7.

72. Hoekman K, Papapoulos SE, Peters AC, et al. Characteristics and bisphosphonate treatment of a patient with juvenile osteoporosis. J Clin Endocrinol Metab 1985;61(5):952–6.

73. Julian BA, Laskow DA, Dubovsky J, et al. Rapid loss of vertebral mineral density after renal transplantation. N Engl J Med 1991;325(8):544–50.

74. Homik JE, Cranney A, Shea B, et al. A metaanalysis on the use of bisphosphonates in corticosteroid induced osteoporosis. J Rheumatol 1999;26(5):1148–57.

75. Reyes ML, Hernandez MI, King A, et al. Corticosteroid-induced osteoporosis in children: outcome after two-year follow-up, risk factors, densitometric predictive cut-off values for vertebral fractures. Clin Exp Rheumatol 2007;25(2):329–35.

76. Bachrach SJ, Kecskemethy HH, Harcke HT, et al. Decreased fracture incidence after 1 year of pamidronate treatment in children with spastic quadriplegic cerebral palsy. Dev Med Child Neurol 2010;52(9):837–42.

77. Shaw NJ, White CP, Fraser WD, et al. Osteopenia in cerebral palsy. Arch Dis Child 1994;71(3):235–8.

78. Apkon S, Coll J. Use of weekly alendronate to treat osteoporosis in boys with muscular dystrophy. Am J Phys Med Rehabil 2008;87(2):139–43.

79. Howe W, Davis E, Valentine J. Pamidronate improves pain, wellbeing, fracture rate and bone density in 14 children and adolescents with chronic neurological conditions. Dev Neurorehabil 2010; 13(1):31–6.

80. Bubbear JS, Gall A, Middleton FR, et al. Early treatment with zoledronic acid prevents bone loss at the hip following acute spinal cord injury. Osteoporos Int 2011;22(1):271–9.

81. Sbrocchi AM, Forget S, Laforte D, et al. Zoledronic acid for the treatment of osteopenia in pediatric Crohn's disease. Pediatr Int 2010;52(5):754–61.

82. Matarazzo P, Lala R, Masi G, et al. Pamidronate treatment in bone fibrous dysplasia in children and adolescents with McCune-Albright syndrome. J Pediatr Endocrinol Metab 2002;15(Suppl 3): 929–37.

83. Isaia GC, Lala R, Defilippi C, et al. Bone turnover in children and adolescents with McCune-Albright syndrome treated with pamidronate for bone fibrous dysplasia. Calcif Tissue Int 2002;71(2): 121–8.

84. Chapurlat RD, Delmas PD, Liens D, et al. Long-term effects of intravenous pamidronate in fibrous dysplasia of bone. J Bone Miner Res 1997; 12(10):1746–52.

85. Lala R, Matarazzo P, Bertelloni S, et al. Pamidronate treatment of bone fibrous dysplasia in nine children with McCune-Albright syndrome. Acta Paediatr 2000;89(2):188–93.

86. Liens D, Delmas PD, Meunier PJ. Long-term effects of intravenous pamidronate in fibrous dysplasia of bone. Lancet 1994;343(8903):953–4.

87. Plotkin H, Rauch F, Zeitlin L, et al. Effect of pamidronate treatment in children with polyostotic fibrous dysplasia of bone. J Clin Endocrinol Metab 2003; 88(10):4569–75.

88. Lane JM, Khan SN, O'Connor WJ, et al. Bisphosphonate therapy in fibrous dysplasia. Clin Orthop Relat Res 2001;(382):6–12.

89. Kim H, Randall TS, Bian H, et al. Ibandronate for prevention of femoral head deformity after ischemic necrosis of the capital femoral epiphysis in immature pigs. J Bone Joint Surg Am 2005; 87(3):550–7.

90. Little DG, Peat RA, McEvoy A, et al. Zoledronic acid treatment results in retention of femoral head structure after traumatic osteonecrosis in young Wistar rats. J Bone Miner Res 2003;18(11):2016–22.

91. Chesnut CH1 III, Skag A, Christiansen C, et al. Effects of oral ibandronate administered daily or intermittently on fracture risk in postmenopausal osteoporosis. J Bone Miner Res 2004;19(8):1241–9.

Five Polyostotic Conditions That General Orthopedic Surgeons Should Recognize (or Should Not Miss)

Saravanaraja Muthusamy, MD, Sheila A. Conway, MD,
H. Thomas Temple, MD*

KEYWORDS

- Polyostotic • Ollier disease • Maffucci syndrome • Multiple exostosis • Fibrous dysplasia
- Paget disease • Skeletal metastases

KEY POINTS

- In history and physical examination, similar lesions should always be looked for in other parts of the musculoskeletal system and additional pertinent findings should be analyzed in review of systems, which might offer clue to the diagnosis.
- Most patients with these diseases are asymptomatic and do not require treatment other than regular clinical and radiographic follow-up. Symptomatic lesions may necessitate further laboratory and radiographic investigation that in rare cases may require biopsy.
- A sudden increase in pain or appearance of swelling may herald pathologic fracture or malignant change. Patients with select conditions should be warned of these rare potential risks and told to seek immediate consultation in the event of worrisome symptoms.
- Skeletal metastasis in the differential in older patients with unexplained bone pain, swelling, and pathologic fracture, especially with a previous cancer history, should always be considered.
- Patients with suspected malignancy should be referred early for further evaluation, biopsy, and expert management.

MULTIPLE ENCHONDROMATOSIS (OLLIER DISEASE AND MAFFUCCI SYNDROME)

Enchondroma is a common benign tumor that consists of mature hyaline cartilage. It can be solitary or multiple. Solitary enchondromas are usually diagnosed incidentally and are commonly observed in the long bones of the hand and extremities. Multiple enchondromatosis (Ollier disease) is rare. Multiple enchondromata associated with soft tissue hemangiomata (Maffucci syndrome) is rarer still. There is no gender predominance for these conditions. Most enchondromata involve the metaphysis

and diaphysis, whereas only 10% are epiphyseal. Enchondromata associated with Ollier disease are commonly found in the femur, tibia, and ilium, followed by phalanges, metacarpals, and metatarsals.[1] Maffucci syndrome is the most severe of all and most commonly involves the hand.[2] Both Ollier disease and Maffucci syndrome are congenital.

Pathology

The cause is unknown, but Ollier disease and Maffucci syndrome are thought to arise from small rests of physeal cartilage entrapped in the

Disclosure: The authors have identified no professional or financial affiliations for themselves or their spouse/partner with a commercial company that has a direct financial interest in the subject matter or materials discussed in the article or with a company making a competing product.
Department of Orthopaedic Surgery, University of Miami Miller School of Medicine, 1400 NW 12th Avenue, Suite 4036, Miami, FL 33136, USA
* Corresponding author.
E-mail address: HTemple@med.miami.edu

Orthop Clin N Am 45 (2014) 417–429
http://dx.doi.org/10.1016/j.ocl.2014.04.004
0030-5898/14/$ – see front matter © 2014 Elsevier Inc. All rights reserved.

orthopedic.theclinics.com

metaphysis of growing bones. These "cartilage rests" grow until skeletal maturity and frequently reside in the metaphysis or diaphysis and over time mineralize in varying degrees. Most cases of enchondromatosis are sporadic, but families with multiple affected members have been reported, possibly suggesting autosomal-dominant (AD) inheritance.[1] There is a controversial and iterative role of one or more mutations in PTHR1 (parathyroid hormone receptor 1).[3] Grossly, the lesions are lobular with a bluish color and microscopically composed of lobules of hyaline cartilage that are relatively hypocellular and matrix-rich. In the hands and feet, enchondromata can appear radiographically aggressive. Microscopically, they are hypercellular with atypical cells but still are considered benign.[4] Also, lesions in young children associated with Ollier disease and Maffucci syndrome are more cellular than solitary enchondromas in adults. Although these features are interpreted as benign in the small bones, similar findings in axial and appendicular long bones in adults could be interpreted as low-grade chondrosarcoma. There is a great deal of variability among pathologists in the interpretation and diagnosis of malignant change in enchondromata. These lesions are variously named as atypical enchondroma, aggressive enchondroma, sarcoma in situ, and grade I chondrosarcoma.

Clinical Features

Most solitary enchondromata diagnosed in adults are asymptomatic and discovered incidentally. Rarely, patients present with pain due to pathologic fracture. Pain in the absence of fracture in patients with a solitary enchondroma suggests another unrelated cause, or rarely, transformation to an active or overtly malignant disease process. The involved bone may also be slightly enlarged. Patients with Ollier disease may be asymptomatic but may present with growth disturbances, enlargement, shortening, and deformity of the affected bones as well as scoliosis.[5] Most patients with Ollier disease have bilateral involvement but may only exhibit unilateral or single limb predominance. This disease is usually diagnosed in younger patients. Maffucci syndrome is characterized by multiple enchondromata with soft tissue lesions, most commonly, cavernous hemangiomas in the subcutaneous tissues, usually affecting the same extremity. The hemangiomas are present at birth in only 25% of affected patients. Most are diagnosed in childhood.

The risk of malignancy is high in tumors that are large and in proximal locations like the pelvis, proximal femur, and proximal humerus. Although malignant transformation in solitary enchondroma is rare, the risk of developing a chondrosarcoma in the setting of multiple enchondromata is high. Malignant change is heralded by progressive pain and the appearance of swelling.[6]

Imaging

Laboratory tests are normal and radiographs are usually diagnostic. On radiographs, enchondromata are centrally located, intramedullary, metaphyseal, or metadiphyseal-based radiolucent lesions with matrix mineralization. Most (95%) demonstrate mineralization variously described as dots, punctuate, stippled, speckled, annular rings, arcs, whorls, flocculent, and popcorn mineralization. The lesions may be completely radiolucent especially in children and in short tubular bones. They may be associated with thinning and expansion of cortex as well as endosteal scalloping, but cortical disruption and periosteal reaction are unusual without pathologic fracture or malignant transformation. In the phalanges, enchondromata may extend to the ends of bones.[7] In hands and feet, these lesions may appear more aggressive radiologically but are generally considered benign. In the long bones, radiolucent streaks or fan-like septations extending from the growth plate into the diaphysis and asymmetric enlargement and flaring of the metaphyses may be present in patients with multiple enchondroma (**Fig. 1**). In the pelvis, and particularly in the iliac bones, these fan-like linear changes are characteristic of Ollier disease. Maffucci syndrome may display phleboliths on radiographs (**Fig. 2**).

On magnetic resonance (MR), the lesions appear as low to intermediate intensity on T1-weighted and high intensity on T2-weighted images with sharp margins. The mineralization appears as punctate or globular dark areas on both T1 and T2 pulse sequences.[5] MR also shows the lobular nature of the tumor (on T2), size, and the intramedullary extent. Computed tomography (CT) is better for identifying the matrix, endosteal scalloping, cortical destruction, and periosteal reaction. Aggressive lesions generally display increased scintigraphic uptake on bone scan but children may also have active lesions that show active and intense uptake. Bone scan or skeletal survey is used to localize the lesions in other bones.

The radiological features suggestive of aggressive behavior are larger lesions, longer than 4 cm, medullary fill of greater than 90%, large unmineralized areas, or faint, amorphous calcification, lysis within a previously mineralized area, a wide zone of transition from normal to abnormal, localized thickening of the cortex, deep endosteal

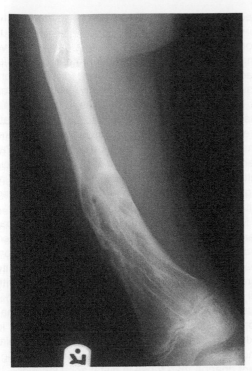

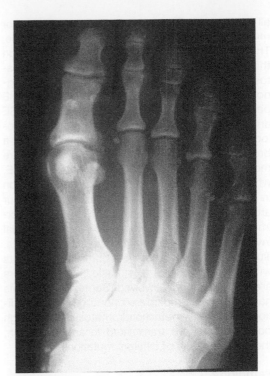

Fig. 1. Anteroposterior (AP) radiograph of a femur in a skeletally immature individual with Ollier disease affecting the right lower extremity. There are linear striations and radiolucent abnormalities as well as a bowing deformity.

Fig. 2. AP radiograph of the foot with radiolucent abnormalities in the second middle phalanx and middle and proximal phalanges of the fourth and fifth toes. There are scattered rounded mineralizations in the soft tissue representing phleboliths in this patient with Maffucci syndrome.

scalloping (greater than two-thirds of cortex), longitudinal scalloping throughout the length of the lesion, cortical disruption, periosteal reaction, and a soft tissue mass. A heterogeneous and increased scintigraphic uptake (greater than the corresponding anterior superior iliac spine) on bone scan is also suggestive of malignant change.

Biopsy can be challenging because it is difficult to differentiate low-grade chondrosarcoma from enchondroma by histology alone; therefore, clinical, radiologic, and pathologic correlation are essential to arrive at a correct diagnosis.

Treatment

Most lesions are asymptomatic and, other than routine radiographic surveillance, surgery is not necessary. For benign symptomatic lesions or for impending pathologic fracture, curetting and bone grafting with or without physical adjuvants can be considered. Internal fixation may be necessary. If a pathologic fracture occurs, the fracture should be allowed to heal before curetting and bone grafting. More aggressive lesions in pelvis and long bones require wide resection. Treatment of patients with enchondromatosis due to Ollier disease and Maffucci syndrome may necessitate

correction of deformities and leg-length discrepancy in addition to careful surveillance, genetic counseling, prompt biopsy, and intervention for suspected malignant transformation.[8]

Prognosis and Follow-Up

In solitary enchondromas, the risk of malignant transformation to chondrosarcoma is less than 1% and is even rarer before skeletal maturity. The risk of malignant transformation of an enchondroma in Ollier disease spirals upward to 25% to 30%[1] and in Maffucci syndrome is up to 56%.[9] Patients with Maffucci syndrome also have the risk of developing acute lymphocytic leukemia, astrocytoma, and gastrointestinal and ovarian malignancies. The risk of skeletal or nonskeletal malignancy in Maffucci syndrome is probably almost certain if patients are followed long enough.[10]

MULTIPLE HEREDITARY EXOSTOSIS (DIAPHYSEAL ACLASIS)

Osteochondroma (osteochondral exostosis) is the most common skeletal tumor, comprising 20% to 50% of benign bone tumors and 10% to 15% of all bone tumors.[11] They occur as either solitary or multiple tumors with a slight male predominance. The solitary exostosis (SE) is much more common than the multiple variant (multiple hereditary exostosis or MHE). Solitary exostoses are generally diagnosed in older individuals (before age 30) and MHE patients are diagnosed before age 10.[12] Both SE and MHE occur in metaphyseal bone and morphologically can exhibit a stalk (pedunculated) or a broad base (sessile). Pedunculated lesions are more often encountered in patients with SE, whereas the sessile morphology is more common in patients with MHE. Solitary exostoses occur around the knee (50%) in the distal femur and proximal tibia followed by proximal humerus. Axial involvement (ie, the flat bones including the scapula, ilium, and clavicle) is much less common. In patients with MHE, the knees, hips, ankles, and shoulders are most commonly involved. Some MHE patients have associated multiple enchondromata, a condition known as metachondromatosis.[13] Although both diseases are transmitted in an AD fashion, they are the result of different mutations.[14]

Pathology

SEs occur sporadically and some are associated with chemotherapy and radiotherapy. Around 90% of the MHE are inherited as AD with 96% to 100% penetrance. Approximately 10% have no family history and represent new, sporadic mutations. The AD variant is associated with tumor-suppressor exostosin genes, EXT I, EXT II, and EXT III, in chromosomes 8, 11, and 19, respectively.[15] The pathogenesis of these lesions is not clear but growth from aberrant ectopic physeal foci is suggested. The growth of individual osteochondromata parallels that of the "normal" growth plate and ceases with skeletal maturity. These lesions have a "cauliflower appearance" with an irregular osseous surface covered by a cartilage cap of varying thicknesses. The cartilage cap resembles physeal hyaline cartilage histologically. The cap is 2 or 3 cm thick in children and usually less than 1 cm thick after skeletal maturity. The stalk is composed of cortical bone with a marrow cavity that is continuous with the underlying native bone. The cartilage cap may mineralize, especially if the tissue undergoes osteonecrosis.[16] A delicate, fibrous membrane known as perichondrium, representing a continuation of the periosteum of the adjacent cortex, overlies the cartilaginous cap.

Clinical Features

Most lesions, in both SE and MHE, are asymptomatic and often found incidentally. Pain and a bump are the most common presenting symptoms. Pedunculated lesions are more symptomatic than corresponding sessile tumors. Pain can result from mechanical irritation of soft tissues, nerve impingement, bursa formation, osteonecrosis, fracture of the stalk, and malignant transformation. Pseudoaneurysm is a rare but known complication of large osteochondral exostoses in the popliteal fossa. Patients with MHE tend to be of short stature and have valgus deformities of the elbows and knees as well as ulnar deviation of the wrists. Patients may also develop joint subluxation if deformities involve the paired bones in the forearm or leg.[15] Lesions in the spine can be associated with neurologic dysfunction.

Malignant change should be suspected in patients with increasing pain, and unexplained growth after skeletal maturity. Malignant transformation is extraordinarily rare in children and quite rare in patients with solitary lesions. Patients with MHE, however, have substantial risk (3%–25%) that requires self-awareness as well as examination and clinical surveillance.[17] Sessile lesions in axial locations (pelvis, hips, shoulders, scapula, and proximal femur) have a greater risk of malignant change than those in distal acral locations.[18] Also, the overlying bursae may develop synovial chondromatosis that mimics malignant change on imaging.

Imaging

The radiographic features are characteristic and diagnostic, revealing pedunculated or sessile lesions arising from metaphysis and growing away from the joint with corticomedullary continuity.[11] In MHE, 90% of the exostoses are sessile and only 10% are pedunculated. A constant radiographic feature is the presence of corticomedullary continuity in contradistinction to entities, such as parosteal osteosarcoma or periosteal myositis ossificans, where the cortex is abutted by the lesion but intact and not in continuity with the medullary canal. The overlying radiolucent cartilaginous cap may be mineralized, a phenomenon that increases with age with corresponding thinning of the cartilage. In MHE, the affected bones are relatively short, whereas the metaphyses are enlarged (**Fig. 3**). There is generalized cortical thinning throughout the body, not only in the regions involved by exostoses. These features contribute to affected patients having a "stocky" appearance with innumerable small bumps. In most individuals with MHE, the femoral neck is short and broad with multiple osseous excrescences, another diagnostic feature of this disease.

Radiologic changes suggesting malignant transformation are progressive thickening of the

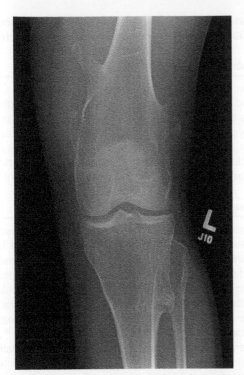

Fig. 3. AP radiograph of the left knee in a skeletally mature individual showing multiple pedunculated exostoses with corticomedullary continuity arising from metaphysis and pointing away from the joint. The radiolucent cartilaginous cap is not visible but the cartilage calcification is visible especially on the tibial lesion. Also note the widened metaphysis and thinned cortex.

cartilaginous cap (>2–3 cm), dispersed calcifications within the cartilaginous cap, lucency in the previously calcified cap, a large soft tissue mass with chondroid matrix, destruction of the stalk, and tumor replacement of marrow fat.[11]

MR and CT are helpful in assessing corticomedullary continuity and cartilage cap thickness. On MR, the cap appears to be high intensity on T2 pulse-weighted sequences with foci of low intensity representing calcification. CT is also useful in demonstrating destruction of stalk and adjacent bone, calcification in the cap, and, to a lesser extent, the soft tissue component.[19,20] Scintigraphic uptake on bone scan generally decreases with skeletal maturity but may become focally intense with malignant change. Sometimes, ultrasound is helpful for measuring the thickness of the cartilaginous cap in superficial lesions.

Treatment

Most osteochondromas (both solitary and multiple) are asymptomatic and do not require treatment. A symptomatic (painful) lesion may require surgical removal.[16] Any lesion suspicious for malignant change, especially after 30 years, should be biopsied and excised appropriately. However, prophylactic removal of asymptomatic lesions is not warranted. In children, the entire lesion, including the cap with its perichondrium, as well as the base and surrounding periosteum should be excised. Physeal arrest can occur with overzealous treatment in a young child. In adults, simple excision is adequate. For patients with spinal lesions and progressive neurologic symptoms, excision and decompression are necessary. Patients with MHE often exhibit skeletal deformities that may require correction.

Prognosis and Follow-Up

Patients with MHE should be seen and evaluated regularly because they are at risk for malignant transformation to chondrosarcoma. Secondary chondrosarcomas are typically low grade, are treated by surgery alone, and generally have a good prognosis.

FIBROUS DYSPLASIA

Fibrous dysplasia (FD) is a benign fibro-osseous tumor in which fibrous tissue with metaplastic immature woven bone replaces normal lamellar bone. It accounts for 5% to 10% of all benign bone tumors. The true incidence is difficult to estimate because many individuals are asymptomatic and undiagnosed. Most (75%) occur before the age of 30 years with no gender or ethnic predilection. Any bone can be involved, but the femur (especially the femoral neck), tibia, pelvis, ribs, skull, facial bones, humerus, and vertebrae are the frequent sites of disease.[21] In most cases (70%–80%), a single bone is involved (monostotic) and in 20% to 30% multiple bones (polyostotic) exhibit disease. Two other polyostotic forms, McCune-Albright syndrome and Mazabraud syndrome, have also been described.[22]

Pathology

FD was classified as a developmental abnormality but is now thought to have a genetic basis. It occurs sporadically and is associated with a missense mutation in the GNAS1 gene on chromosome 20.[23] Grossly, FD is firm and white due to the fibro-osseous component. Cartilage nodules and secondary cystic change with amber or bloody fluid can be observed as well. Microscopically, FD has irregular osseous trabeculae with a "Chinese letter" or "alphabet soup" appearance in a bland fibrous background.[24] The prominent trabeculae are notable for the conspicuous absence of osteoblastic rimming.

Clinical Features

The monostotic form is clinically the least severe and is usually asymptomatic. It most commonly affects the proximal femur and may cause a "Shepard crook" deformity. It may be diagnosed incidentally in young adults by radiographs taken for some other reason. Unlike the monostotic form, the polyostotic form is more severe and is usually symptomatic. It is diagnosed earlier in children and adolescents. The pelvis is the most commonly affected bone. Polyostotic FD has a striking predilection (>90%) for one limb or one side of the body. The two syndrome-associated FDs are even more severe and may even be detected in infancy. In 2% to 3% of affected individuals, polyostotic FD is associated with precocious puberty (males more than females), endocrinopathies (hyperthyroidism, hyperparathyroidism, gigantism or acromegaly, diabetes mellitus, and Cushing syndrome), and café-au-lait spots that stop abruptly at the midline of the body (McCune-Albright syndrome).[25] The café-au-lait spots in McCune-Albright syndrome are irregular and ragged (coast of Maine) in contrast to the smooth margins (coast of California) seen in patients with neurofibromatosis.[26] Rarely, polyostotic FD is associated with multiple soft tissue fibromyxomatous tumors (Mazabraud syndrome). The myxomatous soft tissue mass seen in Mazabraud syndrome may be confused with a primary malignancy.

The most common presenting symptom is bone pain (70%) followed by local swelling in all forms of the disease. Pseudofractures (Looser lines) and progressive bowing deformities may result in pathologic fractures, the most common complication of FD. Skeletal deformities and limb length discrepancy are also common; however, endocrine abnormalities and oncogenic osteomalacia are rare sequelae of this disease.[22] Bone lesions often progress in size until puberty and then become inactive. Pregnancy, though, may result in reactivation of these latent bone lesions. Rarely, malignant transformation may occur and result in osteosarcoma, chondrosarcoma, fibrosarcoma, angiosarcoma, and undifferentiated pleomorphic sarcoma. The risk of malignant transformation in fibrous dysplastic bone in monostotic FD is less than 1% but higher in the polyostotic varieties, especially McCune-Albright syndrome (4%), Mazabraud syndrome, or in the event of prior radiation exposure.[27] Malignant change is heralded by a sudden increase in pain and the appearance of swelling. There are also rare reports of locally aggressive FD and secondary aneurysmal bone cyst formation both of which are associated with cortical destruction and an associated soft tissue mass mimicking overt malignant transformation.

Laboratory Findings

The disease activity can be measured with serum and urine markers of bone metabolism, including the bone formation markers alkaline phosphatase, bone-specific alkaline phosphatase, and osteocalcin. Serum and urine markers for bone resorption include N-telopeptide (NTx) of collagen, pyridinium crosslinks, and deoxypyridinoline crosslinks.

Imaging

Radiographically, FD is an intramedullary based disease located in meta-diphyseal bone. The lesions are usually radiolucent but rarely may appear radiodense, depending on the amount of matrix calcification. There is loss of the normal trabecular pattern within bone that is replaced by a fine granular "ground-glass," "milky," or "smoky" appearance with multiple internal septations (**Fig. 4**).[28] If islands of cartilages are present, "popcorn calcifications" may be observed on radiographs. Sometimes there is a band of surrounding sclerotic bone creating a "rind" sign. The margins are generally

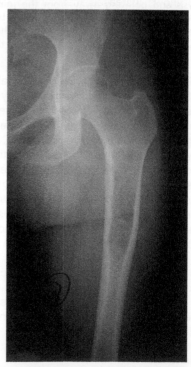

Fig. 4. AP radiograph of the left proximal femur in a skeletally mature individual with a radiolucent lesion in the metadiaphysis. There are deep endosteal scallops and a ground glass matrix that is characteristic of FD.

geographic and may involve the whole bone. Endosteal scalloping is a hallmark of this disease along with cortical thinning and occasional expansion, but no cortical disruption or periosteal reaction. Malignant change is associated with bone destruction and soft tissue disease extension.[29] Multiple pathologic fractures in the proximal femur may lead to a "shepherd's crook" deformity. Occasionally, accelerated growth of a bone or hypertrophy of a digit may be observed. Skull lesions may cause thickening and deformity (leontiasis ossea).

If radiographs are not diagnostic, additional advanced imaging may be useful. The MR appearance is variable depending on the amount and degree of bone trabeculae, collagen, and cystic or hemorrhagic changes. They usually appear low intensity on T1 pulse sequences and hyperintense or sometimes hypointense on corresponding T2 images. The sclerotic rim, if present, appears as low intensity on both T1 and T2 sequences.[30] The lesion enhances with contrast. CT is more sensitive in evaluating matrix mineralization, pseudoseptae, expansion, and thinning of the cortex and pathologic fracture. Bone scintigraphy usually displays intense radiotracer uptake in the involved bones and positron emission tomography (PET) imaging shows increased metabolic activity. In rare cases when imaging modalities fail to characterize the disease, biopsy may be necessary for diagnosis.

Treatment

Asymptomatic lesions do not require treatment other than serial follow-up. The treatment of symptomatic FD is usually nonoperative and involves bisphosphonates and nonsteroidal anti-inflammatory medicines. Bisphosphonates are thought to help control pain and disease progression.[24] Surgery may be required for lesions that are symptomatic, large or progressive, in high-stress locations (ie, proximal femur), and for those patients whose disease does not respond to nonsurgical treatment. The goals of surgery in FD are prevention or treatment of deformity and stabilization of pathologic fractures.[24] Curetting and bone grafting (usually cortical structural allograft) with or without internal fixation may be considered. Particulate graft is quickly resorbed and replaced by fibrous dysplastic bone.[22] Prevention or treatment of deformity and pathologic fractures may require osteotomy and internal fixation.

Prognosis and Follow-Up

The prognosis is better for patients with monostotic FD compared with those with polyostotic FD and syndrome-associated forms of disease. Malignant transformation is associated with a poor prognosis. The lesions can be monitored clinically and with laboratory tests, including imaging for disease progression and malignant change.

PAGET DISEASE OF BONE (OSTEITIS DEFORMANS)

Paget disease (PD) is a focal disease of bone remodeling characterized by accelerated bone resorption coupled with formation. PD is not seen in children and is rare in patients less than 40 years old. It is usually seen in elderly patients and the incidence increases with age. PD has a slight male predominance. It is more common among people of European descent and uncommon in Asian populations. It is prevalent in 2% to 3% of the US population but recent data suggest a decline in both the prevalence and the severity of PD. PD can affect any bone and may be monostotic or polyostotic. The bones most commonly affected are skull, spine, pelvis, and the lower extremities, especially the proximal femur.[31]

Pathogenesis

The cause of PD is unknown, but genetic factors, paramyxoviruses, and exogenous and endogenous factors have been implicated. The osteoclasts play a central role in the pathogenesis. PD is characterized by increased bone turnover. The early stage of the disease is characterized by osteoclastic bone resorption followed by excessive production of woven bone, which causes bone thickening and structural weakness. There is abnormal deposition of both woven and lamellar bone. Histologically, PD displays randomly arranged units of lamellar bone delineated by irregular cement lines forming the pathognomonic "mosaic" pattern. There are numerous, large, multinucleated osteoclasts that actively resorb bone coupled with later osteoblastic bone formation. A highly vascular fibrous connective tissue replaces the normal marrow.[32]

Clinical Features

PD is mostly asymptomatic and, therefore, patients are usually diagnosed incidentally by radiographs or serum alkaline phosphatase levels done for other reasons. Symptomatic patients usually present with pain.[33] Involvement of long bones is characterized by thickening and bone enlargement, progressive and sometimes crippling deformity, resulting limb shortening, secondary arthritis, stress fractures on the convex side of bone, especially the femur (chalk stick fracture), and overt pathologic fracture. Malignant change occurs in 1% of affected patients and is heralded clinically by a sudden increase in pain and the appearance of soft tissue swelling.[34] When malignant transformation supervenes, the femur, pelvis, humerus, and skull are affected in descending order of frequency, but the spine is seldom affected. Benign giant cell tumors have also been reported. Vertebral involvement is characterized by spinal stenosis, spondylolisthesis, disc prolapse, and spinal cord or nerve root compression. Involvement of the skull manifests as a thickened enlarged and deformed skull, compression of the lateral ventricle and brain stem, hydrocephalus, headache, visual disturbances, cranial nerve palsies, and deafness. Involvement of the face, maxilla, and mandible is characterized by facial deformity (leontiasis ossea), proptosis, and disfigurement or dental complications. The increased vascularity may lead to vascular steal syndromes, changes in skin temperature, and high-output heart failure. The metabolic complications associated with PD include hyperparathyroidism, hypercalcemia, osteoporosis, and hyperuricemia.

Laboratory Findings

In laboratory findings, serum calcium and phosphorous levels are usually normal. Serum alkaline phosphatase, however, is characteristically elevated and is a useful marker to assess disease activity as well as the response to therapy. Patients with long-standing disease may have normal serum alkaline phosphatase levels. Other markers of bone formation, such as bone-specific alkaline phosphatase and procollagen type I N-terminal propeptide, may be useful in monitoring therapy. The urinary marker of bone resorption, NTx, also appears to be useful. Urine NTx is the earliest marker of treatment response (reflecting osteoclast activity), whereas the serum alkaline phosphatase value (a measure of osteoblast function) may take months to normalize. Elevated collagen breakdown products, such as N-terminal and C-terminal telopeptides, N-pyridinolines, and hydroxyproline, correspond to bone turnover.[35]

Imaging

Radiographs are usually diagnostic and are also useful in assessing disease progress with treatment.[36] The characteristic features include cortical thickening, bone enlargement with mixed lytic and sclerotic lesions, and coarsened trabeculae (Fig. 5). In long bones, early lesions usually begin in the subchondral region at one end and extend along the shaft for a variable distance, producing

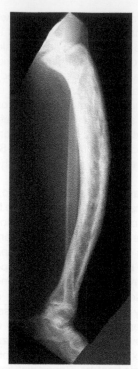

Fig. 5. A lateral radiograph of the tibia showing Looser lines on the anterior cortex, a prominent bowing deformity, thickened cortices and purposeful trabeculae in a patient with PD.

a sharply demarcated, V-shaped lytic area ("flame" or "blade-of-grass" appearance). Weight-bearing bones may bow and small fissure fractures can occur in the cortex, usually on the convex side of the femur. The lesions change over time and the lytic areas revert back with treatment. There are characteristic Pagetic changes in specific areas, such as the "window frame" vertebrae in the spine, protrusio acetabuli and sacroiliac joint ankylosis in the pelvis, and osteoporosis circumscripta and basilar invagination in the skull. Malignant change is indicated by progressive lysis, cortical destruction, and a soft tissue mass. Bone scans are useful in evaluating the extent of disease and response to treatment, but in end-stage disease there is little uptake. In the face of malignant transformation, an area of photopenia is observed scintigraphically. MR and CT are useful in the evaluation of spine, pelvic, and skull lesions as well as malignant change. PET is helpful in evaluating a lesion suspicious for malignancy. Biopsy may be necessary if the diagnosis remains unclear from imaging or if osteosarcoma is suspected.[37] MR imaging and CT are indicated to evaluate spine, pelvic, and skull lesions as well as malignant change. PET is helpful in evaluating a lesion suspicious for malignancy.

Biopsy may be necessary if the diagnosis remains unclear from imaging or if osteosarcoma is suspected.

Treatment

There is no cure and the treatment goals are pain control, preventing disease progression, correcting bowing deformities, and stabilizing pathologic fractures.

Bisphosphonates

These drugs represent the mainstay of therapy and promote sustained clinical remission with improvement in pain, consolidation of lytic lesions, and normalization of serum alkaline phosphatase.[38] A paradoxic increase in pain is observed in a minority in patients (15%). They act by inhibiting osteoclast function via the farnesyl diphosphate synthase pathway and inhibit both resorption and formation. The newer bisphosphonates, such as pamidronate, alendronate, risedronate, ibandronate, and zoledronate, selectively suppress bone resorption. Patients should be treated with vitamin D and calcium concurrently. Resistance to one bisphosphonate is managed by switching over to another bisphosphonate.

Calcitonin

This drug acts to reduce serum alkaline phosphatase with resulting pain relief and stabilization of the skeleton; the effects though are temporal. Calcitonin decreases bone resorption and may be used in conjunction with bisphosphonate drugs in refractory cases. Calcitonin may also be considered in older and debilitated patients for short-term pain relief.[39]

Intravenous bisphosphonates, calcitonin, gallium nitrate, and mithramycin (now called plicamycin) are useful in treating the rare hypercalcemia resulting from fulminant PD.

Supportive therapy

Analgesics, bracing, gait training, walking aids, and physical therapy are also effective ways to manage this disease.

Surgery

Joint arthrosis may supervene in patients as a consequence of mechanical factors related to PD. Patients with hip arthrosis surgery are at risk for excessive bleeding, whereas knee surgery for patients with this disease can be complicated by malalignment.[40] Internal fixation for fractures, osteotomies for severe deformities, and spinal decompression for cord or root compression[41] are other surgical procedures that may be indicated for patients with this disease. Pretreatment with bisphosphonates before surgery reduces bone vascularity, but if continued postoperatively, may delay bone healing.

SKELETAL METASTASES

Bone is the third most common site for metastatic tumors following lung and liver. Multifocal disease is observed in most patients; however, solitary lesions occur in 2% to 3%.[42] The most common primary lesions causing skeletal metastases in descending order of frequency are breast (70% in women), prostate (60% in men), lung, kidney, thyroid, gastrointestinal, and genitourinary tumors.[43] Among common solid organ tumors, lung and kidney cancers metastasize earlier than breast and prostate. In 3% to 4%, the primary is unknown at the time of presentation with bone metastases and, in these cases, lung followed by kidney are the usual sites of primary. The commonest disseminated bone neoplasms in children are neuroblastoma and leukemia.[44] The bones involved by metastases in descending order of frequency are vertebrae (thoracic > lumbar > sacral > cervical),[45] pelvis, ribs, sternum, proximal femur, proximal humerus, and skull.[46] Metastases rarely involve bones distal to the knee and elbow and these usually arise from primaries in the lung and kidney. Usually, the diaphysis and metaphysis in the long bones and the vertebral bodies in spine are affected. Bone metastases occur through either hematogenous (most common) or lymphatic spread.

Clinical Features

Pain is the most common (67%) presenting symptom and is usually dull and insidious in nature and worse at night. Soft tissue swelling may be present especially if the tumor violates the cortex and extends into the soft tissue. When significant bone destruction occurs, pathologic fracture may supervene. Patients with vertebral involvement may present with back pain, compression fracture, deformity, instability, and spinal cord or root compression. Spine involvement is often multifocal and patients often have symptoms related to other sites of disease as well. Skeletal metastasis should be considered in older patients with unexplained musculoskeletal pain or pathologic fracture with a previous history of recently diagnosed or remote cancer. Paraneoplastic syndromes may occur with some tumors and present as sensory neuropathies, enthesopathies, and endocrinopathies. Hypercoagulability can result in deep vein thrombosis and pulmonary embolism. Hypercalcemia is the commonest metabolic abnormality in patients with cancer and is frequently associated with breast, lung, and renal carcinoma, myeloma, and lymphoma. Hypocalcemia and oncogenic osteomalacia rarely occur.

Laboratory Findings

Alkaline phosphatase is the most sensitive marker for bone metastases and is useful in assessing disease progression. Increased urinary hydroxyproline indicates rapid bone turnover associated with destructive bone metastases. Nonspecific markers of osteoblastic activity (bone Gla protein and procollagen 1 carboxy-terminal peptide) and osteoclastic activity (deoxypyridinoline and pyridinolin-crosslinked carboxy-terminal telopeptide) are elevated due to increased bone turnover associated with skeletal metastases. Disease-specific tests include acid phosphatase and prostate-specific antigen (prostate cancer), urinalysis for blood (renal cell or bladder carcinoma), serum and urine protein electrophoresis (multiple myeloma), peripheral blood smears, and bone marrow aspiration (lymphoma and leukemia). Other tests, such as liver enzymes, thyroid function tests, blood urea nitrogen/creatinine, and mammography, may be useful in specific cases. Patients with anemia and altered renal function, although nonspecific, are worrisome for myeloma.

Imaging radiographs

If metastatic disease is suspected, initial imaging should include anteroposterior and lateral radiographs of the entire involved bone. Before destructive bone lesions can be visualized on radiographs, at least 30% to 40% of the bone is involved. The lesion may appear as lytic, sclerotic, or mixed depending on the tumor histology (**Table 1**).[47] In long bones, metastatic deposits usually appear as permeative or moth-eaten destructive lesions with ill-defined margins. Typically, metastatic deposits appear as a diaphyseal-based cortical lucency (shark-bite) (**Fig. 6**). Bone expansion, periosteal reaction, neoplastic bone formation, and soft tissue masses are unusual, unlike primary bone sarcomas. Renal and thyroid tumors may appear as a large expansile metastatic lesion ("blowout" metastasis). A fracture in an elderly patient that occurs with minimal trauma and exhibits radiolucent permeative destruction at the fractured ends of the bone should raise suspicion for a metastatic disease process. In the spine, metastases usually involve the vertebral body at the pedicle body interface initially; the intervertebral disc spaces are generally preserved. Collapse of the vertebral body and kyphotic deformity may occur with progressive disease. The absence of a pedicle ("wink" sign) on the anteroposterior radiograph is characteristic of metastases.

MR

MR may be useful to assess additional lesions in an affected bone that may not be apparent on radiographs. Aside from marrow replacement, the diagnosis of a soft tissue component and its interface with normal tissue is best seen on MR. The signal characteristics and overall appearance of metastatic tumors are nonspecific. In spine, MR is ideal for evaluating cord compression.

CT

CT, especially quantitative CT,[48] is superior in defining cortical disruption and predicting pathologic fracture in select patients.

Bone scintigraphy is used to detect subclinical disease that is not apparent on radiographs, but more importantly, to assess the skeleton for multiple sites of disease.

Whole body MR imaging and *PET/CT* are important adjuncts for detecting subclinical metastatic deposits and to assess the effects of chemotherapeutic intervention.

Biopsy is indicated for patients first presenting with presumed metastatic disease with a proximal history of a primary organ tumor and for those individuals with or without a history presenting with a "solitary" lesion.[45]

Differential Diagnosis

The differential diagnosis for patients with multiple bone lesions and presumed skeletal metastases includes primary bone sarcomas, multiple myeloma, lymphoma, Langerhan cell histiocytosis, osteomyelitis, and in children, leukemia and neuroblastoma. Although the clinical findings may be

Table 1
This table shows the radiological appearance of metastases from different primary cancers

Primary Tumor	Usual Appearance	Unusual Appearance
Breast	Mostly lytic or mixed	About 10% are blastic
Prostate	Mostly blastic or mixed	Rarely purely lytic
Lungs	Majority are lytic	Rarely blastic
Renal, bladder	Almost always lytic	Rarely blastic
Thyroid	Usually lytic	Rarely blastic
Gastrointestinal tract	Usually lytic	Rarely blastic
Genital tract	Usually lytic	Rarely blastic

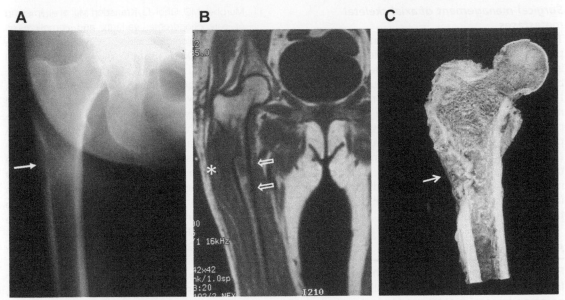

Fig. 6. (*A*) AP radiograph of the right proximal femur in an elderly woman with hip pain showing a cortically based radiolucency (*solid arrow*). (*B*) MR coronal T1 pulse weighted image showing marrow replacement (*open arrows*), cortical breakout (*asterisk*), and a soft tissue mass. (*C*) Resected specimen demonstrating cortical destruction (*arrow*) and medullary tumor infiltration.

somewhat helpful, biopsy is often necessary to confirm the diagnosis. As a rule, every biopsy specimen should be sent for culture also.

Treatment

A comprehensive discussion of the different treatments available and their indications is beyond the scope of this article. In general, the goals of treatment are pain control, prevention or treatment of pathologic fracture, improving function, and rarely, cure.[45]

Nonsurgical treatment

Nonsurgical treatment is considered in small asymptomatic lesions and patients with very advanced disease. Treatment includes bracing, pain management, and radiotherapy to relieve local pain and slow tumor growth. Chemotherapy, hormone therapy, immunotherapy, systemic radiopharmaceuticals, and targeted therapy are used to control local disease as well as distant micrometastases. Bisphosphonates decrease skeletal complications of metastases and may prevent skeletal metastases. Steroids are helpful in spinal cord compression.

Surgical treatment of appendicular skeletal metastases

Most patients with bone metastasis are treated nonsurgically. The most common sites of skeletal metastasis causing complications and requiring surgery are the pelvis, femur, and humerus.[49] The femur is the commonest site of pathologic fracture; 50% of the fractures occur in the femoral neck.[50] Surgery is performed to decrease pain in an effort to prevent or treat pathologic fractures. The risk of pathologic fracture of long bones is assessed by Mirels score, which takes into account the site, size of the lesion, type of lesion (blastic or lytic), and presence of pain. Factors, such as life expectancy of at least 1 to 3 months, functional status, extent of disease, and histology, are considered in deciding whether surgery is beneficial. For destructive lesions around major joints, wide excision and prosthetic reconstruction should be considered. This strategy is also important for patients with tumors that are not sensitive to radiotherapy or systemic strategies, such as renal cell carcinoma, select patients with melanoma, and thyroid carcinoma. For lesions in long bones, intramedullary nail placement spanning the entire bone is preferred over plates and other fixation methods. Pathologic fractures due to breast and prostate metastases have good healing potential generally because patients survive for longer periods of time compared with patients with lung carcinoma metastatic to bone. Internal fixation may be combined with intralesional excision and cementing.[50] Preoperative embolization may be useful in vascular tumors, such as renal, thyroid cancers, and multiple myeloma, to reduce blood loss. Amputation is rarely indicated in metastatic disease and is occasionally done for lesions involving hand and foot, fungating tumors, infection, and intractable pain.[51]

Surgical management of axial skeletal metastases

The risk of pathologic fracture is more difficult to predict in the spine. Indications for intervention include pain, pathologic fracture, deformity, instability, presence of progressive neurologic symptoms, and radio-resistant tumors. There are multiple surgical options available and the basic principles are to remove as much tumor as possible, decompress the cord and roots, and align, stabilize, and fuse with instrumentation. Vertibroplasy and kyphoplasty are percutaneous methods used to treat vertebral body compression fractures, especially in patients with breast metastases and multiple myeloma.[52]

Prognosis and Follow-Up

Prognosis and survival depend on various other factors and is 18.8 months overall. Of the most common tumors, prostate and breast metastases have the best prognosis. Renal and thyroid metastases have an intermediate prognosis, and lung metastases have the worst prognosis.[45]

REFERENCES

1. Silve C, Jüppner H. Ollier disease. Orphanet J Rare Dis 2006;1:37.
2. Casal D, Mavioso C, Mendes MM, et al. Hand involvement in Ollier disease and Maffucci syndrome: a case series. Acta Reumatol Port 2010;35(3):375–8.
3. Superti-Furga A, Spranger J, Nishimura G. Enchondromatosis revisited: new classification with molecular basis. Am J Med Genet C Semin Med Genet 2012;160C(3):154–64.
4. Zhou J, Jiang ZM, Zhang HZ, et al. Clinicopathologic study of Ollier's disease and its chondrosarcomatous transformation. Zhonghua Bing Li Xue Za Zhi 2009;38(10):673–7.
5. D'Angelo L, Massimi L, Narducci A, et al. Ollier disease. Childs Nerv Syst 2009;25(6):647–53.
6. Muramatsu K, Kawakami Y, Tani Y, et al. Malignant transformation of multiple enchondromas in the hand: case report. J Hand Surg Am 2011;36(2):304–7.
7. Cerny M, Rudiger HA, Aubry-Rozier B, et al. Clinical images: enchondromatosis (Ollier disease). Arthritis Rheum 2013;65(11):2886.
8. Dening J, van Erve RH. Increasing leg length discrepancy in multiple enchondromatosis. Ned Tijdschr Geneeskd 2011;155:A2188.
9. Ruivo J, Antunes JL. Maffucci syndrome associated with a pituitary adenoma and a probable brainstem tumor. J Neurosurg 2009;110(2):363–8.
10. Schwartz HS, Zimmerman NB, Simon MA, et al. The malignant potential of enchondromatosis. J Bone Joint Surg Am 1987;69(2):269–74.
11. Murphey MD, Choi JJ, Kransdorf MJ, et al. Imaging of osteochondroma: variants and complications with radiologic-pathologic correlation. Radiographics 2000;20(5):1407–34.
12. Jensen BG, Neumann L. Multiple cartilaginous exostoses. Ugeskr Laeger 1989;151(47):3140–3.
13. Fisher TJ, Williams N, Morris L, et al. Metachondromatosis: more than just multiple osteochondromas. J Child Orthop 2013;7(6):455–64.
14. Jennes I, Pedrini E, Zuntini M, et al. Multiple osteochondromas: mutation update and description of the multiple osteochondromas mutation database (MOdb). Hum Mutat 2009;30(12):1620–7.
15. Kok HK, Fitzgerald L, Campbell N, et al. Multimodality imaging features of hereditary multiple exostoses. Br J Radiol 2013;86(1030):20130398.
16. Kitsoulis P, Galani V, Stefanaki K, et al. Osteochondromas: review of the clinical, radiological and pathological features [review]. In Vivo 2008;22(5):633–46.
17. Sansón-RíoFrío JA, Santiesteban N, Bahena RI, et al. Differential diagnosis of multiple hereditary exostosis: presentation of a clinical case with secondary chondrosarcoma and literature review. Acta Ortop Mex 2009;23(6):376–82.
18. Pannier S, Legeai-Mallet L. Hereditary multiple exostoses and enchondromatosis. Best Pract Res Clin Rheumatol 2008;22(1):45–54.
19. Shah ZK, Peh WC, Wong Y, et al. Sarcomatous transformation in diaphyseal aclasis. Australas Radiol 2007;51(2):110–9.
20. Bovée JV. Multiple osteochondromas. Orphanet J Rare Dis 2008;3:3.
21. DiCaprio MR, Enneking WF. Fibrous dysplasia. Pathophysiology, evaluation, and treatment. J Bone Joint Surg Am 2005;87(8):1848–64.
22. Parekh SG, Donthineni-Rao R, Ricchetti E, et al. Fibrous dysplasia. J Am Acad Orthop Surg 2004;12(5):305–13.
23. Schreiber A, Villaret AB, Maroldi R, et al. Fibrous dysplasia of the sinonasal tract and adjacent skull base. Curr Opin Otolaryngol Head Neck Surg 2012;20(1):45–52.
24. Chapurlat RD, Orcel P. Fibrous dysplasia of bone and McCune-Albright syndrome. Best Pract Res Clin Rheumatol 2008;22(1):55–69.
25. Zacharin M. The spectrum of McCune Albright syndrome. Pediatr Endocrinol Rev 2007;4:412–8.
26. Leslie WD, Reinhold C, Rosenthall L, et al. Panostotic fibrous dysplasia. A new craniotubular dysplasia. Clin Nucl Med 1992;17(7):556–60.
27. Riddle ND, Bui MM. Fibrous dysplasia. Arch Pathol Lab Med 2013;137(1):134–8.
28. Lädermann A, Stern R, Ceroni D, et al. Unusual radiologic presentation of monostotic fibrous dysplasia. Orthopedics 2008;31(3):282.
29. Collins MT, Singer FR, Eugster E. McCune-Albright syndrome and the extraskeletal manifestations of

fibrous dysplasia. Orphanet J Rare Dis 2012; 7(Suppl 1):S4.

30. Bulakbaşi N, Bozlar U, Karademir I, et al. CT and MRI in the evaluation of craniospinal involvement with polyostotic fibrous dysplasia inMcCune-Albright syndrome. Diagn Interv Radiol 2008; 14(4):177–81.

31. Ralston SH, Layfield R. Pathogenesis of Paget disease of bone. Calcif Tissue Int 2012;91(2):97–113.

32. Sabharwal R, Gupta S, Sepolia S, et al. An insight in to Paget's disease of bone. Niger J Surg 2014; 20(1):9–15.

33. Cundy T, Reid IR. Paget's disease of bone. Clin Biochem 2012;45(1–2):43–8.

34. Horvai A, Unni KK. Premalignant conditions of bone. J Orthop Sci 2006;11(4):412–23.

35. Ralston SH. Clinical practice. Paget's disease of bone. N Engl J Med 2013;368(7):644–50.

36. Cortis K, Micallef K, Mizzi A. Imaging Paget's disease of bone–from head to toe. Clin Radiol 2011; 66(7):662–72.

37. Theodorou DJ, Theodorou SJ, Kakitsubata Y. Imaging of Paget disease of bone and its musculoskeletal complications: review. AJR Am J Roentgenol 2011;196(6):S64–75.

38. Bolland MJ, Cundy T. Paget's disease of bone: clinical review and update. J Clin Pathol 2013;66(11): 924–7.

39. Seton M. Paget disease of bone: diagnosis and drug therapy. Cleve Clin J Med 2013;80(7):452–62.

40. Gabel GT, Rand JA, Sim FH. Total knee arthroplasty for osteoarthrosis in patients who have Paget disease of bone at the knee. J Bone Joint Surg Am 1991;73(5):739–44.

41. Ralston SH, Langston AL, Reid IR. Pathogenesis and management of Paget's disease of bone. Lancet 2008;372(9633):155–63.

42. Rubin P, Brasacchio R, Katz A. Solitary metastases: illusion versus reality. Semin Radiat Oncol 2006; 16(2):120–30.

43. Scutellari PN, Antinolfi G, Galeotti R, et al. Metastatic bone disease. Strategies for imaging. Minerva Med 2003;94(2):77–90.

44. Toma P, Defilippi C. Bone tumours and neuroblastoma in children. In: Adam A, Dixon AK, Grainger RG, et al, editors. Adam: Grainger & Allison's diagnostic radiology. 5th edition. Philadelphia: Elsevier Churchill Livingstone; 2008. p. 1639–51.

45. Eastley N, Newey M, Ashford RU. Skeletal metastases - the role of the orthopaedic and spinal surgeon. Surg Oncol 2012;21(3):216–22.

46. Xu DL, Zhang XT, Wang GH, et al. Clinical features of pathologically confirmed metastatic bone tumors–a report of 390 cases. Ai Zheng 2005;24(11):1404–7.

47. Söderlund V. Radiological diagnosis of skeletal metastases. Eur Radiol 1996;6(5):587–95.

48. Kaneko TS, Bell JS, Pejcic MR, et al. Mechanical properties, density and quantitative CT scan data of trabecular bone with and without metastases. J Biomech 2004;37(4):523–30.

49. Harrington KD. Orthopaedic management of extremity and pelvic lesions. Clin Orthop Relat Res 1995;(312):136–47.

50. Harrington KD. Orthopedic surgical management of skeletal complications of malignancy. Cancer 1997;80(8):1614–27.

51. Wittig JC, Bickels J, Kollender Y, et al. Palliative forequarter amputation for metastatic carcinoma to the shoulder girdle region: indications, preoperative evaluation, surgical technique, and results. J Surg Oncol 2001;77(2):105–13.

52. Schaser KD, Melcher I, Mittlmeier T, et al. Surgical management of vertebral column metastatic disease. Unfallchirurg 2007;110(2):137–59.

Index

Note: Page numbers of article titles are in **boldface** type.

Orthop Clin N Am 45 (2014) 431–434
http://dx.doi.org/10.1016/S0030-5898(14)00097-2

Moving?

Make sure your subscription moves with you!

To notify us of your new address, find your **Clinics Account Number** (located on your mailing label above your name), and contact customer service at:

Email: journalscustomerservice-usa@elsevier.com

800-654-2452 (subscribers in the U.S. & Canada)
314-447-8871 (subscribers outside of the U.S. & Canada)

Fax number: 314-447-8029

Elsevier Health Sciences Division
Subscription Customer Service
3251 Riverport Lane
Maryland Heights, MO 63043

*To ensure uninterrupted delivery of your subscription, please notify us at least 4 weeks in advance of move.